Walk Around Arundel

52 Places to Hike with Your Dog

(and Other Best Friends)

Walk Around Arundel
52 Places to Hike with Your Dog
(and Other Best Friends)
by Jefferson Holland

Copyright © 2024
by Jefferson Holland
All Rights Reserved

Editor
Sandra Olivetti Martin
New Bay Books
Fairhaven, Maryland
NewBayBooks@gmail.com

Cover and interior design by Suzanne Shelden
Shelden Studios
Prince Frederick, Maryland
sheldenstudios@comcast.net

A Note on Type:
Cover and section heads are set in
Minion Std Black and Myriad Pro
The text font is Garamond Premier Pro

Library of Congress
Cataloging-in-Publication Data

ISBN 979-8-9882998-5-1

Printed in the United States of America
First Edition

Early Praise from Holland Readers

Jeff Holland is our renaissance man: poet, musician, environmentalist. Go hiking with him (and his pup) in and around the Chesapeake Bay. Pure fun!

    —Terrance Smith, journalist and author of
Four Wars, Five Presidents: A Reporter's Journey from Jerusalem to Saigon to the White House.

Letters to the Editor of the *Annapolis Capital:*

I always enjoy reading Jeff Holland's columns about where to hike and stroll. His use of words is so visual: "spouts of daffodils pushing up through the crunchy snow" or referring to saplings as "hors d'oeuvres for the deer." This can put you walking beside him.

    —Barbara Cantor, Annapolis

Please thank Jeff Holland for all of his guidance on local and almost local trails. Four of us, two in our 70s and two in our 80s, are having a ball following his lead.

    —Karla Goodbridge, Annapolis

What a jewel we have in Anne Arundel County in the person of Jeff Holland. His enlightening walks with Millie, the pooch, delight readers of the Sunday *Capital* and provide a positive alternative to what makes news today. We hope Mr. Holland will consider putting his stories into a guidebook that will attract hikers to explore new and rewarding trails.

    —Max and Suzanne Ochs, Severna Park

I always look forward to reading Jeff's hiking tales. They are a Sunday morning treat! I especially enjoy the way Jeff reveals the hidden gems and secret entrances he discovers. It's like Jeff's right there with me, sharing a coffee, giving me a personal tour through the twists and turns of the forests. Each adventure reveals bits of history, culture, nature, wildlife...and the charming characters he and Millie befriend along the way.

—Thomas Guay, Author,
Chesapeake Bound: An Annapolis Novel

Executive Citation:

The Citizens of Anne Arundel County, Maryland, salute Jeff Holland in recognition of your dedicated service to the Anne Arundel County Department of Recreation & Parks: "Your selfless efforts as an outstanding volunteer are evident in your tireless work during the Covid-19 Pandemic where you have promoted our parks and trails, public health, and encouraged people to participate in outdoor sports. Your contributions to County, State, and Federal Government stand on their own merit and serve as a record of your unwavering commitment to our community. We extend to you our sincere appreciation and best wishes in all your future endeavors.

—Steuart L. Pittman, County Executive
January 31, 2021

Preface

The Viral Isolationist Song
(to the tune of "Modern Major General"
from the *Pirates of Penzance* by Gilbert & Sullivan)

I was the very model of a viral isolationist,
I used my down-time wisely, now indulge me while I share my list:
I mastered Kiswahili and some other feats linguistical
And delved into theology, both biblical and mystical
I catalogued my photos, twenty thousand forty-three in all,
And scrubbed away the mildew building up inside my shower stall
I binge-watched every episode of Friends and Mary Tyler Moore
And scrapped the crap contaminating my refrigerator door

(Chorus:
He scrapped the crap contaminating his refrigerator door
Scrapped the crap contaminating his refrigerator door
Scrapped the crap contaminating his refrigerator-rator door)

I painted all my toenails puce, and monitored the growth of them
Of Moby Dick and War and Peace, I thought of reading of both of them,
Of course, it made me bonkers, still in any case I must insist
I was the very model of a viral isolationist.

(Of course, it made him bonkers, still in any case we must insist
He was the very model of a viral isolationist).

JEFFERSON HOLLAND

This book is a product of the COVID pandemic. It all started in January, 2020, when I got together with Rick Hutzel for a cup of coffee. Rick was the editor of the *Annapolis Capital* newspaper at the time, and he was kind enough to listen while I pitched him a few story ideas. The one pitch he thought had merit was simple in concept: I would take a walk in a park with my dog and write about it.

Little did either of us know that right after the column started to run, the world shut down and just about the only healthy thing anybody could do was to take a walk in the park with their dog. Visitation to public parks in Annapolis and Anne Arundel County flourished, and while I can't take full credit for that, I'd like to think I gave some readers inspiration to grab a leash and get out walking.

I use the term "guide" loosely, because this isn't a common guidebook. I've left out a lot of details that can best be accessed with up-to-date smart phone apps like AllTrails, PeakVisor, Strava, REI's Hiking Project, and Seek by iNaturalist.

Most of these places are within Anne Arundel County, though I've included a couple from nearby Baltimore County and Queen Anne's County. I have included information on how to find each site, where to call or look on line for more information, and whether there's an admission fee. Most are free; others have discounted passes for seniors, handicapped individuals or those in the armed services. Some of the more established parks have flushable toilet facilities, while others might or might not have a portable toilet available.

I've also noted whether dogs are welcome. Most places allow dogs on a leash. You might get the impression that I prefer the company of well-behaved dogs and that I get irritated by owners who insist on dragging their anti-social pets out in public where they're certain to have unpleasant confrontations.

Most of these walks are easy, since most of Anne Arundel County is relatively flat. Sometimes there will be hills to climb, in which case, I've noted that the site requires some moderate effort to negotiate the topography.

But mainly, this is a collection of essays inspired by my experience at each site I visited along with a good dog and a good friend or two, all the while negotiating the challenges of the arc of the COVID-19 pandemic.

What inspires me is natural history and cultural history of the place, and I'm fascinated by the origin of place names. Basically, I'm a storyteller, and I hope the stories of these places give you pleasure in their reading and inspire to go visit them on your own. With a good dog and a good friend along, of course.

—JH

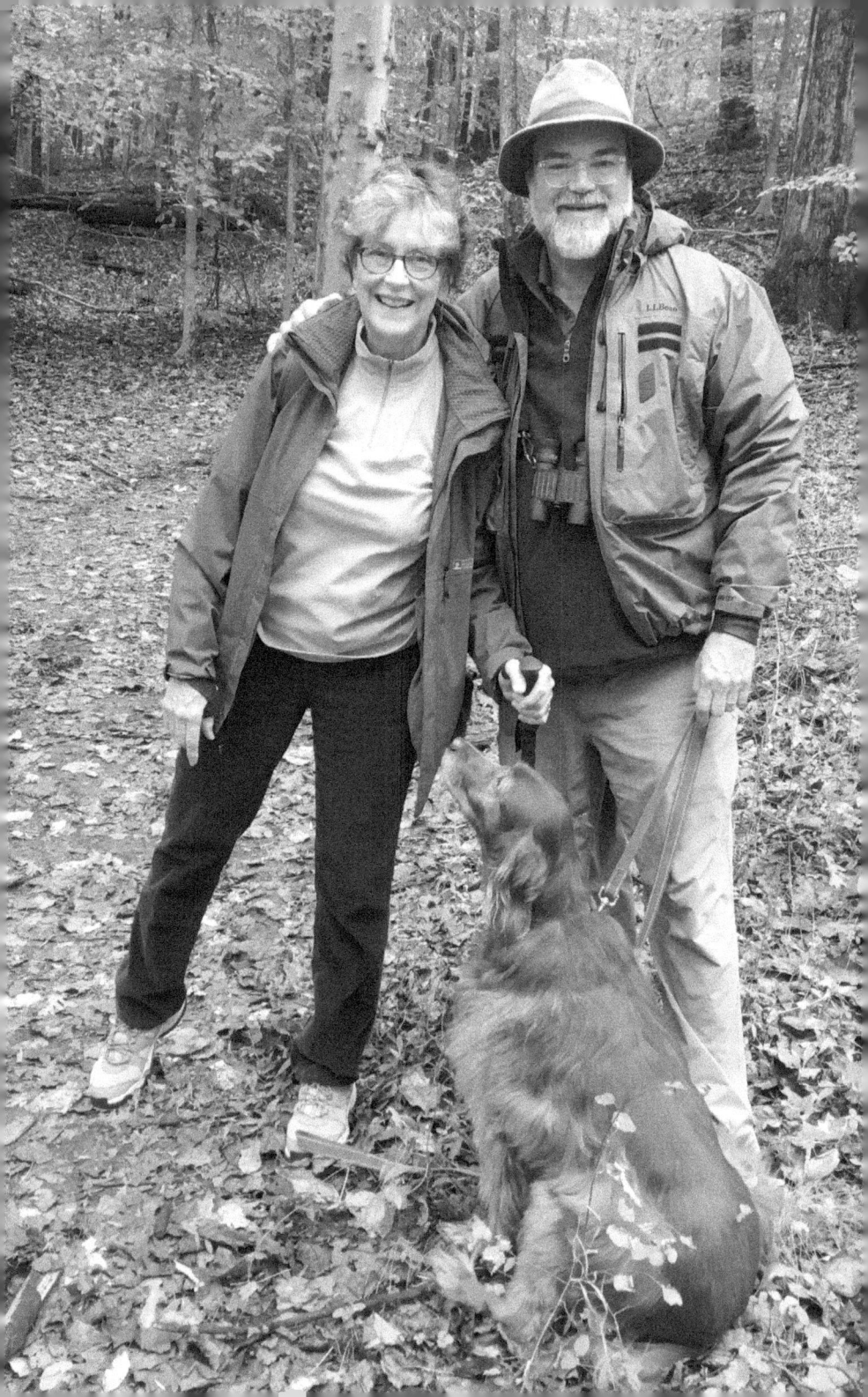

Dedicated to Louise, love of my life

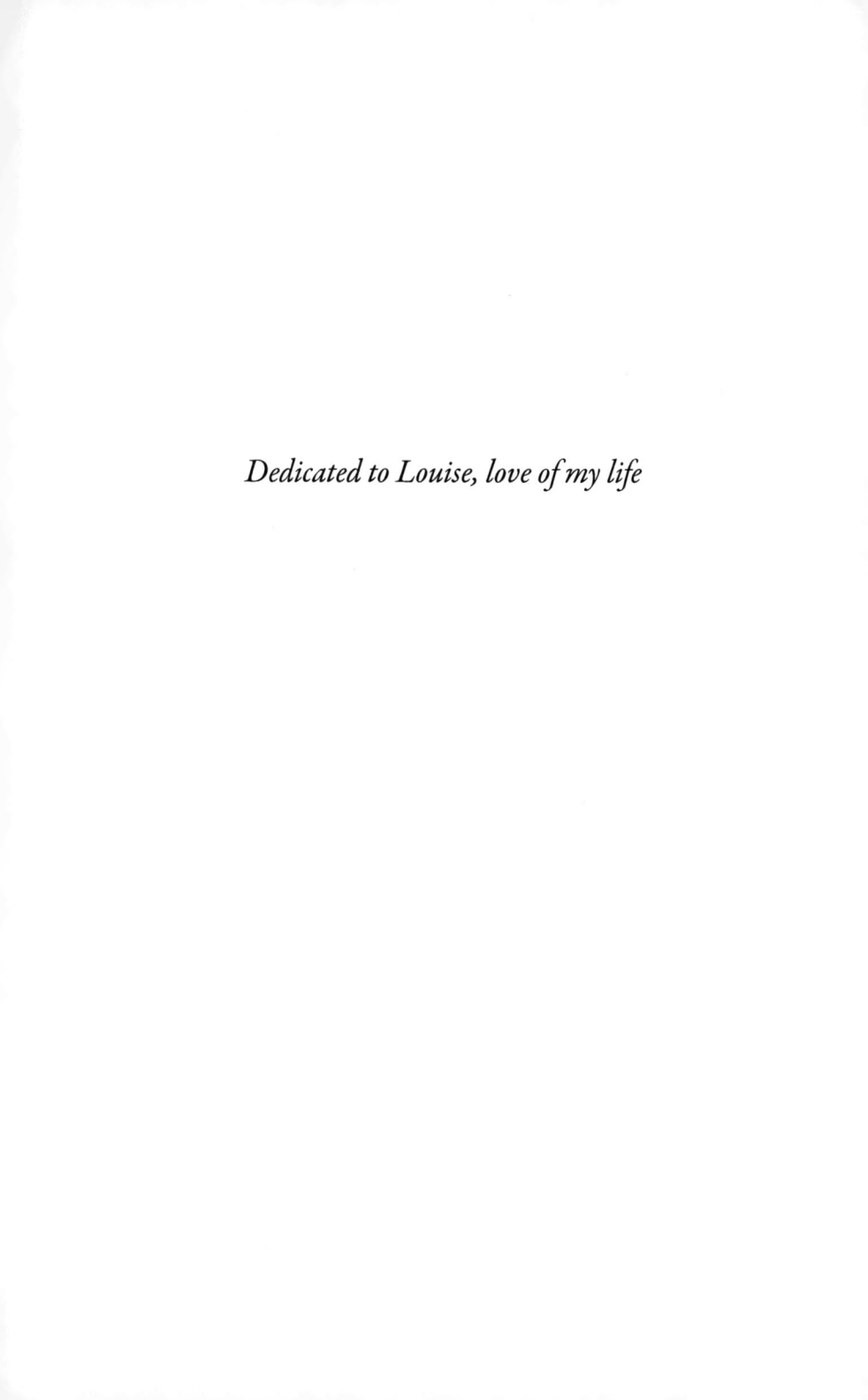

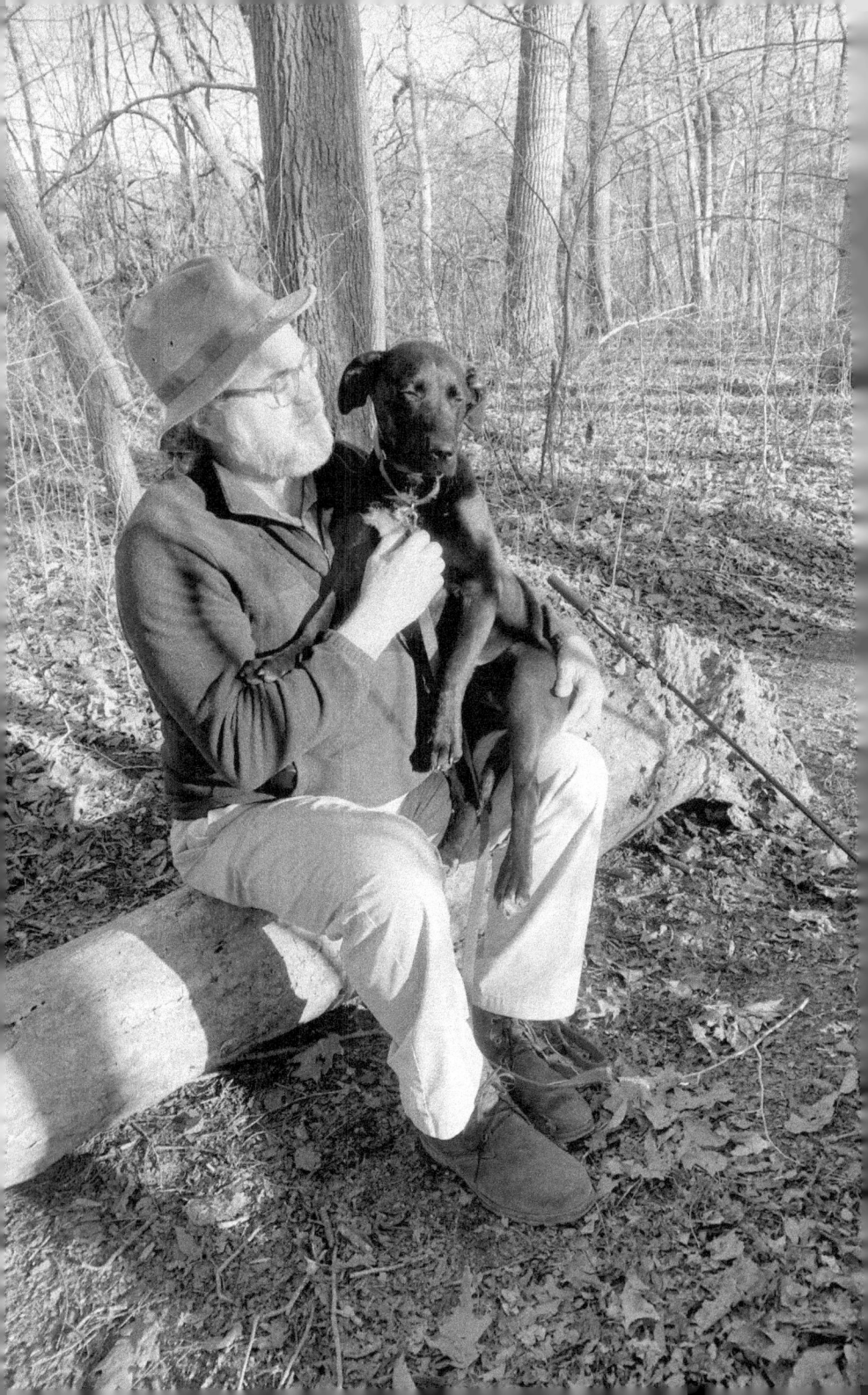

Foreword

Every week or so Jeff Holland sets out with a notebook, his "emotional support dog" Millie, and his custom walking stick (ahem, made by me). Sometimes his emotionally supportive wife, the incomparable Louise, comes along.

To find out where he went, you need to check out The *Annapolis Capital* newspaper on periodic Sundays. There, illustrated with a large photograph, will be his wonderful column about the parks and natural spaces in our county and state.

And you won't need a guidebook, either, because Jeff is better informed and a whole lot more interesting. As he ambles along wooded paths or quiet beaches, some of them seldom seen, he comments not only on what he observes but also on what he knows. His considerable research skills as well as wide life experience are invaluable here.

At various times, he has been a county Riverkeeper and head of the Annapolis Maritime Museum. He is a published author, a poet and founder of the swingin' Them Eastport Oyster Boys.

Jeff is an avuncular-looking guy who, as they say, has been around. You can tell by what he packs into his accounts: a bit of local history, a good bit of environmental lore and facts about special attractions in the parks. Even better is the wry wit he sprinkles around his commentary.

In a column typically full of information, in this case about Fort Smallwood Park, you can learn diverse things like when to see osprey, the origin of the name Patapsco, and why the fort was built there. In other columns you can find out how to build a breakwater and where to find the site of a 3,000-year-old oyster roast.

I always look forward to seeing what Jeff has to say about where he's been. I've known him for years, and when I read his words I can hear his voice and the voices of the many local people (some of them experts) he talks to on his pleasant wanderings.

As I said, this book is better than any guidebook and way more fun.

—Eric Smith, Cartoonist: *Annapolis Capital*

Contents

Walk 1   Scoping the Scoters at Thomas Point Park 1

Walk 2   Winter Wandering at Franklin Point State Park 6

Walk 3   Sauntering Around the Odenton Natural Area 13

Walk 4   Fort Smallwood Park: An Ageless Attraction 19

Walk 5   Ease Your Anxiety with a Good Walk at
Annapolis Waterworks Park 25

Walk 6   Walkin' in the Rain at Beverly Triton Nature Park 32

Walk 7   Discovering a Pocket Wilderness in Arnold 39

Walk 8   You Don't Know Jack Creek 46

Walk 9   Riding Baby Elephants at Patuxent Research Refuge . 53

Walk 10   A Solitary Beach Walk at Sandy Point State Park 60

Walk 11   Requiem for a Red Dog at Quiet Waters Park 67

Walk 12   Delving into the Historic Depths
at Wooton's Landing Wetlands Park 73

Walk 13   Hooking Sea Monsters at South River Farm Park 81

Walk 14   Discovering Sources at Severn Run
Natural Environmental Area 87

Walk 15   Spritely Whimsy of Spriggs Farm Park 93

Walk 16   Keeping Broad Creek Trail Safe from Bears 101

Walk 17   Trekking Through Truxtun Park 109

Walk 18   Waterworks Park Redux 115

Walk 19   Chillin' Out with Max at Bacon Ridge 121

JEFFERSON HOLLAND | xiii

Walk 20	The Goddess of Glendening Nature Preserve at Jug Bay	129
Walk 21	Dogless on the Hog Island Trail at Smithsonian Environmental Research Center	136
Walk 22	What's Towering over Greenbury Point	143
Walk 23:	Thank Volunteers for Beachwood Park	149
Walk 24	Mushing on Morning Choice Trail	155
Walk 25	Walking with Giants at Corcoran Woods	162
Walk 26	Meet Millie at Davidsonville Park	171
Walk 27	Back Creek Nature Park: A Hidden Gem in Annapolis	177
Walk 28	Taking a Turn Around Terrapin Nature Park	184
Walk 29	Searching for Palm Trees at Weinberg Park	191
Walk 30	Nursing a Broken Heart at Valentine Creek Trail	197
Walk 31	Patrolling the Yard at the United States Naval Academy	203
Walk 32	Kinder Farm Park: A Literal Kinder-garten	208
Walk 33	St. Luke's Restoration of Nature	215
Walk 34	Magothy Greenway Natural Area: a Wonderful Wilderness	221
Walk 35	Exploring Franklin Point State Park with Senator Sarah	227
Walk 36	What's Up at Downs Memorial Park	234
Walk 37	Millie Runs Happily Amok at Matapeake Dog Park	241
Walk 38:	Stroll Horn Point on the Eastport Walking Tour	247

Walk 39	Doggie Parks for the Dog Days of Summer	257
Walk 40	Hooray for Butterflies at Tawes Garden	262
Walk 41	Tour a Restored Stream at Broadneck Trail	268
Walk 42	Smelling the Begonias at Historic London Town and Gardens	276
Walk 43	Who's Who at St. Anne's Cemetery	282
Walk 44	A Free Morning at Annapolis City Dock	291
Walk 45	Paddling the Rhode River	299
Walk 46	Elktonia Beach: Walking a New Park with a New Walking Buddy	304
Walk 47	Chasing the Chill at Chesapeake Bay Foundation	310
Walk 48	Discovering History at Jonas and Anne Catharine Green Park	315
Walk 49	Ferry Point Park and Fried Oysters: A Winning Combination	321
Walk 50	Encountering Genius at Benjamin Banneker Historical Park & Museum	327
Walk 51	Back Creek by Kayak	333
Walk 52	Old Critters Endorse New Living Shoreline at Franklin Point State Park	340

About the Author ... 347

Photo Credits ... 349

Location Maps ... 355

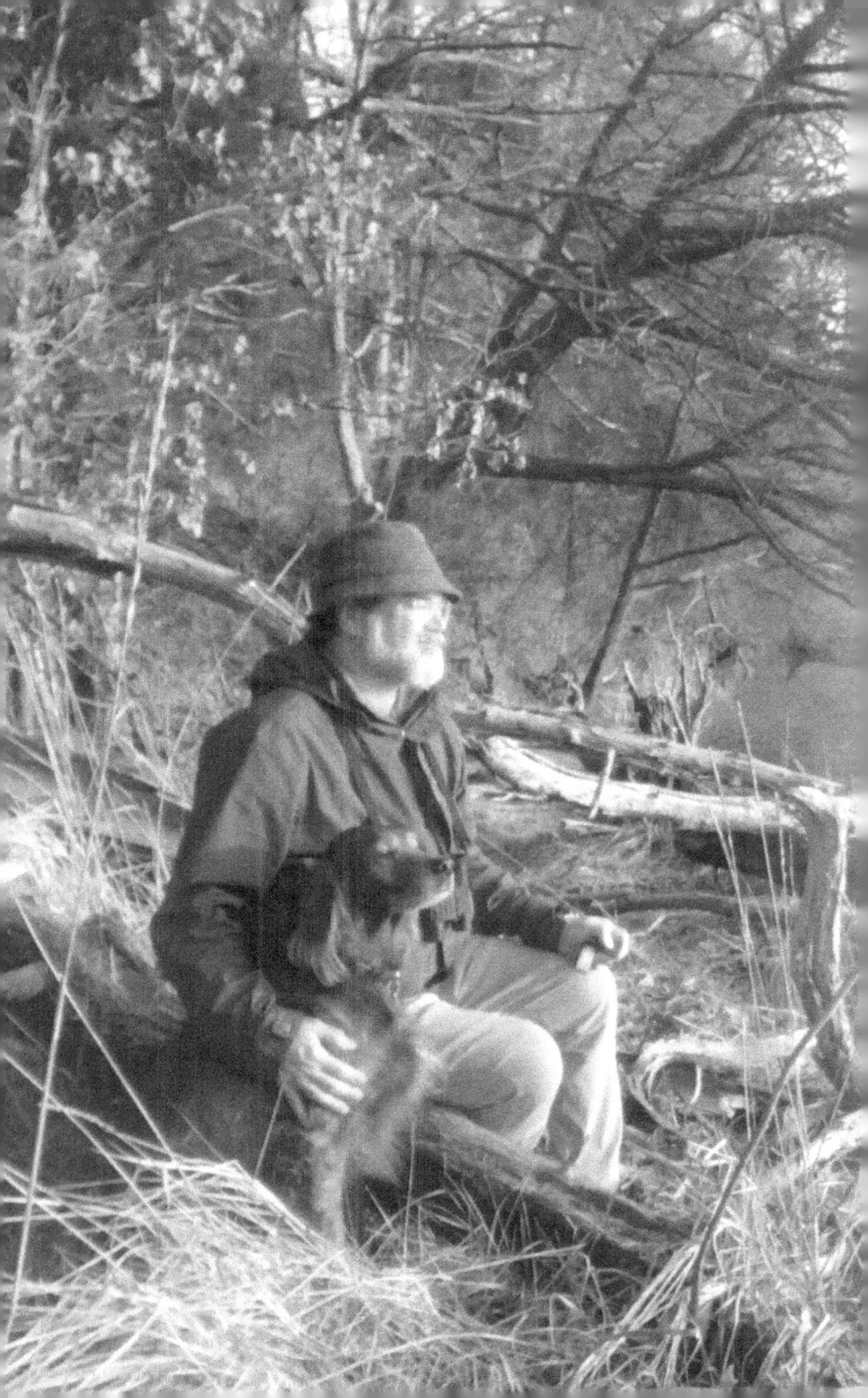

Walk Around
Arundel

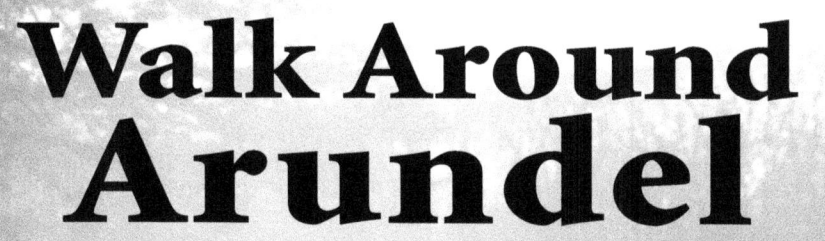

52 Places to Hike with Your Dog
(and Other Best Friends)

by Jefferson Holland

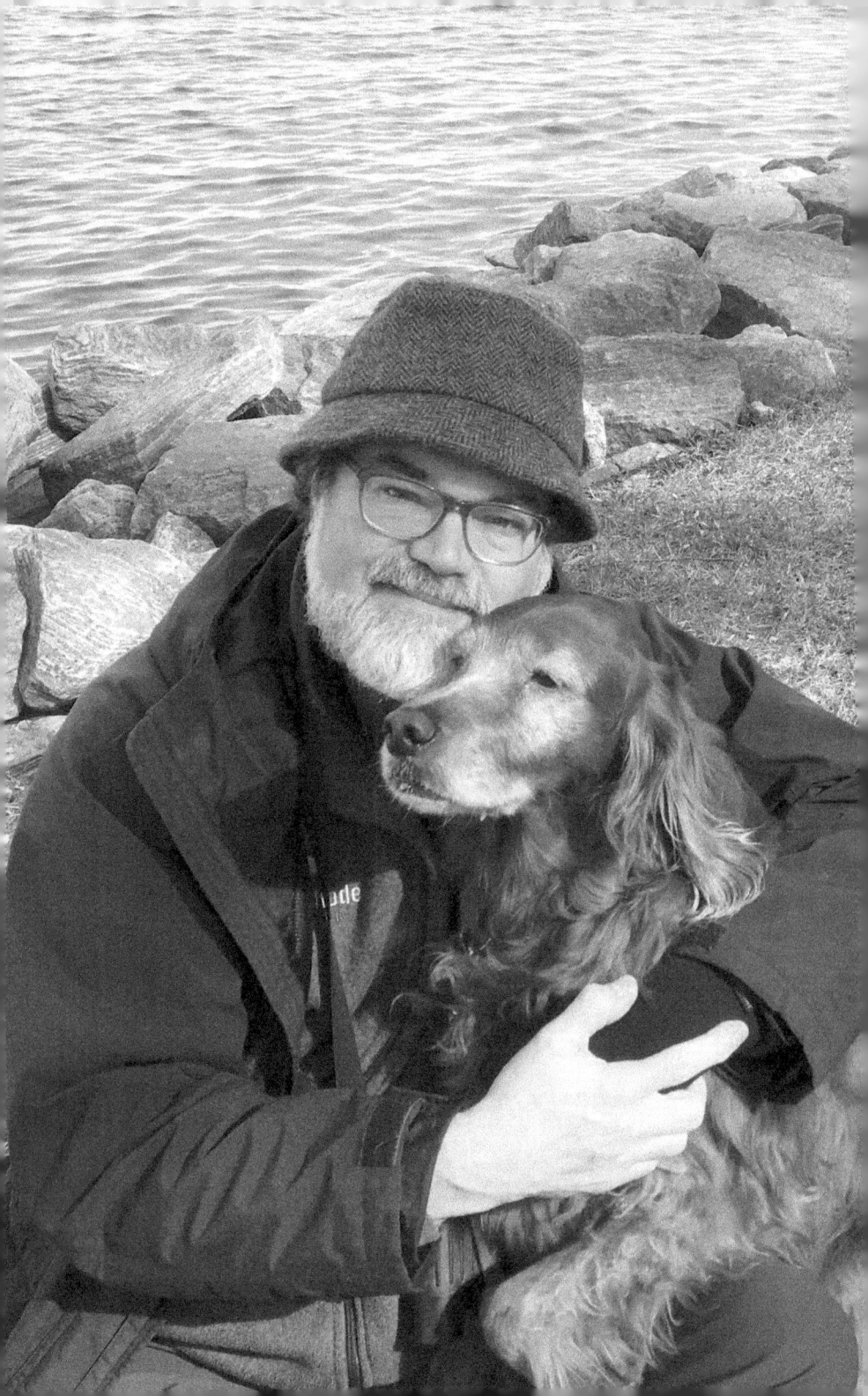

Walk 1

Scoping the Scoters at Thomas Point Park

Our Irish setter, Bonnie, was not a trained service dog, but she did have the instinctive ability to sense when my lower limb muscles were beginning to atrophy, when my oxygen level needed a boost, and when my mood would swing lower than low tide in a November nor'easter. She communicated her alarm with intense eye contact and a positively eerie interspecies mode of ESP. She stares at me and I know exactly what she's thinking: "Time for a walk!"

On President's Day in 2020, a sunny day with a bit of a nip in the air. Bonnie and my emotional-support spouse, Louise, went for a favorite cold-weather stroll in Thomas Point Park at the end of Arundel on the Bay Road. We bundled up, following the British advice that *There's no such thing as inclement weather, only inappropriate attire.*

Thomas Point is one of Anne Arundel County's smallest parks but one of the best for gawking at migratory waterfowl and the panoramic scenery of the Chesapeake Bay.

Thomas Point Park makes for an ideal winter walk if only for one practical reason: It's open without charge from 8 a.m. until about 5 p.m. every day between November 1 and March 31, except for Thanksgiving and Christmas. The rest of the year, you need to get a $6 day permit at the Quiet Waters Park gatehouse. Since Thomas Point Park is so small—just over a half-mile from the gate to where the tip of the peninsula pokes out into the Chesapeake Bay—only a limited number of permits are sold each day. A mere 75 monthly permits are available on a first-come, first-served basis on the last Thursday of the prior month for $30.

This is a very easy walk, all flat on unpaved road or forest path, and, as I mentioned, only about a mile to the end and back. But you're rewarded with a view sweeping from the Chesapeake Bay bridges to the north, all the way down to Curtis Point at the end of the Shady Side peninsula to the south. Curiously, on this day, there were no ships at anchor in the middle of the Bay.

On the day we were there, we shared the park with just one jogger, one dog walker, one young couple hugging an inexplicably inapt concrete statue of a brontosaurus, one trio of bird watchers speaking in a language that sounded like Estonian, one wildlife photographer, a family with a baby, and a retired guy from the Bay Woods community in Annapolis named James Harrison, who had launched a drone to take aerial videos of the Thomas Point Shoal Lighthouse. He said he's on a quest to get aerial views of all the active lighthouses on the Bay.

Mr. Harrison showed me the image on the screen of his hand-held controller. The drone was hovering directly above the lighthouse, showing the red tin roof of the hexagonal cottage. This is remarkable, since the lighthouse is 1.21 miles from the end of the point.

You can barely see the lighthouse without binoculars, but there it is, the last screw-pile lighthouse left in its original location, keeping passing vessels safe from running aground in the shallow waters between it and Thomas Point proper. It's been there since its iron pilings were manually screwed into the muddy bottom of the Bay in 1874. The rock piles you see on the north and south sides are an anachronism in this age of global warming. They were put there to protect the lighthouse from massive ice floes that caused the demise of many of the other 40-some such structures that once festooned the Bay.

You can get a closer look at similar lighthouses that have been moved to the maritime museums in St. Michaels and Solomons Island, or you can take a guided tour by boat of the Thomas Point Light offered by the volunteers from the Chesapeake Chapter of the U.S. Lighthouse Society starting each summer in June.

While we met so few people on our walk, we were delighted by the vast number of migratory waterfowl we encountered. The peninsula that is the park is shaped like a boomerang jutting out into the Bay, with the mouth of South River on one side and Fishing Creek on the other. As you enter through the iron gate (be sure to close it after you), the neck is barely wider than the road. We saw a large flock of tundra swans on the south side and a smaller flock on the north side.

We parked in the lot at the crook of the point, by an old log cabin that once served as the ranger's quarters. It's a pleasant walk along a trail through the mature oak forest. We popped out at the end of the point, where we found an armada of clown-faced surf scoters, more than I've ever seen together in one spot. Other diving ducks, mostly buffleheads and canvasbacks, bobbled in between. If you've never seen a surf scoter, look them up. They might remind you of a puffin that lost a bout with a pugnacious penguin. Definitely worth a visit to Thomas Point Park.

There's evidence of people visiting this site more than 2,000 years ago. Archaeologists have found ancient piles of oyster shells, indicating that this was an ideal spot for an oyster roast long before Capt. John Smith sailed by here on his voyages of discovery in 1608 and 1609. In fact, there's a blip on his map of 1612 that just might be this very point. In the mid-1600s, the surrounding area was owned by Phillip Thomas, one of the earliest English settlers. It was bequeathed to Anne Arundel County by the Lee family in the early 1960s.

When you visit Thomas Point Park for your winter walk, please heed the request of one nearby neighbor we met while walking her Australian labra-doodle: when you're driving along Thomas Point Road, slow way down where the road narrows. There are kids and dogs and cyclist and other wildlife that need your consideration.

Close the gate behind you, and don't neglect to pick up after your pup!

Thomas Point Park
3890 Thomas Point Road
Annapolis, MD 21403

410-222-1777

aacounty.org/locations-and-directions/thomas-point-park

Open 8 a.m. until ½ hour before dusk

Free admission between November 1 and March 31; $6/vehicle April 1–October 30 (see web site for discounts)

Plenty of parking on site

Portable toilet is available in the parking lot at the end

Sociable dogs on leash are welcome; bring your own doggy bags

Easy going

Walk 2

Winter Wandering at Franklin Point State Park

It was Sunday morning. I was planted in my comfy chair, sipping on a cup of coffee and reading the paper, when a wet nose poked up from under the letters to the editor and a furry chin pressed on my knee, emphasized by a fervently perched paw.

My beautiful red-haired companion, Bonnie, was subtly trying to get my attention. She is my Irish setter hike-along pal, the motivational force for hauling my lethargic hulk out of the house and into the woods for a breath of fresh air and a stretch of the legs. This day, when she stared up at me with those liquid brown eyes, I interpreted her interspecies ESP to mean, *Let's take a walk at Franklin Point!*

Franklin Point State Park is an undiscovered gem set on the Bay shore in southern Anne Arundel County. The best time to visit is in the winter, and so we went there on a sunny Sunday afternoon in late February 2020.

What makes this park special is not just its 477 acres of marsh, forest and field with saltwater ponds that open up onto the Chesapeake Bay, but also the inspirational tale of its salvation from development. Once a family-owned air park, similar to Lee Airport in nearby Edgewater, this property was doomed for development in the 1990s until a group known as the

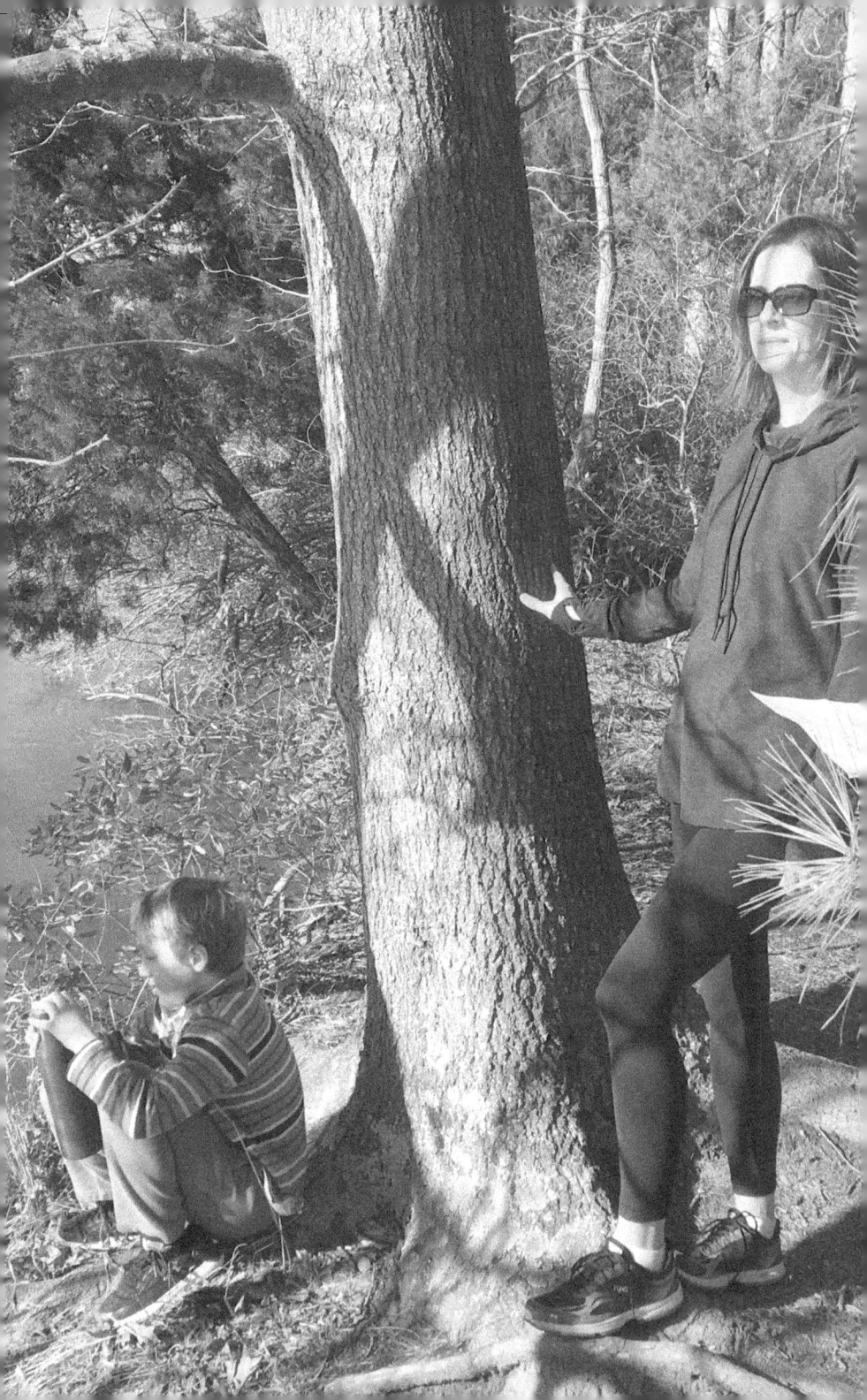

South Arundel Citizens for Responsible Development (SACReD) fought for its rescue.

Eventually, the state of Maryland took it over; it's managed by the staff at Sandy Point State Park. But lacking the resources to do anything with it, they padlocked the gate and let it lie fallow for 20 years. In 2015, Mike Lofton, the head of what became the Anne Arundel County Public Water Access Commission, encouraged the West & Rhode Riverkeeper organization to enter into an agreement with the Maryland Park Service to provide the volunteer people power to open the park to the public.

I had the privilege of serving as the Riverkeeper at that time, and I was blessed with a great team of volunteers led by local resident Dick Worth to do all the necessary work. They got busy cleaning up the site, creating trails, and providing monitors to keep an eye on the place. It opened to the public in 2017 and is now open every day, all year long, sunrise to sunset, and free of charge.

The park itself is in two parts, separated by a shallow estuary called Flag Pond. On one side, the actual peninsula called Franklin Point extends south along the Bay shore from the end of Columbia Beach Road.

You'll want to access the park on the mainland entrance off Shady Side Road. There's a sign for the park on the main road, but you have to keep an eye out for the turn onto Dent Road. Two dogleg turns will lead you to the newly renovated parking lot. As you approach, slow down and keep an eye out for the local kids on bikes and other wildlife.

There's a gate across the road leading beyond the parking lot to the boat launch on Deep Creek Pond. You can log onto the park service web site and get a combination for the lock so you can drive to the pond to launch your canoe or kayak. The launch site is just an opening in the low bank, but the bottom is fairly hard and it's an easy place to put in. Ironically, Deep Creek is only about 18 inches deep in the middle channel, so you have to check the tide tables if you don't want to shovel mud with your paddle blades.

Paddlers will have a lot of fun riding the tide, weaving through the reeds along the narrow channel out onto the open Bay. But you won't want to try that until the water temperature climbs up above 70 degrees, or you'll risk hypothermia if you dump.

The main trail leads you across the old landing strip and along a grassy path through the new growth of sweet gum trees and under a tunnel formed by overarching branches of an old stand of long-leaf pines. At the end of this half-mile-long path, you'll have a view of the channel leading from Deep Creek Pond out to the open Bay. A side trail will lead you through the mature oak forest and out onto the marsh. Here you can see the how the low native shrubs and grasses are being overrun by the tall invasive reeds from Eurasia called phragmites.

You can generally expect to see tundra swans, Canada geese, and great blue herons on the pond this time of year, and at least one glimpse of the pair of bald eagles nesting in the park, as well as throngs of songbirds and even a big flock of wild turkeys.

We met up with the Hinsch family. Mom, Dad and their two tween-age boys were visiting from Crownsville. We got acquainted as we strolled along the trails. We talked about the flora and fauna at the park, and about how county archaeologists have discovered ancient piles of oyster shells called "middens" in the park, indicating that there were people living here and feasting on the succulent bivalves nearly 3,000 years ago.

The Hinsch family did not bring a dog, but Bonnie was happy to be theirs for the time being. She likes kids a lot. In fact, when it came time for us to part paths, Bonnie was bound to go home with them. It took considerable negotiating to get her to follow me back to our car. I did not take offense. Not much.

Keep in mind that this is still a relatively new and pristine park; in other words, it's primitive. The sole facility of comfort, besides a couple of picnic tables by the water, is one handicap-accessible portable toilet in the parking lot.

Since this is coastal lowland, the trails can be muddy in spots even on the driest day, so be sure to wear sturdy, waterproof boots. The trail volunteers have lined up planks over some of the soggiest spots. The trails are well marked by bright white rectangles blazing the trees. Be sure to pick up one of the hand-drawn trail maps from the dispenser on the information kiosk at the parking lot.

There are some challenges, like lots of ticks in the summer, so wear your gaiters or white socks. But if you're looking for miles of solitude with walks through an interesting variety of habitats, from open marsh to dense hardwood forest, this place is well worth exploring.

Franklin Point State Park
End of Dent Road
Shady Side, MD 20764
410-974-22149
dnr.maryland.gov/publiclands/pages/southern/franklinpoint.aspx
Log on for combination to gate lock if launching
car-top boats
Plenty of parking in the lot to the left before the gate
Open dawn to dusk, seven days a week
Free admission
Portable toilet in the parking lot
Polite dogs on leash are welcome; bring your own doggy bags
Easy going, with some soggy bits and lots of summer bugs

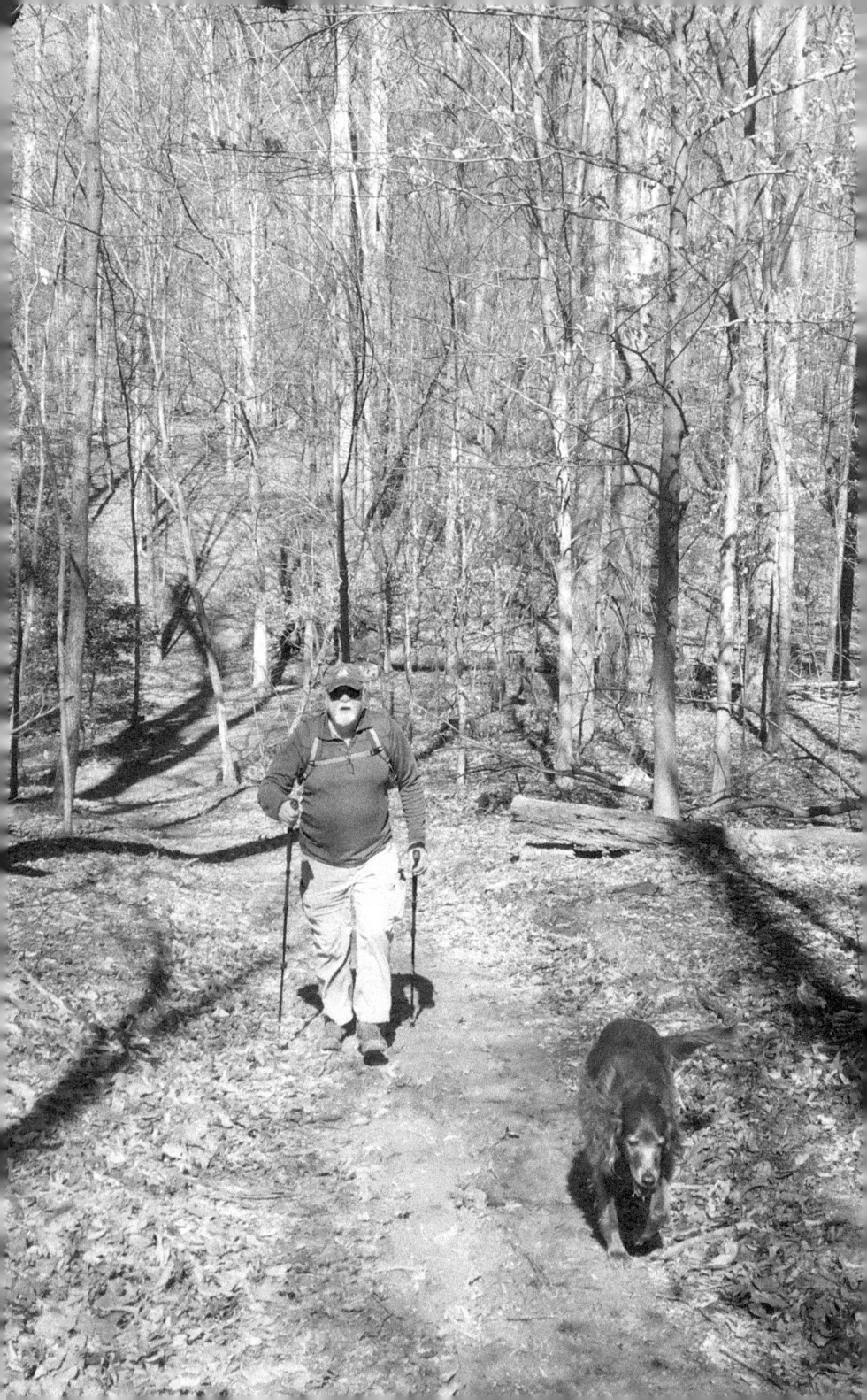

Walk 3

Sauntering Around the Odenton Natural Area

John Muir, the Father of the National Parks, hated "hiking." "People ought to saunter in the mountains—not hike!" he declared. He noted that the verb "to saunter" had its origins in the Middle Ages, when people would go on pilgrimages to the Holy Land, or "A la sainte terre."

"Now these mountains are our Holy Land," Muir said, as quoted by Albert W. Palmer in *The Mountain Trail and Its Message* in 1911, "and we ought to saunter through them reverently, not 'hike' through them."

One spring Sunday in 2020, I took a reverential saunter through the valley of the Odenton Natural Area with my friend Dave Isbell. Of course, Bonnie, my Irish setter walking companion, came along with us.

While it was not mountainous like Muir's beloved Sierras, there was some undulating topography, and we spent a pleasant couple of hours rambling amicably through the forest of lofty gray beech, white oak, and yellow poplar trees.

Dave retired from a career in the Coast Guard and now splits his time between building authentic Aleut kayaks in his basement, setting off on challenging paddle adventures in the upper reaches of Canada or through the Florida Everglades, and sharing his expertise at Annapolis Canoe and Kayak in Eastport.

He found the Odenton Natural Area on a smartphone app called AllTrails. The area is located in the watershed of Towsers Branch, a rivulet tributary to the Patuxent River tucked in between Fort Meade and the Sunrise Farm, formerly known as the Naval Academy Dairy Farm. Since it was news to both of us, we decided to give it a go.

We parked at Arundel Middle School, which seemed to be the best place to gain access. There's a broad wooden staircase leading down to the trailhead. The area is part of a spur of the county's WB&A trail, the nine-mile paved recreational trail that runs along the old Washington, Baltimore and Annapolis Railroad right-of-way between Odenton and the Patuxent River. The park is managed by the Anne Arundel County Department of Park and Recreation.

On the AllTrails app, there's a broad green trail looping around the site. Down in the valley there is a nice beaten path, but it's not terribly well marked and didn't seem to sync with what showed up on our cellphone screens. There are big white arrows spray-painted on random trees, but then there are other arrows marking cross trails as well as small green signs that must be somebody's inside joke. Perhaps these are mementos of cross-country runs or other events over time. To us, they only added to the adventure. After all, we weren't hiking to get anywhere; we were just sauntering.

I must note here that Dave knows his way around a chart. He has taught classes in celestial navigation. He has sailed the oceans by the stars. But here, in this valley, with a three-inch screen showing a map that had little relationship to what we found on the ground, he was a bit befuddled. "It's easier out on the water," he muttered.

We chatted as we sauntered. We talked about upcoming kayak adventures. Dave cautioned me not to launch too soon in the season. "If you fall into cold water," he said, "the biggest problem is the gasp reflex. Suck in icy water and you're a goner instantly. If you survive that, the cold water makes your hands and limbs useless, making it harder to rescue yourself. After a short time, you succumb to hypothermia." He later sent me a link to the National Center for Cold Water Safety. They say that you should "treat any water colder than 70 degrees Fahrenheit with caution." I will certainly do so from now on.

We hardly saw anyone the whole time we were there, except for a group of middle-school kids, a young couple from Crofton, and a father and daughter walking with their yellow Lab. This last trio baffled us. First, they veered off onto a side path to our right, and then not much later, we saw them again high up on top of the hill to our left. Or maybe we got turned around in the meantime. Still, it didn't matter. We were enjoying the brilliant sunshine filtering down through the bare treetops and the ratcheting sound of the woodpeckers in the distance as we walked and talked.

This is a particularly dog-friendly place, but you need to bring your own doggie bags, as any responsible dog person would do. I generally bring another plastic bag just for litter, but we didn't see any, and the creek was refreshingly devoid of trash and running clear.

Bonnie is an exceptionally well-behaved dog and responds to my slightest whistle. The county requires a leash, but in this instance, I followed my own strict rule, which is to always have your dog on a leash while there's anybody watching. Generally, even when she's not on the leash, she walks right with me as though she's attached anyway. Whenever we encounter wildlife, like deer, she freezes, not like a pointer but like a deer. A deer in the headlights, that is.

Both Dave and I had hiking staffs. I've got one, but Dave prefers using a pair of them. His double as tent poles when he goes on overnight hikes. Mine was particularly helpful on the downhill scoots along paths covered with fallen leaves. While it hadn't rained much lately, there were some muddy spots in the lower portions of the main trail, so I was glad I was wearing my waterproof walking shoes.

The app shows the main trail runs about 2.4 miles. When we got back to the car, we had logged 2.1, so I guess we didn't see everything there was to see, but what we did see was quite pleasant for a sunny winter Sunday afternoon. We spent nearly two hours there. That's what I call sauntering.

Odenton Natural Area
517 Higgins Drive
Odenton, MD 21113

Plenty of parking at Arundel Middle School, 1179 Hammond Lane

410-222-7317

aacounty.org/locations-and-directions/odenton-natural-area

Open dawn to dusk, seven days a week

Free admission

No toilets on site

Polite dogs on leash are welcome; bring your own doggy bags

Moderate going, with some topography

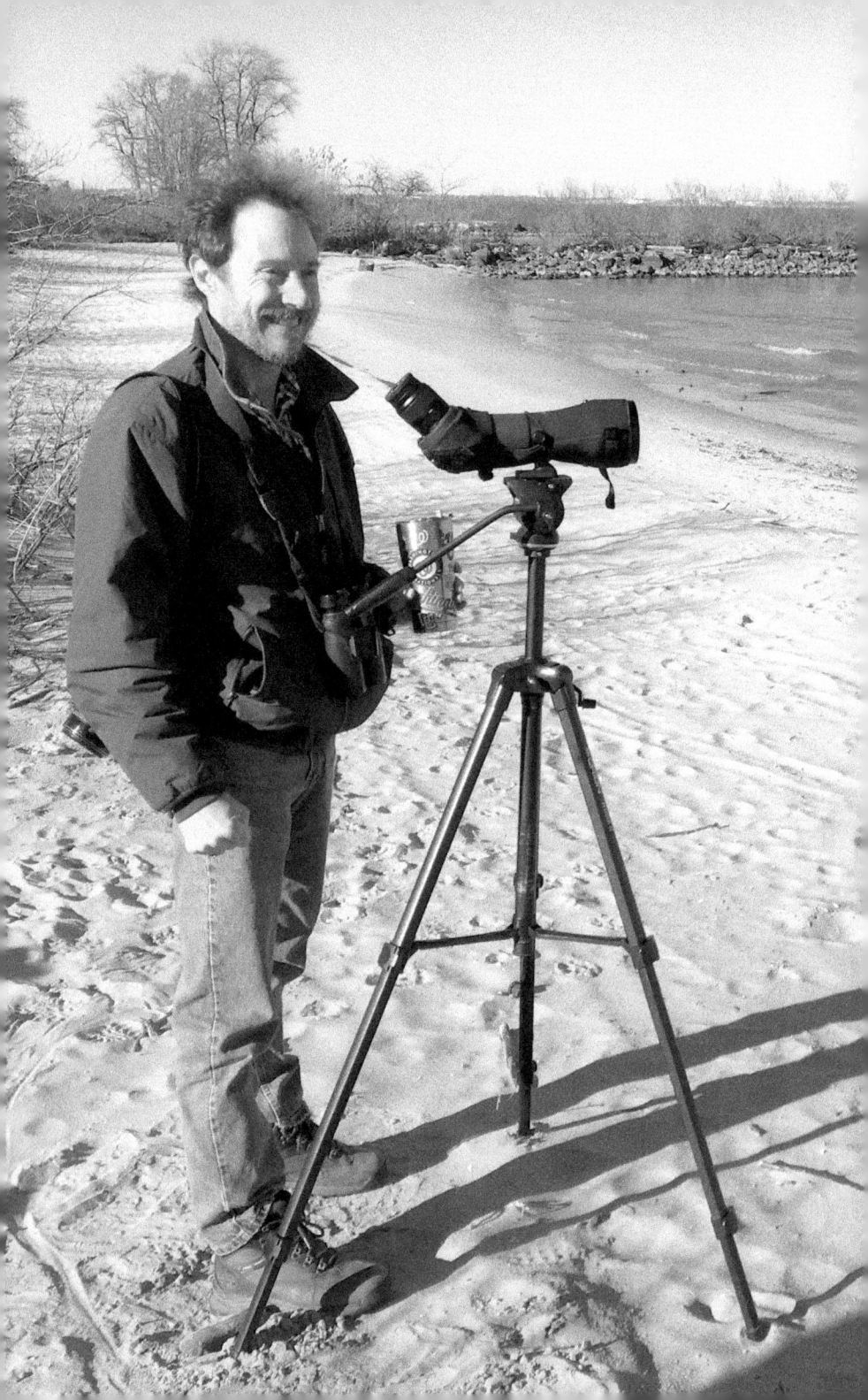

Walk 4

Fort Smallwood Park: An Ageless Attraction

Jack Benny had it right. "Age is strictly a case of mind over matter," he said. "If you don't mind, it doesn't matter."

Me, I like being my age. In some stores, cashiers take one look at my gray beard and give me senior discounts without my even asking. I can get a fishing license from DNR for just five bucks. And the minute I turned 60, I splurged a whole $40 to buy my Lifetime Senior Citizen Permit that gets me into any Anne Arundel County park as often as I like. And I like to use it a lot.

One Saturday in early March 2020, I checked out Fort Smallwood Park with my walking buddy, Bonnie, the eight-year-old Irish setter who, like me, is a bit gray around the muzzle, but always eager to find a new place to go for a good walk. The pass got us through the gate. For those of you who are not so privileged with seniority, there's a daily parking fee $6 per vehicle. If you have an MVA handicapped tag, the fee is $5. Those in the military, veterans, or their families get in for free.

Named for a Revolutionary War general, Fort Smallwood was built in 1890 as a coastal battery protecting Baltimore from attack. It sits strategically on Rock Point at the mouth of the Patapsco River at the very northeastern tip of Anne Arundel County.

The cement hulk of a gun battery still exists. A map of the fort from 1921 shows two batteries, each mounting two large guns. The surviving structure is Battery Hartshorne, which, until 1927, mounted two six-inch guns. Each gun could hurl a 108-pound shell more than eight miles across the mouth of the river or into the Chesapeake Bay.

There was a second fort on the opposite side, at North Point, and a third upstream near the south end of the Key Bridge.* Between these three forts, the triangulated cannon fire could destroy any enemy fleet foolish enough to try to enter the river. If those forts had been there a hundred years earlier, we'd have had to find a different national anthem.

When the fort was decommissioned in 1928, it became a Baltimore City park. Bonnie and I met a photographer named Derrick Camper, who remembers playing around the old barracks and the battery when he was a kid, tagging along with his father, a recreation guide who would bring groups of inner-city children here for a breath of fresh air. A resident of Woodlawn, Derrick likes to come here with his telephoto lens to take panoramic pictures of the Baltimore skyline when he's not marketing medical textbooks.

Anne Arundel County took command of Fort Smallwood in 2006 and made it into one of its crown-jewel regional parks. Fort Smallwood Park covers about 90 acres along the river's edge, with open, grassy fields and stands of tall sweet gum trees.

Walking along the shoreline, you can see Derrick's view of Baltimore's skyscraper skyline beyond the brontosaurus skeleton of the Key Bridge.* In the foreground, you see something you'll hardly find anywhere else on the Chesapeake Bay: rocks.

New England is famous among sailors for its rocks. They make a sickening *crunch* when your hull connects with them, which is a good incentive for never running aground in New England cruising waters. Here in the Chesapeake, it's different. It's shallow, which means the chances of your running around are good, but the bottom is mostly soft mud, which means your hull doesn't go crunch as much as it goes *whoomph*. And even then, sometimes it takes you awhile to realize you've stopped going anywhere fast. And that's not so bad. You just have to wait until the tide turns, or, if worse comes to worse, you get out and wade home.

But here are these huge white rocks, plunked down near the mouth of the Patapsco. Even John Smith noted them on his voyage of discovery in 1608. They're likely the source of the river's name. A scholar of the Algonquian family of languages, a guy named William Wallace Tooker, was quoted in "Indian Place Names in Maryland," published in a 1907 volume of the *Maryland Historical Magazine*. He claimed to have sussed out the true meaning of the word *Patapsco*. Tooker said that "Pota-" means "to jut out;" "-psk" means "a ledge of rock;" and "ut" means "at." So "Potapsk-ut" means this very point, "at the jutting ledge of rock."

They're called the White Rocks, but it's not because of what you think. There are birds hanging out there, but the white color is not from guano. It seems that they are comprised of hard white sandstone from the Cretaceous period, deposited here eons before the glaciers receded 20,000 years ago, forming the Chesapeake Bay.

Bonnie and I walked around the pond, which for some curious reason is protected by a high cyclone fence. I'm not sure whether it's there to protect me from the water or to protect the wildlife—great blue heron, geese and even beavers— in the water from me and Bonnie. There are several small crescents of sandy beach on the Bay side with no protection at all, not even lifeguards.

There we met Fred Shaffer of Crofton, peering through his spotting scope perched on a tripod stuck in the sand. He was looking at the diving ducks bobbing off in the Bay. An avid birder, Fred likes to come to the park often. "This is a great spot," he said. "It's always good for seeing waterfowl."

He was eager to share his latest sighting: "I saw my first osprey today," he grinned, noting that the raptors seem to be migrating back to the Bay at least two weeks earlier than usual. He's working on a book of all of the gull species in North America and has traveled from the West Coast to Alaska for his research.

Fred's a big fan of the park for another reason. He recently retired from the Prince Georges County planning department, where he created parks and trails. "People need access to the outdoors," he noted. "People want to get outside and be by the water. I always thought that trails were one low-cost thing governments can do to improve people's quality of life."

In addition to the walking and bike trails and paths crisscrossing the grounds, Fort Smallwood Park's recreational amenities include a new trailerable boat ramp, the 380-foot Bill Burton Fishing Pier, a colorful children's playground, volleyball courts, and the original barracks. If you want to entertain 99 of your closest friends, say, for your next birthday party, you can rent the historic Cedar Pavilion.

* The Key Bridge was felled by an errant container ship on March 26, 2024.

Fort Smallwood Park
9500 Fort Smallwood Road
Pasadena, MD 21122

410-222-0087

aacounty.org/departments/recreation-parks/parks/fort-smallwood/

Open 5:30 a.m. to dusk, seven days a week

Admission: $6 per car (see web site for discounts)

Plenty of parking on site

Toilet facilities on site

Happy dogs on leash are welcome; doggie bag dispensers available

Easy going

Walk 5

Ease Your Anxiety with a Good Walk at Annapolis Waterworks Park

You can't catch anything from trees except tranquility.

Okay, there's all that pollen. So you might get a little hay fever, but a walk in the woods will cure your cabin fever. And your viral anxiety.

It was late March 2020, just as the pandemic pandemonium was settling in. After several days of hand washing—and hand wringing—my wife Louise, with whom I was co-isolating–and since there are two of us, I guess you could call it "bi-solating"—suggested that the dog needed a walk.

Upon reflection, I think Louise was actually trying to get rid of me for a few hours. I consulted the Center for Disease Control guidelines on the web, but didn't find anything to contraindicate a good walk outdoors, as long as I kept a respectful distance from anybody trying to be social with me.

Just then a text popped up from my pal Dave Isbell, saying he was on his way to check out the trail at Annapolis Waterworks Park. "Wait for me!" I replied, and whistled for the dog. Bonnie appeared at the head of the stairs, eager to go anywhere. Right now. Anywhere. Now. Fortunately, I had everything I needed already waiting out in the car, being prepared like the good scout I used to be.

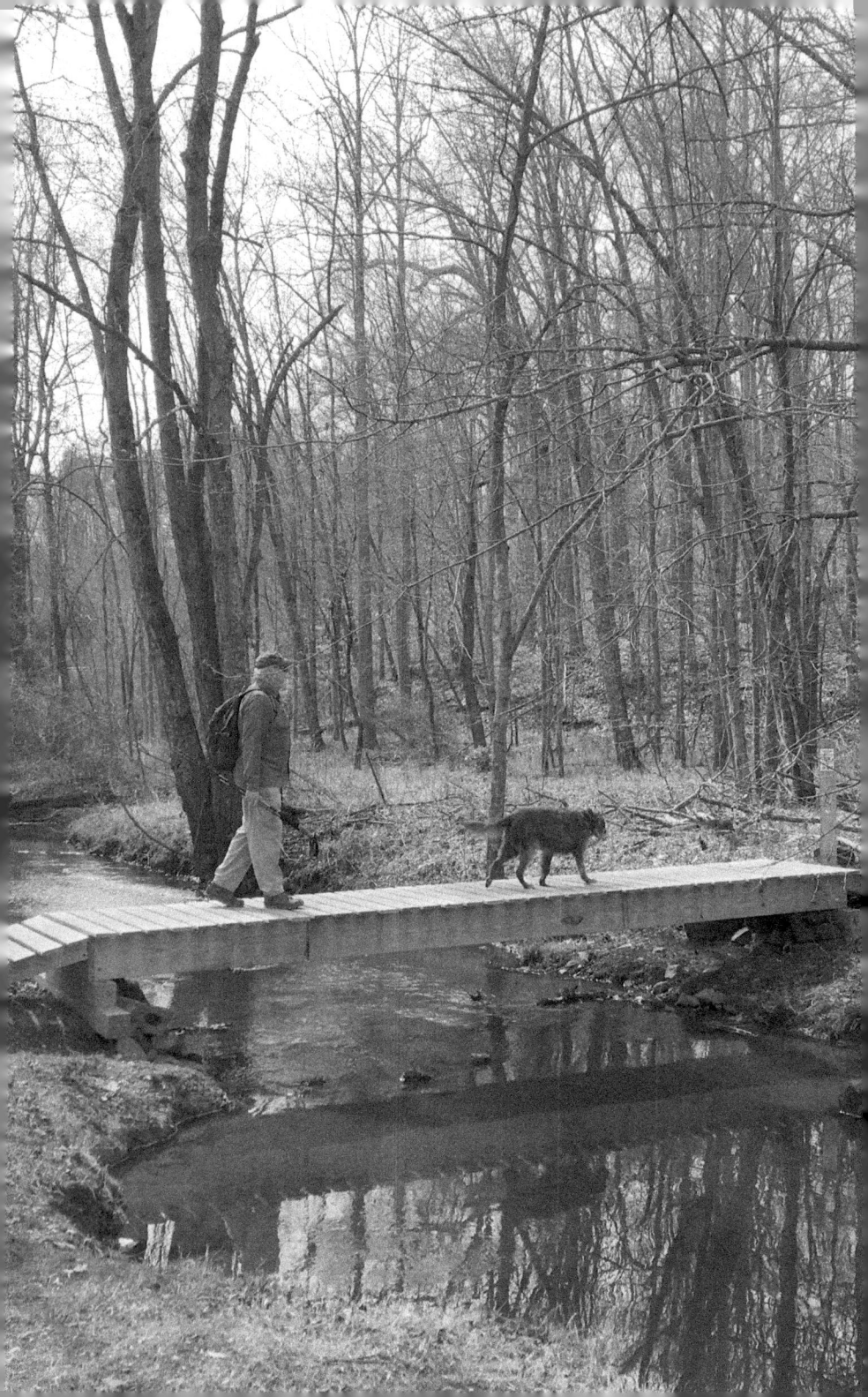

I've got a daypack, water bottle, binoculars, hiking shoes, hat, and walking stick in the back of the Forester, along with a leash, doggie bags, a water bowl, and a box of dog biscuits. I use a Thermos for a water bottle, rather than any of the 23 designer bottles we've collected over the years. I am always mystified by alleged water bottles that are designed more like infants' sippy cups, or more accurately like gag-gift dribble glasses. One might think that a key goal in designing a water bottle is to make it so that it actually holds water.

My dad was ahead of his time, always recommending that we kids dress in layers for the outdoors, and that's how I'm dressed most of the time now, no matter where I'm going. This was on a bright, clear day, a little on the cool side, but a light fleece was plenty of protection. Bonnie jumped in the back, and we were off.

Dave had told me about the trails at the Annapolis Waterworks Park, and I was eager to investigate. You'd never believe that there are 11 miles of trails winding through 600 acres of dense hardwood forest in an area tucked between General's Highway and Defense Highway. I met Dave at the trailhead on Housley Road. There's a wide berm along the road near the Stone Point Apartments where a dozen or so cars can park. Since it was a weekday, there was plenty of space for our cars, but I've seen all the spots taken on busy weekends.

This single-file hard-packed trail runs through property managed by the city of Annapolis Recreation and Parks Department. It starts out along the deep gully of the headwaters of Broad Creek and winds through a forest of oak and holly mixed with huge yellow poplars and beech trees.

Volunteers from the nonprofit group Mid-Atlantic Off-Road Enthusiasts and TrailWerks Cyclery in Millersville blazed these trails the year before. They comprise four loops and five connector trails over steeply rolling terrain. One loop takes you across a little footbridge over the outfall of the dam at Waterworks Park and up around the 80-acre field of solar panels that covers the old Annapolis landfill. From there, it goes all the way up to Honeysuckle Lane. You can go on even farther to connect with Anne Arundel County's Bacon Ridge trails in Crownsville.

Since the trail was single-file, Dave and I were able to keep our respectful distance while we walked and talked. The trails are narrow, but they seem ideal for avid mountain bikers, and we saw tire tracks in the dirt but no actual cyclists that day. Dave peered down one sheer hillside about 100 feet to the creek and wondered drolly if we might see any bodies crumpled up in a heap of bike bits at the bottom.

This was a Monday, and perhaps it was an off day, early in the season, but still, we met few fellow trekkers, other than one woman walking her two little dogs while chatting on her cell phone and a couple of happy-looking moms shepherding a scraggle of kids, glad for now not to have to be in school. The littlest one jumped and cheered, "It's a Corona day!"

We were surprised to run across our friend and kayaking buddy Rick Leader, who recently moved back to Annapolis and now lives in the nearby Stone Point Apartments.

"It's great to have all this in my back yard," he grinned. Until recently, Rick served as the executive director of Scenic Rivers Land Trust, a nonprofit group that has protected more than 3,000 acres of Anne Arundel County open space like this over the past 30 years, including 630 acres in the Bacon Ridge Natural Area and 574 acres of the Contee Farm on the grounds of the Smithsonian Environmental Research Center in Edgewater.

Dave, Bonnie, and I enjoyed the challenge of a brisk walk up and down the hillsides. We admired the splendid views of the creek valley below, more visible while the trees were still in their leafless winter mode. For years, I've driven past a Maryland historical marker on Defense Highway that says this area was part of a plantation patented to the Dorsey family in 1664 called "Hockley-in-the-Hole," and I've always wondered about that odd name.

It probably refers to a neighborhood in London infamous for the sports of bull and bear baiting, but it's not hard to believe that one of the Dorsey brothers was reminded of the word "hole" while looking down into the deep valley of Broad Creek.

The trail is well marked with directional plaques mounted on four-by-four posts at the crossroads. We followed the creek and wound up on the hill overlooking the dam at the Waterworks Park. This part of the park is accessible by car from Defense Highway. You can fish in the three freshwater fishing ponds behind the dam. It's catch-and-release only, and you'll need a license unless you're 16 or younger.

Another historical marker notes that the Annapolis Water Company dates back to the Civil War. The Maryland General Assembly chartered it in 1863 after a fire broke out in the State House. When it was completed in 1866, the water works could pump clean, potable water from this reservoir about three miles to Annapolis through then-innovative concrete pipes. The availability of abundant water might also have helped persuade the Naval Academy to return from Newport, Rhode Island, where it had decamped for the duration of the war.

In 1939, Annapolis drilled its first drinking water well and began mixing that with the water from the reservoir. Today, the city pumps its water from eight wells ranging from 250 to 1,000 feet deep. The wells tap into three aquifers: Magothy, Upper Patapsco, and Lower Patapsco. We walked behind the cisterns of the city's water treatment plant, situated at the top of the hill overlooking Defense Highway. This plant delivers more than 1.5 billion gallons of water to residents and businesses every year.

Off on a distant hilltop, we could see the glint of some of the 55,000 solar panels in that solar field the city had built over its old landfill in 2018. One of the loops of the Waterworks trail leads up around there and beyond, but we decided to save that for another day.

Instead, we looped back toward Housley Road. Checking my apps back at the car, I saw that we'd logged 3.3 miles in about two hours, having enjoyed a good adventure in a place that promises a lot more adventures until it's safe to shake hands again.

Annapolis Waterworks Park, Waterworks Trailhead
2607 Housley Road
Annapolis, MD 21401

410-263-7958

annapolis.gov/DocumentCenter/View/449/Waterworks-Park-Brochure-PDF?bidId

Limited parking along Housley Road near Stone Point Apartments

Open dawn to dusk, seven days a week

Free admission

No toilets on site

Obedient dogs on leash are welcome; bring your own doggy bags

Moderate going, some topography

Walk 6

Walkin' in the Rain at Beverly Triton Nature Park

Face it, Bonnie is a wuss. She hates getting wet. If it's raining, she'll hold her bladder as long as it takes for the grass to dry so she won't get her dainty paws bedewed. Maybe it's her breeding. She's an Irish setter, an upland bird dog, not like all of our former dogs, bred to retrieve waterfowl. And tennis balls.

The other dogs, like me, not only endured getting wet, but required it, like salamanders. Or better yet, like manatees. But not Bonnie. So when I decided I needed a walk on a recent rainy day, I knew that for just this once, I had to leave my best walking buddy behind.

It had been a while since I'd been to one of my favorite spots, Beverly Triton Nature Park, so I headed for the end of the Mayo peninsula all by myself on a damp, dank day in late March 2020. When I arrived at the park, there was only one other car in the parking lot, while on a nice day, it can be quite full. I like this place because of its unmanicured, natural setting along the Bay shore at the mouth of West River. It has quite an interesting history, another victory of public access over private development.

According to an article published in 2019 in the *Annapolis Capital* newspaper, Beverly Triton Nature Park was once part of a beach resort for whites only that closed

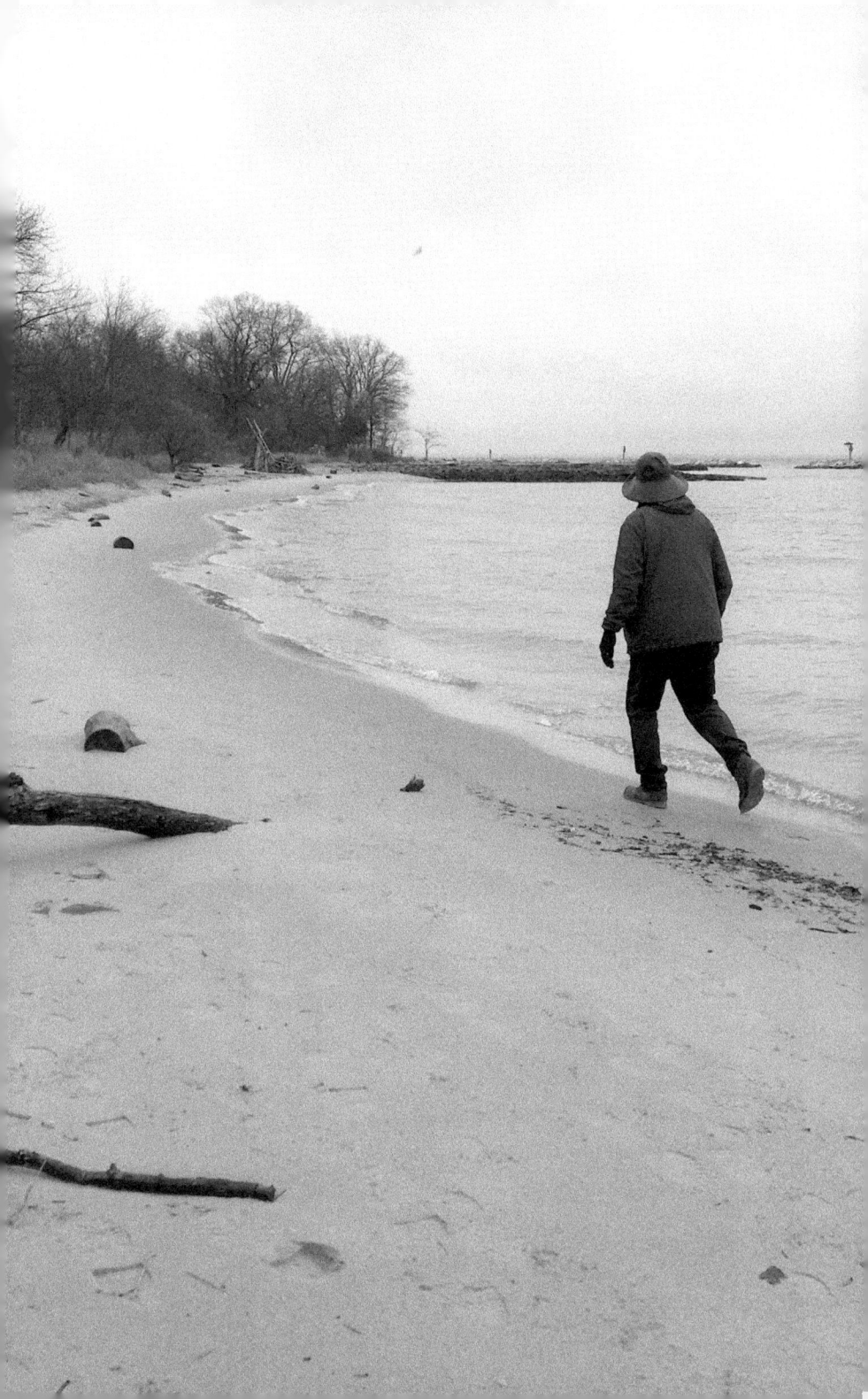

in 1968 when a court ruled that the resort could no longer be segregated.

In the 1980s, a plan to build more than 2,000 luxury units went bust after the developer couldn't get the county to provide sewer service. In 1985, under the leadership of then County Executive O. James Lighthizer and Council President Virginia Clagett, the county procured $3.2 million in Program Open Space funding to buy the property. This is a program managed by the Maryland Department of Natural Resources, designed to provide funds to acquire outdoor recreation and open space areas for public use.

At the time, Lighthizer focused the county's resources on developing Quiet Waters Park in Annapolis and let Beverly Triton go fallow. It has only recently become accessible to the public.

Beverly Triton Nature Park comprises 340 acres of oak-and-holly forest surrounding large tidal ponds. It's set at the end of the Mayo peninsula, where the West River meets the Chesapeake Bay. About five miles of trails wind through the park. I hadn't done the whole length of the trail around the ponds, so that's the one I took.

I had dressed for the occasion in my usual foul-weather gear: pants, parka, boots and gloves, all made with breathable, waterproof Gore-Tex linings. You can keep the rain off with a plastic garbage bag, but you'll still get wet. The plastic will keep the rain out, but it will also keep condensation and perspiration in, creating a vapor that will make you just as damp and uncomfortable as if you'd been wearing a burlap sack. Gore-Tex isn't perfect, but it is designed to let tiny particles of vapor seep out through the fabric while repelling the larger water droplets.

Under my parka, I layer with a quick-dry wicking polo shirt and a lightweight fleece. I prefer a good hat to the parka hood. My favorite rain hat is a classic Black Diamond sou'wester, rubber on the outside and lined with flannel. It keeps the rain off my face and keeps it from dripping down the back of my neck. It doesn't obstruct peripheral vision like a hood, and best of all, lets me keep the top of the parka open to vent the vapors, while the hood just keeps all that moisture building up inside.

The Pond Trail is well marked with orange blazes painted on tree trunks and color-coded arrows on waymark posts at the intersections. It starts out as a hard-packed gravel road. It's important to consider the surface of the path when you're walking in the rain. Try to choose trails that are paved, graveled, mulched, boardwalked, or otherwise well-groomed. If you churn up mud, you're leaving it in a mess for the rest of us when it dries. This trail is a curious mix of all of the above, graveled in odd stretches, planked in others.

I managed to circumvent the mud puddles as I circumnavigated the ponds, spooking great blue herons and white-tailed deer that seemed astonished to see any humans out and about on a day like this. Osprey were busy reclaiming the nests they had abandoned last fall. I kept a keen eye out for the otters that are rumored to hang out around here but had no luck spotting them.

It was delightful walking in the intermittent rain, filling my lungs in the early spring air and watching the forest come to life, while the only green yet showing came through in the abundant holly leaves and the bright emerald splotches of moss along the banks of the ponds. The habitat changes dramatically as you approach the Bay shore, the massive oaks and holly trees giving way to salt-loving pine, sedge, and myrtle.

I traced the graceful arcs of sandy beach with my boot prints, admiring the pyramids of driftwood sculptures left behind by artistic visitors. There was only one boat in view, a red-and-white tugboat steaming out of the West River from the Smith Brothers yard in Galesville. Curtis Point, on the far side of the river's mouth, was just a gray smudge in the mist. At the north end of the park, you're close to Saunders Point at the mouth of the South River. You can see the posts of a waterman's pound net stretching out into the Bay.

In the summer, this stretch of the beach can be busy with wading kids, kayakers and kite boarders. The web site cautions that the park can reach its capacity in the afternoons, and visitors might be turned away. But not on this day.

The only other rain-walkers I met were a jolly rotund retriever named Molly and her human companion, Brook Walsh. They live in Davidsonville but come here at least once a week, no matter the weather. "The wetter the better," Brook grinned, giving Molly a hug. "This is the perfect park for dogs, between the ponds and the beach."

Brook serves as South River High School's soccer coach, and while she regretted not being able to work with her teams when the viral crisis had closed all the schools, she did appreciate the county's keeping the parks open. "This is our No. 1 park, for sure," she said, "especially when the weather's bad, and because we have it all to ourselves."

Back at the car, I noted that I'd covered about three miles in a little over two hours, and while I was a bit cold and damp, I felt elated. On the way back home, I stopped by one of the little shopping centers along Central Avenue in Mayo and got some Pho to go. I would describe Pho as a Vietnamese version of your grandmother's chicken noodle soup. When I got home, I lit a fire and warmed my feet on the hearth and slurped that astonishingly good broth and rice noodles to warm my innards, too.

Bonnie wagged her greeting and then curled up in front of the fire, warm and dry.

Beverly Triton Nature Park
1202 Triton Beach Road
Edgewater, MD 21037

410-222-7317

aacounty.org/departments/recreation-parks/parks/beverly-triton/

Note: On weekends and holidays May 25 until September 2, park patrons will be required to reserve a free "reservation pass" in addition to paying the daily entry fee. Visit yourpassnow.com to get your reservation or visit Reservation Pass at Beverly Triton Nature Park page for more information

Open 7 a.m. to dusk daily

Admission: $6 per vehicle (see web site for discounts)

Parking can be limited in summer months; otherwise plentiful

Toilet facilities are available in the new bathhouse

Well-mannered dogs on leash are welcome; doggie bag dispensers available

Easy going

Walk 7

Discovering a Pocket Wilderness in Arnold

"I have never been lost," Daniel Boone once said, "but I will admit to being confused for several weeks."

I imagine him in his coonskin hat, wandering through the uncharted forests of the Appalachians, searching for the gap through the mountains that would open up the West for all the other pioneers. That vast wilderness is long gone for us Easterners, but we here in Anne Arundel County are lucky there are a few small open spaces, what I call "pocket wildernesses," where you can roam for a few hours, and for a bit of time anyway, lose yourself in the woods.

One of those spaces is tucked in between suburban developments in Arnold. It's a small forest hidden behind Broadneck Elementary School covering the watershed of one of the tributaries to Forked Creek on the Magothy River.

Like everyone, I had been hunkered down in our home during this viral crisis. I was blessed to be in isolation with my emotional-support spouse, Louise White. And, of course, our Irish setter, Bonnie. We also have two peculiar cats, but I'm not sure how blessed we are to have them around.

We had been adhering faithfully to Governor Larry Hogan's edict, doing our part to combat the spread of

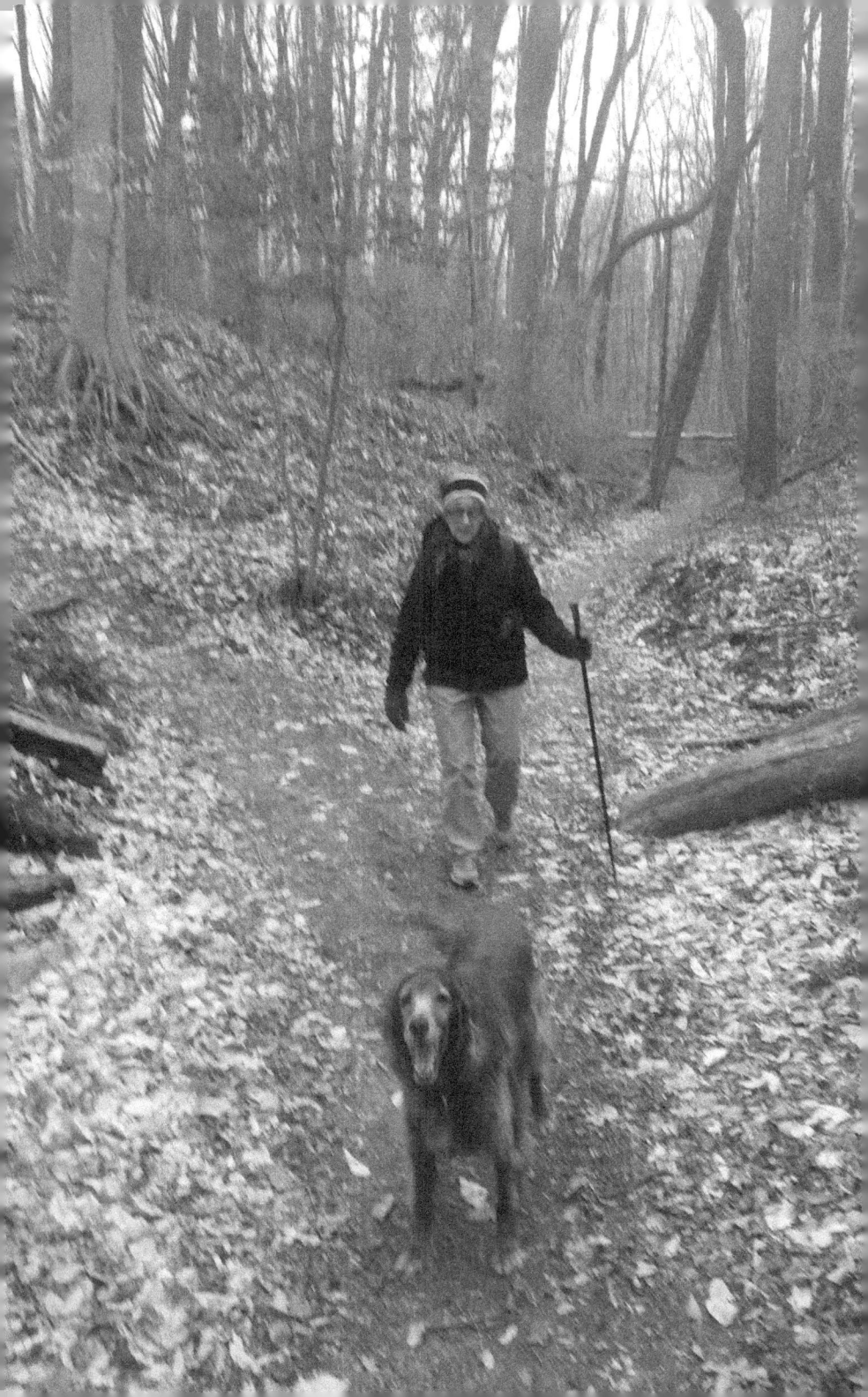

the virus by staying homebound. However, we happily noted that one exception to the rule is that you can get out to take a walk with those with whom you have been co-isolating. Or in our case, "bi-solating." One day in early April 2020 we decided to take advantage of a gap between spring showers and go stretch our legs.

The Forked Creek Trail popped up on the AllTrails app. We headed there, not knowing what to expect. My impression of Arnold is that it's fairly suburban, a blend of apartment complexes, townhouse developments and residential subdivisions spanning the Broadneck peninsula between the Severn River and the Magothy. I had a premonition of a boring paved walkway bordering people's backyard fences. I was pleasantly surprised by what we found.

In past columns, I have scoffed at the AllTrails app, but this time it proved to be fairly accurate and quite helpful. Curiously, the main trails are well marked with color-coded blazes spray painted on tree trunks, but the trail head is not. We parked in the visitor's parking lot at the school, the only car there, and then searched the hillside until we discovered a dirt path disappearing into the woods near the southwest corner.

It was a cool, overcast day; in other words, perfect walking weather. We donned parkas over fleeces, leashed up the dog and slipped inside the forest. The map on the app shows the red trail looping around the perimeter of the area, with several blue trails crisscrossing the interior.

We followed the red trail around to the right, through the tall oak and beech trees.

The path is a single-file, hard-packed trail, well maintained, that follows the steep contours of the hollow of the stream valley. We were glad we brought our walking sticks to help negotiate the slopes. Fallen trees have been chain-sawed to clear the path, and well-built footbridges span most of the gaps. One crossing of the creek, an improvised bridge had blown out in a recent storm.

This early in spring, the trees had yet to sprout their leaves. The small beeches showed slender shiny buds at their twig tips, each one starting to push off last year's withered leaf. The underbrush, mostly blackberry bushes and vines, was just beginning to show new green growth. There were mature ferns nearly everywhere emerging from their winter blanket of fallen leaves, with some delicate fiddleheads popping up here and there. We made a note to come back in a couple of weeks to see everything in its full spring resurgence. The lush carpet of ferns must be amazing.

Along the way, my partner and I talked about how lucky we are and how heart-broken we are for all the suffering in this world. We talked about the new heroes of our time, not just the brave people working in the hospitals and clinics, but also the men and women staffing the grocery stores, our mail carrier, everyone who is out there confronting the pandemic every day for the benefit of complete strangers.

After a while, we were grateful to have a hike like this to take our minds off everything that was happening beyond the periphery of the forest. We were also grateful for the volunteers who do such a good job grooming these trails.

Now and then we caught a glimpse of civilization through the trees. When the leaves come out fully, those views of parking lots and townhouse blocks will fade into the foliage. We heard very little traffic noise, perhaps because there was so little traffic to hear.

We hardly saw anybody else along the trail. A jogger with his curious German shepherd. A young biker dawdling to let his little sister and their dad catch up on foot. A young woman with her new pup, too rambunctious to stop and say hello.

We did meet one woman who lives nearby, Jennie Kinsfather, who was walking with her dog, Lucy, a diminutive chocolate Lab with a little gray in her muzzle—though not as much gray as either Bonnie or me. Jennie is spending her down time researching diseases affecting the immune system and hopes to write a series of articles to help people afflicted with them. She uses walking as therapy, both physical and mental. "I'm here almost every day," she noted. "Not many people know about this place."

I had always wondered about the origin of the place name of Arnold. According to the Arnold Preservation Council web site, a veteran of the War of 1812 named John Arnold bought 300 acres along the Severn River's northern bank. His eldest son, Elijah Redmond Arnold, married Matilda Hammond and built a store that still stands where Old County Road meets Baltimore and Annapolis Boulevard. Arnold's Store became a post office in 1852. In 1880, their son, Edgar F. Arnold became postmaster, and "the name was changed from Arnold's Store to just plain Arnold."

Louise, Bonnie, and I got about three quarters of the way around the red trail loop. It was getting chilly and the next bout of rain was looming, so we found a blue trail that cut across the middle and took us back to where we started. We had covered about two and a half miles in a little less than two hours. The AllTrails app kept us from getting lost, though there have been some new trails marked in white and others in green that haven't been uploaded onto the app's map yet. Despite all the markings, we had a few moments when we were a might confused, though pleasantly so. We found our way back to the car, legs well stretched and minds refocused on what's most important in life.

We had found a delightful pocket wilderness in "just plain Arnold" that we'll return to again and again.

The Arnold Trails Loop
470 Shore Acres Road
Arnold, MD 21012

Accessible from the parking lot at Broadneck Elementary School

Open dawn to dusk

Free admission

No toilets

Mannerly dogs on leash are welcome; bring your own doggy bags

Moderate going, with some topography

Walk 8

You Don't Know Jack Creek

Early in 2014, when I was still a neophyte Riverkeeper for the West and Rhode Rivers, I knew I needed to learn more about my new environs in the southern regions of the county. Like many Annapolitans, I thought of the State House as the center of the universe. The map in my head of the territory beyond the South River Bridge was like those ancient nautical charts that had vast blank spaces dotted with sea serpents and mermaids.

I studied a modern map and was surprised to find a site called Jack Creek Park on the end of the Shady Side peninsula. Since I didn't know jack about Jack Creek Park, I drove down Muddy Creek Road and followed it south until it curved around the end of West River and became Shady Side Road, then north through "downtown" Shady Side, then east along Snug Harbor Road toward the open Chesapeake Bay.

From my home near Quiet Waters Park, this can take 45 minutes by car. It takes far less time to cut across the mouth of South River by boat. I know. Since then I've done it both ways many times.

When I got to the park back then, there wasn't much to it, just a path bushwhacked through the scrub grass that led about a half-mile to the water's edge. There you could see the brunt of the Chesapeake Bay scouring away at the embankment. The shoreline was a tangle of toppled trees

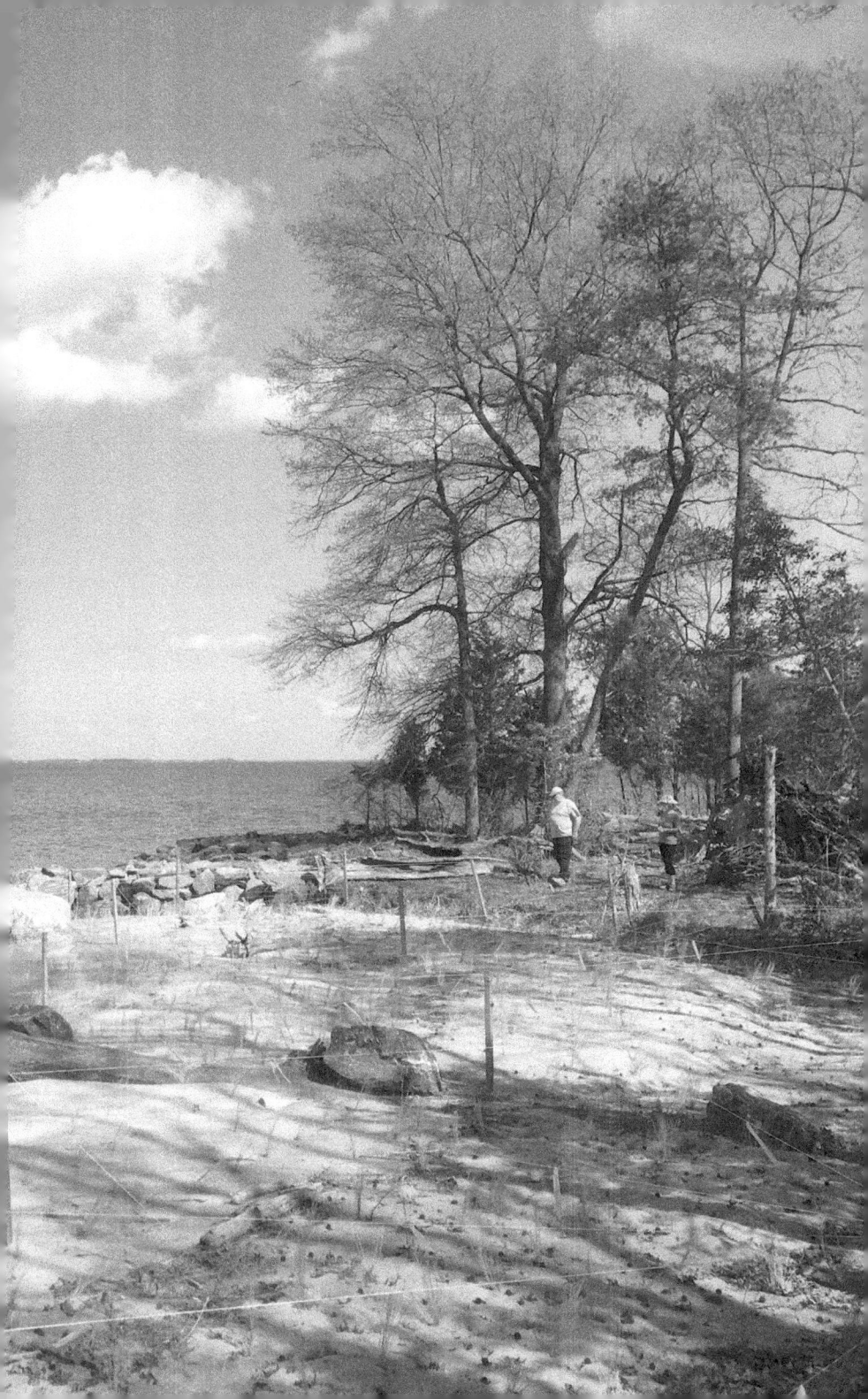

dangling over the side, roots waving at the sky. At this site, the shore is exposed to the south, and the Bay has about a hundred miles to build up the power in the wind and the waves that smash against this bank. The Bay had eaten up more than six acres of land in the past 20 years alone.

I checked with Mike Lofton, who served as chair of the Anne Arundel County Public Water Access Committee at the time. He filled me in on the background of the park. Apparently, the county purchased the property about 24 years ago with a little over $1 million in Program Open Space funding. Chris Trumbauer, who was the Riverkeeper before me, had worked with Anne Arundel County to make the park accessible to the public in 2013.

Four years later, I heard that the county had new plans for the park and hosted an informational meeting to introduce those plans to the community.

Over the next two years, the county's Department of Public Works and the Department of Parks and Recreation teamed up to deliver the newly renovated Jack Creek Park. It was due to open with aplomb in March 2020, but the pandemic pandemonium put a kibosh on the ceremony.

A month later, we visited the park, my wife Louise and I, and of course, our Irish setter, Bonnie. There are now two parking lots, one just inside the gate and another at the end of the new access road. There's a lock on the gate, but you can call the county or log onto the web site to get the combination, although you don't have to drive past the gate unless you're going to launch a canoe or kayak or need to use the accessible parking space at the far end. We parked in the nearest lot off Snug Harbor Road and sidled past the gate.

The rough path has been replaced by a permeable gravel access road. We saw a lot of bicycle tire tracks in the gravel, so it's bike-worthy as well as ADA compliant. Being permeable, the roadway will allow rainwater to soak through into the subsoil rather than run off, causing pollution. The road runs along the northern edge of the 58-acre park, along an expansive meadow.

You wouldn't know it by looking at it, but buried below three acres of the meadow, underneath the native shrubs and grasses, lie tons of silt. It was dredged from local rivers and creeks in recent years to keep the channels open for recreational boaters and working watermen alike. The silt had been tested to assure that it's free of pollutants like heavy metals, pesticides, and PCBs.

The dredged material had been stored in a drainage site on nearby Idlewilde Road. That site filled up with silt over time and needed to be emptied to allow for future dredging projects. You can't dredge unless you have someplace to store the silt you dredge up. If you can't dredge, channels fill up with silt and boats can't navigate. The dried silt had to go somewhere, and this is the result: acres of meadow planted with native trees, shrubs, and grasses, providing habitat for songbirds and butterflies.

We walked the half-mile to the end of the road. It was on a warm, summery day when the leaves on the trees were just about to burst open and the redbuds were already in full bloom.

The second parking lot at the far end of the access road features a permeable grassy surface with room for 20 cars, including one handicapped space. A wooden fence structure marks the space where two portable toilets will eventually be placed. We could have driven out here, but we needed the walk, all three of us.

A path from the parking lot leads out to the centerpiece of the park, a small, sandy beach with an expansive vista of the Chesapeake Bay. Bonnie enjoyed a bask in the sun while we took in the view. Since the world had shut down for the pandemic, there were few cars, trucks, and planes to pollute the atmosphere, and the sky was so clear you could plainly see the low white arc of the Bay bridges on the horizon, 14 miles to the north. We watched the osprey and kingfishers sweeping above the mouth of Jack Creek, a shallow tidal nook fringed with phragmites.

What had been all steep banks and fallen trees the last time I had been here was now a living shoreline protecting about 1,500 linear feet around the point of the park. A living shoreline protects the shore from erosion while still providing habitat for all the wildlife that needs to get in and out of the water, like terrapins, horseshoe crabs, and kids.

Instead of a solid wall of rock, the engineers created stone breakwaters with wide gaps between the rows of stone. They backfilled the rocks with sand, then planted the sand with shoots of marsh grass. The roots of the grasses will help keep the sand from washing away, while the rock barriers protect the shoreline from being eroded by the force of the waves.

When we were there, a grid of wooden stakes had been pounded in the sand, each connected by a web of string. This netting was meant to keep geese from turning the newly planted marsh grasses into a gourmet salad bar. All told, the newly planted marsh will cover an area the size of a football field. The grasses will not only secure the sand but also provide habitat for all kinds of critters. They'll suck up carbon dioxide, exhale oxygen, and filter out sediment and trash washing in with the tide.

As a Riverkeeper, I helped manage a living shoreline project a few years ago at YMCA Camp Letts on the Rhode River. The day after the contractors pulled out all of their heavy construction equipment, we saw a horseshoe crab shuffling up the new beach to lay her eggs. Build it and they will come.

The open beach created in the gap between two of the nearest breakwaters will serve as a soft canoe and kayak launch once the water gets warmer. I can't wait to try it out. For now, we walked along a narrow path through the pines along the water's edge. The path looped back around to the access road.

Along the way, we met just three other couples. We struck up a conversation—from a polite and healthy distance—with Mark and Randye Williams, who live off

Idlewilde Road. He's a financial officer with a nonprofit group in Baltimore, and she's a registered nurse working at a local adult day care center. They take a walk here almost every day and love the park's renovations.

"This is a big difference since I started coming here," Mark said. He noted that the ticks and bugs used to be fierce before the access road got graveled.

"I grew up in Snug Harbor, just around the corner from here," Randye said. "This reminds me of the beach like it used to be when I was growing up."

So now we have a newly renovated park with access to the Chesapeake Bay. Going there for a walk would be a wonderful way to celebrate the anniversary of Earth Day.

Jack Creek Park
1600 Snug Harbor Road
Shady Side, MD 20764
410-222-7317
aacounty.org/locations/jack-creek-park
Open dawn to dusk
Free admission
Parking: Log on for combination to gate lock
Portable handicap toilets in parking lot
Civil dogs on leashes are welcome; doggie bag dispenser available
Easy going

Walk 9

Riding Baby Elephants at Patuxent Research Refuge

I miss the part where I was the dad of a three-year-old girl. That's why it was such a delight to come across Greta Marie and her mom and baby brother on a trail in the North Tract of the Patuxent Research Refuge one day in early May, 2020. Greta Marie was sitting astride a fallen log in her little blue jeans and pink fleece vest.

Greta Marie informed me that she was riding her new pet elephant. Not just any elephant, but a baby elephant. It was a well-behaved elephant, all smooth and gray. No ears, though. Her mom, Genevieve Mason, was balanced on top of another log, with the six-month-old baby Hugo nestled in a front pack. Mom was grinning at the elephant, but Hugo was glaring at me, wondering where in the world I had come from and why was I barging in on their family outing.

I had come from Annapolis, for once without my dog, Bonnie, who let me know that an old frolicking injury had flared up in this cold, damp weather and that she preferred resting at home.

The Mason family had also made the 38-minute drive from Annapolis. Each of us had picked this spot randomly as a place to get out of the house and into the woods. This arbitrary choice paid off with a delightful afternoon of exploration.

A while back, I wrote about a pocket wilderness of less than a hundred acres tucked in between housing developments in Arnold. The Patuxent Research Refuge, it turns out, is a true wilderness of 12,841 acres tucked in between Washington, D.C., and Baltimore, just south of Fort Meade. And we had much of it all to ourselves, in all its spring beauty.

The Patuxent Research Refuge was established in 1936 by President Franklin D. Roosevelt. There are now 555 refuges among the 50 states managed by the U.S. Fish and Wildlife Service, but this is the only one dedicated to wildlife research. The territory covers bits of the Patuxent River and Little Patuxent River watersheds.

There are three sections to the refuge: North Tract, which offers hunting, fishing, a wildlife observation area, trails, and interpretive programs; Central Tract, where the U.S. Geological Survey biologists conduct much of their work at the Patuxent Wildlife Research Center; and South Tract, where the National Wildlife Visitor Center and its trails are located. The National Wildlife Visitor Center and North Tract are the only areas open for visitors, and the trails are open to the public every day except for federal holidays.

The North Tract is the most recent addition to the refuge, and it's entirely tucked into the western corner of Anne Arundel County between Fort Meade and Route 197. This section covers more than 8,000 acres of upland hardwood forest, meadow, and marsh.

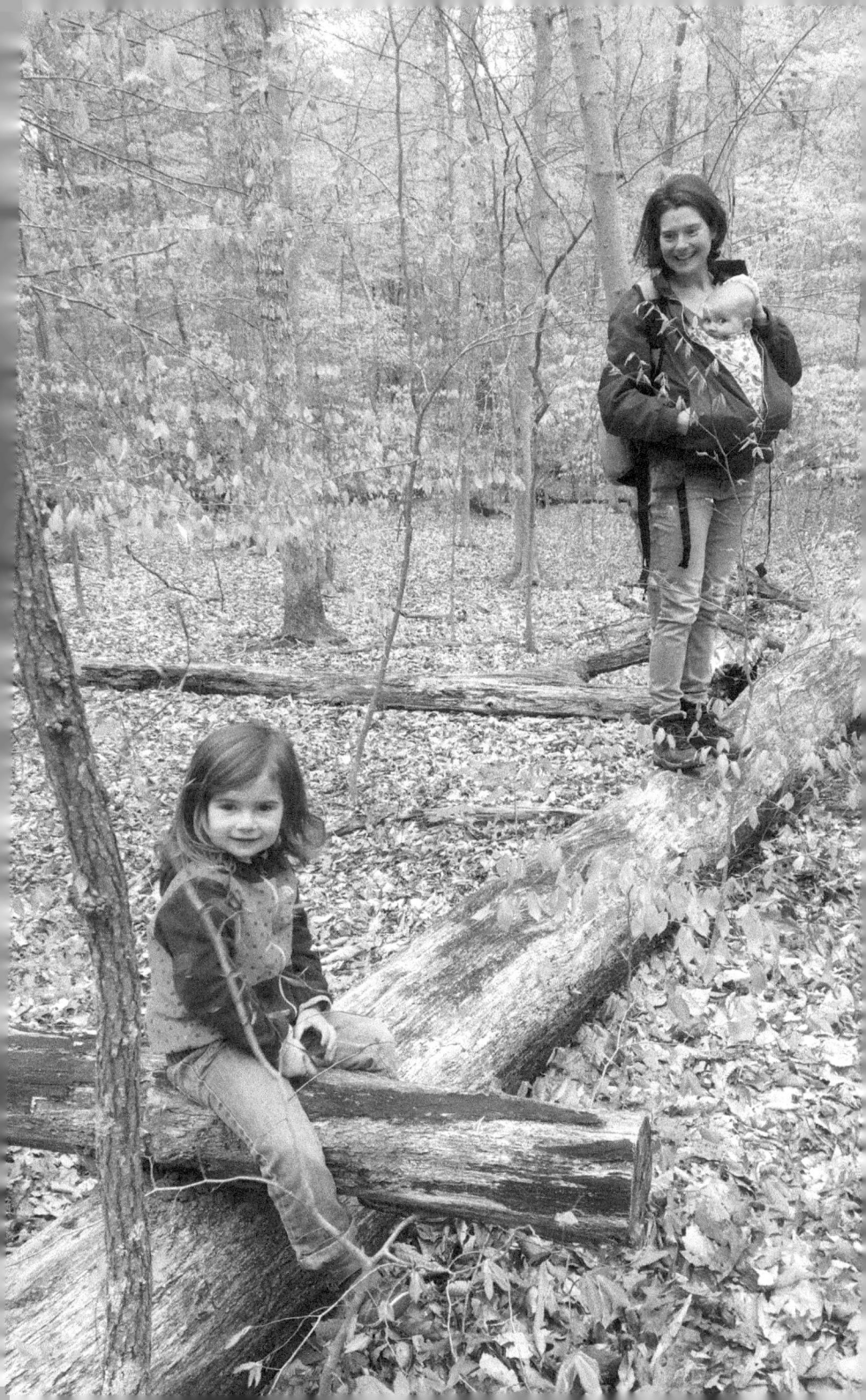

You'd never believe it when you wander through the mature beech, oak, red maple, and yellow birch trees that this area was deforested by the earliest European settlers starting in the mid 1600s. Woodsmen chopped down all the trees to supply fuel for pig iron smelters and to clear fields for tobacco and row crops well into the 1800s. The trees we see here now started growing back after the Civil War.

In the 20th century up to 1990, the U.S. Army used the property to train soldiers for fighting in both world wars and other conflicts. There were firing ranges everywhere. In fact, today there are numerous signs warning you not to mess with any unexploded ordinance you might trip over if you stray from the trails. Other parks tell you to stay on the pathways; this park gives you an incentive to obey that rule.

U.S. Fish and Wildlife Service procured the property in 1992 and created the North Tract of the Patuxent Research Refuge. In 1994, Baltimore Gas and Electric constructed a 5.5-mile high-voltage transmission line across the property, compromising some of the wetlands. To make up for this, BGE created 42 acres of habitat at the site of former firing ranges to create the refuge's Wildlife Viewing Area. The area has two trails, a pollinator garden, and an observation tower.

There are nine miles of gravel and dirt roads for hiking, biking, horseback riding, and even cross-country skiing if we ever get snow again this far south.

The three-quarter-mile Pine Trail follows an abandoned roadway from Wildlife Loop Road to the old St. Peter's Church Cemetery, where you can still read the names etched in the tombstones of some of the families who once farmed here.

The Little Patuxent River Trail follows the riverbank for about three quarters of a mile, providing pleasant views of this scenic river. I met a couple jogging along the boardwalk trail. They stopped to catch their breath and we chatted from a prescribed distance. He was Alex Robertson, who serves as a policeman in Washington, D.C. She was Gabby Morrin, a behavioral health specialist. We agreed that they were engaged in very healthy behavior here in this bucolic setting. They both live in nearby Laurel, and usually visit the South Tract for their exercise, but this was their first time in the North Tract. "We like to find new places to run," Alex said.

The spot where I met the little girl on the baby elephant was on the Forest Trail, which loops about two and a half miles through the second-growth hardwood forest. The leaves on the trees had just recently sprouted bright green, with the white blossoms of the dogwoods providing a lacy backdrop.

Greta Marie's mom, Genevieve, said that they had been to the South Tract a few times, but this was their first time on this section of the refuge. "We live off Forest Drive in Annapolis," she said, "and we sometimes go to Quiet Waters Park, but it's hard on Greta Marie when she sees the playgrounds all taped up so she can't play on them." The little girl didn't seem to be missing the swing set here. Genevieve also said she prefers the lack of crowds and the unspoiled nature of the wildlife refuge to the more manicured feel of the Annapolis park.

This trail leads off from the North Tract visitor contact station, where you need to sign in to get a day pass. There are real rest rooms there, as well as pamphlets with maps of the trails and lists of all of the flora and fauna you might happen to meet along the way. The refuge does an excellent job of providing interpretive panels and signage there and along the trails.

I made my way back to the station along one of the old dirt roads, with a wonderful feeling of freedom, walking down this lonely country road and nearly forgetting that I was in the middle of some of America's most populous urban sprawl.

I listened to the songs of the birds I could identify—red-winged blackbird, northern flicker, white-throated sparrow—but then one I didn't recognize coming from far off in the woods, a high-pitched, trilling hoot, almost like a little girl's shriek of laughter—and I realized what it was, without even reaching for my bird book: Greta maria pachydermus, the rare pink-vested elephant rider.

Patuxent Research Refuge, North Tract
280 Bald Eagle Drive, Laurel

301-497-5580

www.fws.gov/northeast/patuxent/

Visitor Contact Center and grounds daily from 8 a.m. to 4 p.m. except federal holidays

Plenty of free parking on site

Free admission

Toilets available at the visitor center

Civil dogs on leash are welcome; bring your own doggy bags

Easy going

Walk 10

A Solitary Beach Walk at Sandy Point State Park

I thought I was doing okay after six weeks of hunkering down for the coronavirus pandemic emergency, going for occasional walks, and doing my part to "level the curve," in other words, reduce the rate of infection. But when Governor Larry Hogan announced that he was finally lifting some restrictions and allowing people to go boating, fishing, and walking on Maryland beaches, I confess I broke down in unexpected sobs of relief.

Imagine my surprise when I got to the recently re-opened Sandy Point State Park one morning in mid-May 2020 and found I practically had the whole 786-acre park all to myself. There were 17 pick-up trucks with empty boat trailers parked by the boat ramps, a mere sprinkle of vehicles in a lot that could hold hundreds. On my solitary walk along a mile of beach, I met just two fishermen, one turkey vulture, six herring gulls, and an upturned horseshoe crab.

Not that I was disappointed to be able to indulge in such solitude; I was just surprised that more Marylanders weren't exercising their right to access this wonderful public asset. The park features picnic groves, fishing on dedicated piers, rock jetties, picnic areas, shelters, bathhouses, playgrounds, boat rentals, a marina in a protected lagoon, and more boat ramps than there are screens at your local cineplex.

But the signature asset is the beach, stretching more than a mile around Sandy Point proper. When you're standing on the beach, off to the right you can see the twin spans of the Chesapeake Bay Bridge swing across to the Eastern Shore, while the silhouette of the historic Sandy Point lighthouse marks the horizon on your left. This gives you a magnificent view of the Bay.

I parked by the boat ramps shortly after the park opened for the day. It was still cool for mid-May, and corrugated clouds arched across the sky. Since pets are restricted between May 1 and September 30, I had to leave Bonnie behind. I walked through a grove of huge, gnarled trees that looked like part of the setting of an old Errol Flynn movie. I later identified them as chinkapin oaks. I have always wondered how Chinquapin Round Road in Annapolis got its name, and why it's spelled with a QU and not a K. There are few trees along that road these days, let alone majestic oaks. I'm happy to have finally met real chinkapins; next time, I'll bring my rope swing and green-feathered cap.

I started my beach walk at the jetty that protects the channel leading from the Bay to the lagoon. The channel, in turn, parallels the off-ramp from the east-bound bridge. The Bay was calm, with soft ripples lapping up onto the sand. I had the whole beach to myself. A lone tug pushed a barge loaded with coal up the middle of the Bay, and one

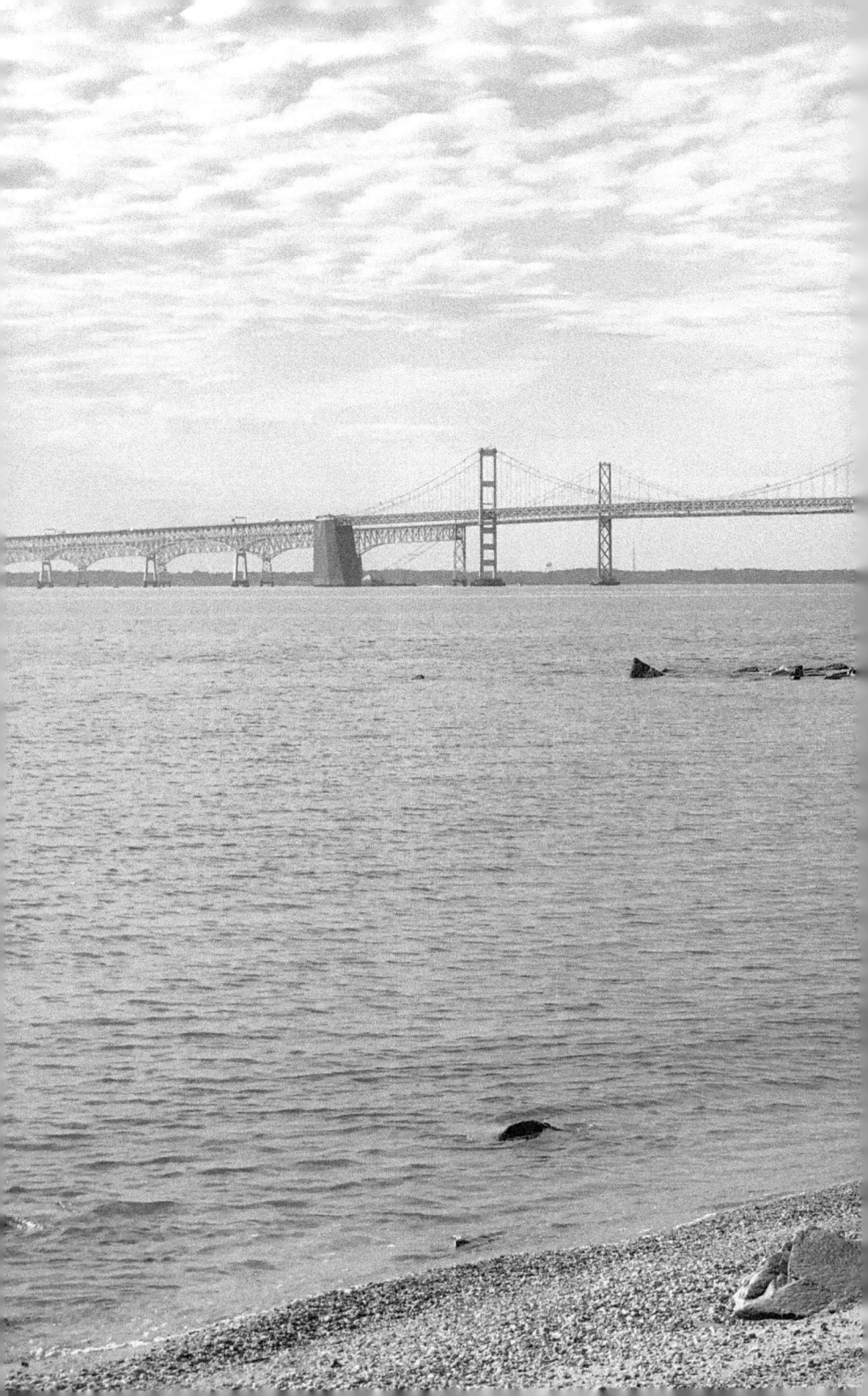

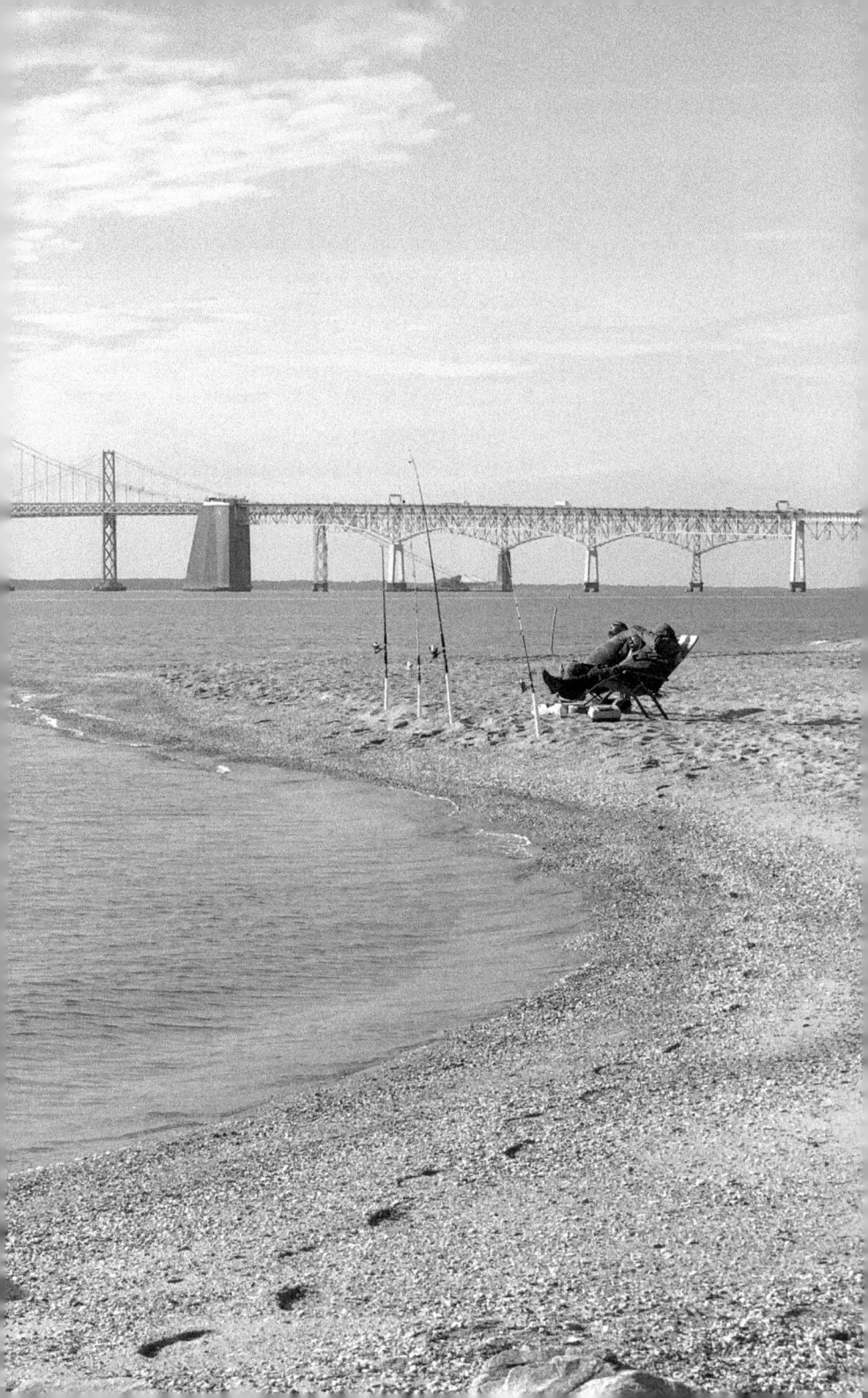

powerboat plowed by in the other direction. Not another boat to be seen.

Along the way, I came across a horseshoe crab that had turned turtle at the high tide mark, its pointy "tail" or "telson" waggling at the sky. These are amazing creatures. They've been around for eons. Fossils of horseshoe crabs have been found that date back 455 million years. In all that time, for every spring between the full moon in May and the full moon in June, the females have found beaches like this one that they can crawl up to lay their eggs in the sand. Sometimes you can see little green BBs when you're building sandcastles. Those are future horseshoe crabs, and they're vital food for certain birds, so don't mess with them if you do find them.

Horseshoe crabs congregate on the beaches in Delaware Bay by the tens of thousands. I felt lucky to find this one here, and happy to be able to be of assistance. I gently picked it up by the shell and set it in the water. They're not actual crabs, so they don't have any claws to harm you, and you don't want to pick them up by the telson; it might snap off and they need it for navigation and to help set themselves upright if the waves tip them over.

You probably don't know it, but you very likely owe your life to a horseshoe crab. The blood has a rare protein called limulus amebocyte lysate (LAL). Biomedical industry scientists use the blood to test pharmaceuticals and medical devices for toxic contaminants that could make you sick or even kill you.

So horseshoe crabs are important to humans, and they need beaches like this to propagate. That's one reason why it's so important to preserve these habitats. Horseshoe crabs can't make their way to shore through a solid wall of rock or wood or metal. Living shorelines provide the gaps between the breakwaters that these and other critters need to get in and out of the water.

I have one more tale about Sandy Point. Looking at the bridge always reminds me of an iconic black-and-white photograph by the late Annapolis photographer Marion E. Warren, whom I consider the Ansel Adams of the Chesapeake Bay. You might have seen this picture: It shows the first span of the bridge, just completed in 1952, the same year as the founding of Sandy Point State Park. It's a night shot, and the headlights and taillights of the cars and trucks string together to form neon tendrils along the roadway. The full moon hangs in a haze.

Before his passing in 2006, Marion told me the story behind that shot. He had a rival, *Baltimore Sun* photographer Aubrey Bodine. They would often shoot the same subjects. Marion had this one shot of the bridge in mind, and took pains to make sure Aubrey wouldn't be able to duplicate it.

Marion knew that once the bridge was completed, the ferryboats would no longer be needed. He waited until the day before the old two-story ferry building, located near where the bridge tollbooths used to be, was slated for demolition. He got permission to set up his tripod on the roof of the building, waited for the moon to rise just right, and snapped the picture. The next day, the building was razed and Marion had his unduplicable photograph.

Sandy Point State Park
1100 East College Parkway, Annapolis
410-974-2149 (Office) • 410-974-4699 (Marina)
dnr.maryland.gov/publiclands/pages/southern/sandypoint.aspx
Open daily, 7 a.m. to sunset except 5 p.m. November and December
Boating: 24 hour access year-round
Fishing: 24 hour access January to mid-November
Dogs are welcome only October 1 to April 30, unless in the boat ramp area while boarding boats
Admission: $5 per person on weekends and holidays and $4 per person on weekdays
Toilets available
Easy going

Walk 11

Requiem for a Red Dog at Quiet Waters Park

One day I will write a book about all of the dogs in my life, and the opening line will read: "Don't worry, nobody dies in the end." But dogs do die, and I'm sad to report that my sweet Irish setter, Bonnie, did so just before I wrote this column in late May 2020. With all the human suffering in the world these days, I'm not going to dwell on the fate of one small animal. But this one was important to me and part of my family for eight years. And she was my favorite walking companion.

To commemorate her passing, I brought her memory along with me to the place we loved the best: Quiet Waters Park. Our last walk there was on one of her good days, when the cherry trees and dogwoods were still in bloom. We always enjoyed meeting people along the paved trails, when Bonnie would invariably be fawned over by small children and their parents alike. Everyone would remark on how beautiful she was, and she would modestly accept the compliment, knowing it was true.

But our favorite jaunt was off the paved track. There's a path marked with a red blaze spray painted onto the tree trunks. It winds its way along the bank of Harness Creek, from where it emerges as a trickle through the skunk cabbage, then climbs to a bluff where you can see its tidal expanse merge with South River.

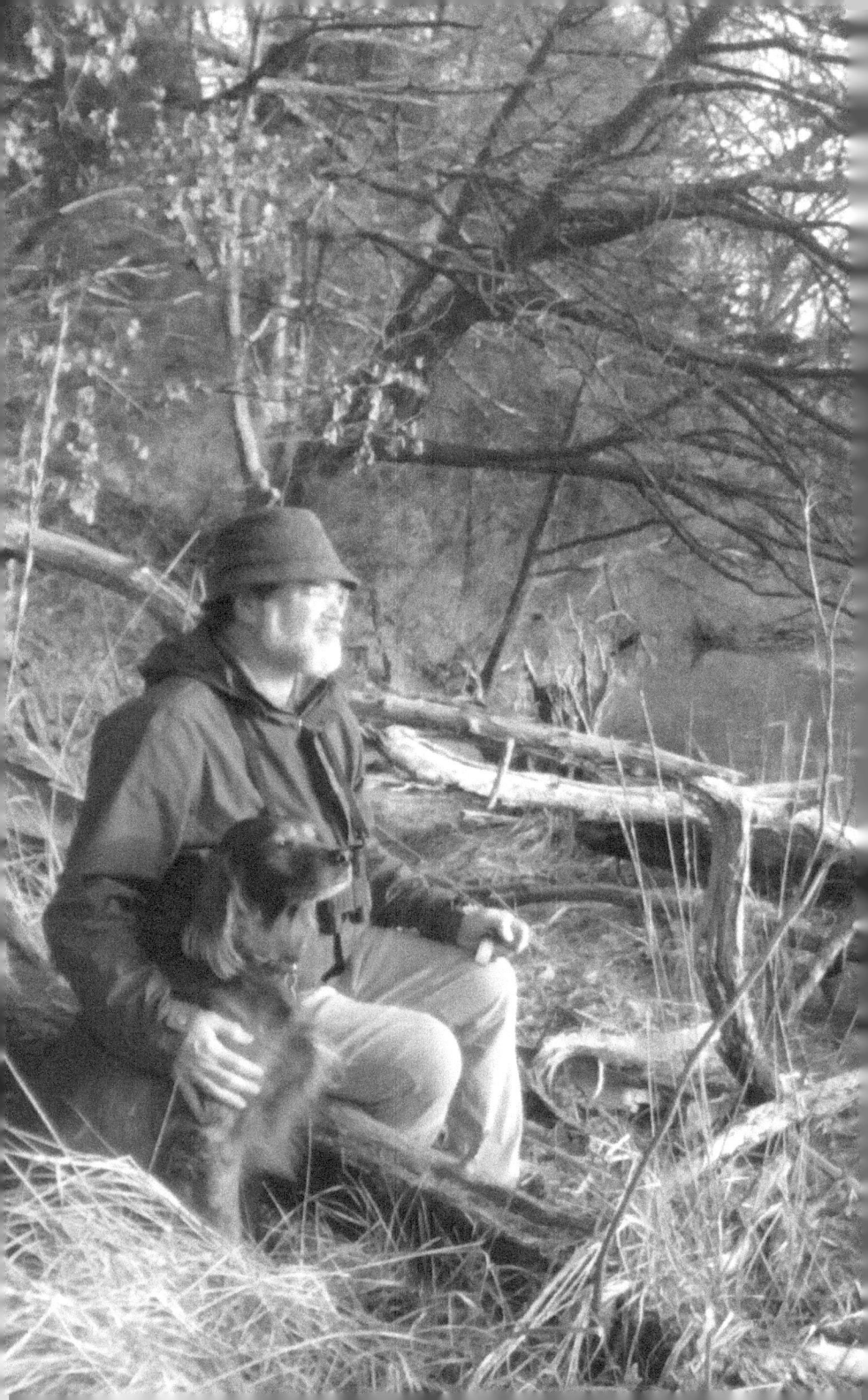

This trail has some splendid topography, touching the creek in spots and then rising to reveal inspiring views of the cove where sometimes you'll see a sailboat or two anchored peacefully. This time of year, osprey screek overhead and red-bellied woodpeckers cackle among the treetops.

Now and then you'll find oyster shells high up on a bluff and wonder how they got there. The answer is that people left them there after feasting on them, long, long ago. Archaeologists at the Smithsonian Environmental Research Center on the Rhode River, just a few miles away as the osprey flies, have carbon-dated such shells. Some of them are nearly 3,000 years old.

Every time I discover one of these discarded collections of ancient shell, called "middens" by the archaeologists, I look around and see that it's in a delightful place to camp out and hold an oyster roast, as it must have been way back then. The people who lived here at that time had it made, at least until we showed up.

One leg of the path winds its way around to the kayak rental pier; the next goes from there around the cove to the overlook near the amphitheater. On one of those winter days when the north wind blows all of the water out of the creek, you can follow the shoreline all the way to the river. All in all, you can walk three or four miles through the woods, then backtrack along the paved trail.

Bonnie always wanted to lead the way. She knew it well. I will miss her.

I've long been curious about the name of Harness Creek. According to Anne Arundel County's web site, it's named after William Harness, who patented the acreage on the park side of the creek in 1652. Eventually, it became a farm that was owned by different families over the centuries.

Here's a fascinating update with information I didn't learn until just before the publication of this book: One of the owners of the property that eventually became Quiet Waters Park was a remarkable gentleman named Truxtun Beale, a wealthy diplomat who served as ambassador to Persia, Greece, and other countries in the early years of the 20th century.

In 1926, Beale purchased as his country home an estate comprising 333 acres on the South River known then as Thunder and Lightning Point. It was also known as Laurel Bank Farm, which is appropriate, since today the trails tunnel through several dense groves of mountain laurels. Beale's town home in Washington, D.C. was the historic Decatur House, situated not far from the White House. The Laurel Bank property included a 12-room mansion and numerous outbuildings in addition to a fully functioning dairy farm.

Beale had no way of knowing it, but he signed the deed on the property the same day that his only child, Walker, was mortally wounded in combat in France. Despondent, he turned to philanthropy. Among his many achievements in benefitting the public, he bought an undeveloped parcel on Spa Creek and arranged to donate it to the city of Annapolis through the Annapolis Rotary Club, of which he was an honorary member. That property is now Truxtun Park. It's not named after Beale, but his great-grandfather, Commodore Thomas Truxtun, a naval hero in the Revolutionary War and later the commander of the USS *President*, the last of the six original frigates in the United States Navy.

Beale's niece recalled that he liked to go on long canoe rides well into his later years. I can imagine him paddling Harness Creek as I have, he with his favorite dogs, Micky and Dora, me with mine. He died at the mansion at Laurel Bank Farm in 1936 at the age of 80.

I discovered all of this information in a book by Annapolis author William H. Cooke, *The Gun-Wielding Philanthropist and the Adventuress Socialite: the Charming and Eccentric Lives of Truxtun and Marie Beale, 1856–1956*. You'll just have to read the book to grasp the subtle nuances implied by the title.

The county bought the property in 1987 during O. James Lighthizer's administration. Quiet Waters is one of the crown jewels of the county's park system, with more than five miles of paved trails for walking, jogging, and biking. There's a skating rink that's open in the winter. You can enjoy the visitor center and the Blue Heron Center, where the Friends of Quiet Waters Park hold art exhibits and festivals, summer concerts in the amphitheater, and picnics in the many pavilions.

There's not just one but two separate fenced-in dog parks, one for big dogs and a separate one for small dogs. And for the web-footed and aquatically inclined, there's even a short expanse of beach where you can let your retriever loose in his natural habitat.

For some time, the doggy beach was closed due to erosion, so the fenced-in dog park was busier than usual when Bonnie and I went one day. In one corner of the park, there's a spigot where there were several large pans to provide water for the dogs. It was a hot day, and one huge Labrador retriever, aching for a swim, put a paw in one pan, then the other paw in another pan, and then he had all four paws in four separate pans, ankle deep in water, and I swear he gave a wistful sigh.

Quiet Waters Park
600 Quiet Waters Park Road
Annapolis, MD 21403
410-222-1777
aacounty.org/departments/recreation-parks/parks/quiet-waters/
Open 7 a.m. to dusk
Admission: $6/vehicle (see web site for discounts)
Toilets available in the Visitor Center
Good dogs are welcome on leash or off leash in two fenced-in doggie parks; doggie bag dispensers available
Moderate, some topography

Walk 12

Delving into Historic Depths at Wooton's Landing Wetlands Park

You've seen the sign a thousand times while you're driving on the highway and about to cross a bridge. The sign says that the river you're about to cross is not just any river; it's been designated a "scenic river."

So of course, after miles and miles of boring highway, you're delighted that you're about to be treated to something worth seeing. But no, the traffic engineers know that you'll be so impressed by the beauty of the scenery below, you'll be distracted from looking ahead and cause a massive chain-reaction pile-up, so they raise the side barriers to make it impossible for you to see whether the river is actually scenic or not.

This precaution works in reverse for me, because I always want to see any river, so I can't help taking extra pains to get a glimpse, which typically causes my emotional-support spouse in the passenger seat to stomp on the phantom passenger brake and clutch at the door handle in case of the need for an emergency ejection.

So when I get a chance to take a walk along a river, scenic or not, I take it.

The Maryland General Assembly designated the Patuxent River as one of the state's nine scenic rivers in 1968. The Severn, as you can see when you pass the sign as you cross the Route 50 bridge, is also a scenic river.

JEFFERSON HOLLAND | 73

The Patuxent is the longest river whose watershed lies entirely within the state of Maryland. Curiously, it originates in the "Four Corners" of the state, where Howard, Frederick, Montgomery, and Carroll counties come together, just half a mile from the source of the south fork of the Patapsco River. The Patuxent then flows 115 miles to where it meets the Chesapeake Bay at Solomons Island. It marks the western border of Anne Arundel County. There are several sites in the county where you can walk along the Patuxent and be impressed by how beautiful it really is, safely and without scaring your spouse.

I started my trek at the Patuxent Wetlands Park at Wayson's Corner, where Route 4 crosses the river. This is a good place to see part of the tidal section of this river. I chatted with several fishermen at the pier in the shadow of the highway overpass. One had caught a fair-sized catfish earlier, but this was mid-afternoon on a warm day, and the others hadn't had much luck. I scrambled under the highway, over the muddy rocks and found a dirt path leading south along the river's bank. It was disappointingly trashed with litter left by other fishermen. Still, I followed it about a quarter of a mile to where it petered out in a marsh choked by huge-leafed plants Native Americans called tuckahoe.

I stopped and made a few casts with my fly rod and marveled at the vast expanse of the marsh to the south and east, and the lazy, murky sweep of the river rolling toward the Chesapeake with the wind and tide. Just about a mile

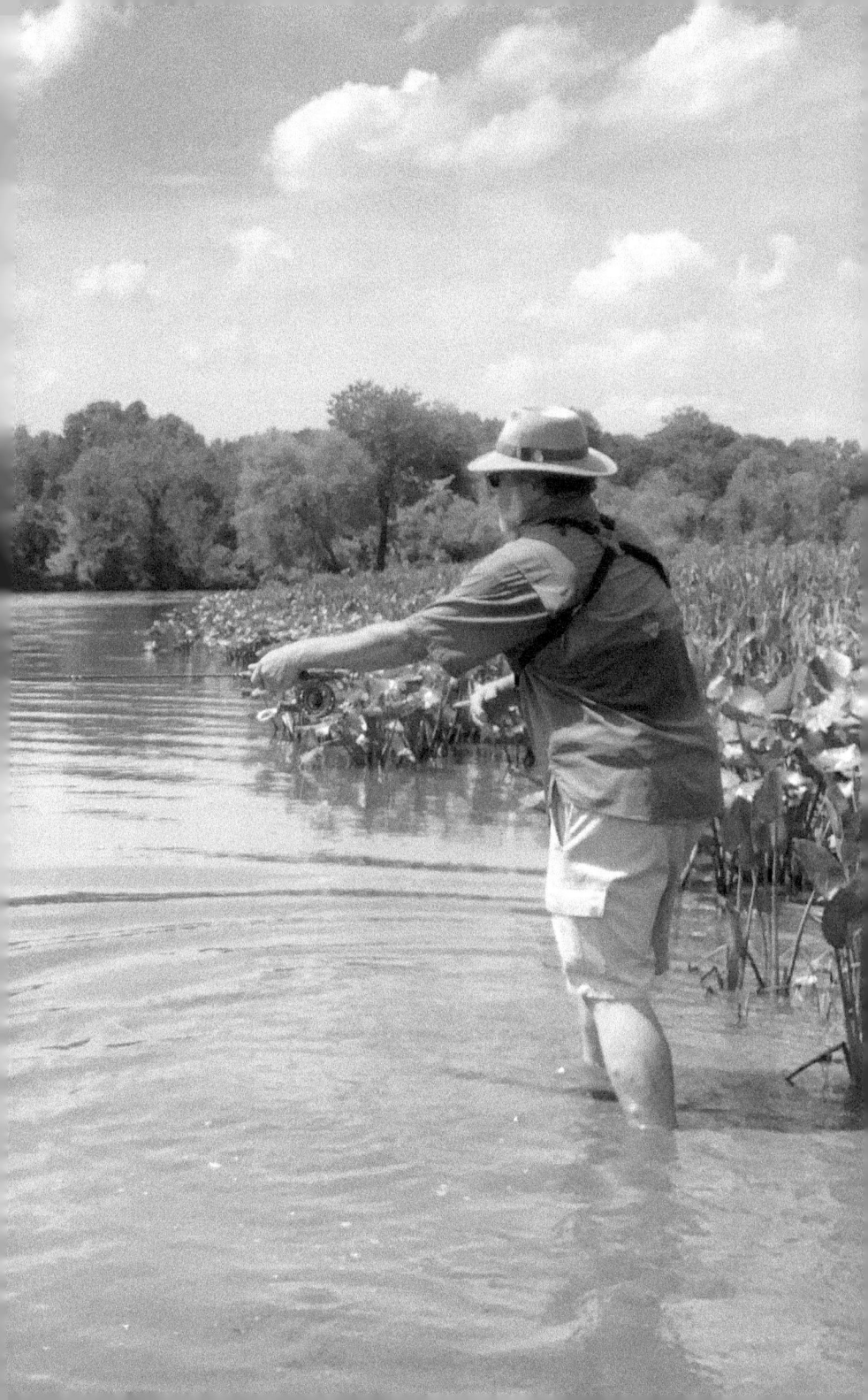

south of here lies Pig Point, which has an astonishing historical significance.

County archaeologists have been studying the site since 2009, and they have discovered evidence of thousands of people living there for thousands of years. They've uncovered no fewer than 14 sites within a mile of the original Pig Point dig site, unearthing arrowheads and other projectile points that date back 6,500 years and older. I couldn't help thinking that there must have been other guys fishing long ago in the same spot where I was fishing, and no doubt they had better luck than me.

I reeled in my line, slogged back to my car, and drove three and one-half miles north along Sands Road to Wooton's Landing Wetland Park. It's a bit of walk from the parking lot to the river, and a walk was what I was looking for. There's a locked gate, but can you get in on foot. If you want to drive down to launch a canoe or kayak, you can access the code to the padlock by logging onto the Anne Arundel County web site.

The gravel road leads to a grove along the riverbank. You can fish or launch a small boat from the floating dock. The river here is relatively narrow. My ancestors of the Hyatt family settled along this stretch of the river back in the early 1700s. One of them founded Hyattsville. Another emigrated to Pittsburgh, where my great-grandfather, George Hyatt, became a railroad telegrapher in the early 1900s. His daughter, Gaynell, was my father's mother.

And somewhere very near this spot, Commodore Joshua Barney scuttled his fleet to keep it from being captured by the British Royal Navy in August of 1814.

Barney had proved his mettle, serving heroically in the Continental Navy during the Revolutionary War. Congress assigned him the duty of protecting the Chesapeake Bay in the War of 1812. In April 1814, he assembled a flotilla of 18 ships: seven 75-foot barges, six 50-foot barges, two gunboats, one row galley, one lookout boat, and his flagship, the USS *Scorpion*, a 49-foot sloop-rigged, self-propelled floating battery armed with two long-range cannon and two short-range carronades.

The smaller boats each had a cannon in the bow and a carronade on the stern, and each was manned by a crew of 40 to 60 men. The crewmen included U.S. Navy sailors, white Chesapeake Bay watermen, free Blacks, and runaway slaves. The idea was to have a small fleet of heavily armed small boats, fast and maneuverable in shallow water, that could harass the British fleet comprised of larger and less maneuverable ships.

The flotilla fought several battles against the British fleet as it made its way up the Patuxent to land the army at Benedict. American authorities were afraid that Barney's flotilla would be captured. The first plan was to haul the boats overland and launch them on the South River, but then Barney was ordered to scuttle them in the Patuxent.

I looked up a first-hand account of the scene before me now, written by British Admiral Cockburn in his report to General Cochrane on August 22, 1814, just two days before the general attacked nearby Washington, D.C.

As we opened the reach above Pig Point, I plainly discovered Commodore Barney's broad pendant in the headmost vessel, a large sloop and the remainder of the flotilla extending in a long line astern of her. Our boats now advanced towards them as rapidly as possible, but on nearing them, we observed the sloop bearing the broad pendant to be on fire, and she very soon afterwards blew up. I now saw clearly that they were all abandoned and on fire with trains to their magazines, and out of the seventeen vessels which composed this formidable and so much vaunted flotilla sixteen were in quick succession blown to atoms, and the seventeenth, in which the fire had not taken, [was] captured.

That happened right here, two hundred years ago. In 2010, underwater archaeologists from the state of Maryland, the U.S. Navy, and the Maryland Historical Trust discovered the wooden hull of a sunken ship in the river near here and they're pretty sure it's Joshua Barney's flagship, the *Scorpion*.

I mused over that spectacle as I wandered down a country lane past beaver ponds and marshes sprouting cattails and the big yellow buds of the cow lilies just about to bloom. I listened to the twirl of the red-winged blackbirds and felt cooled by the shade of the lowland trees, the river birches, cottonwoods, and ash. Overall, you can walk three or four miles along the river bottom, though not always within sight of the scenic Patuxent River.

Wootons Landing Park
4550 Sands Road
Harwood, MD 20776
410-741-9330
aacounty.org/locations-and-directions/wootons-landing-park
Open dawn to dusk daily
Plenty of parking on site
Free admission
No toilets
Courteous dogs on leash are welcome; bring your own doggy bags
Easy going

Patuxent Wetlands Park
1426 Mt. Zion Marlboro Road,
Lothian, MD 20711
410-222-7317
aacounty.org/locations-and-directions/patuxent-wetlands-park
Open dawn to dusk daily
Plenty of parking on site
Free admission
Mannerly dogs on leash are welcome; bring your own doggy bags
Easy going

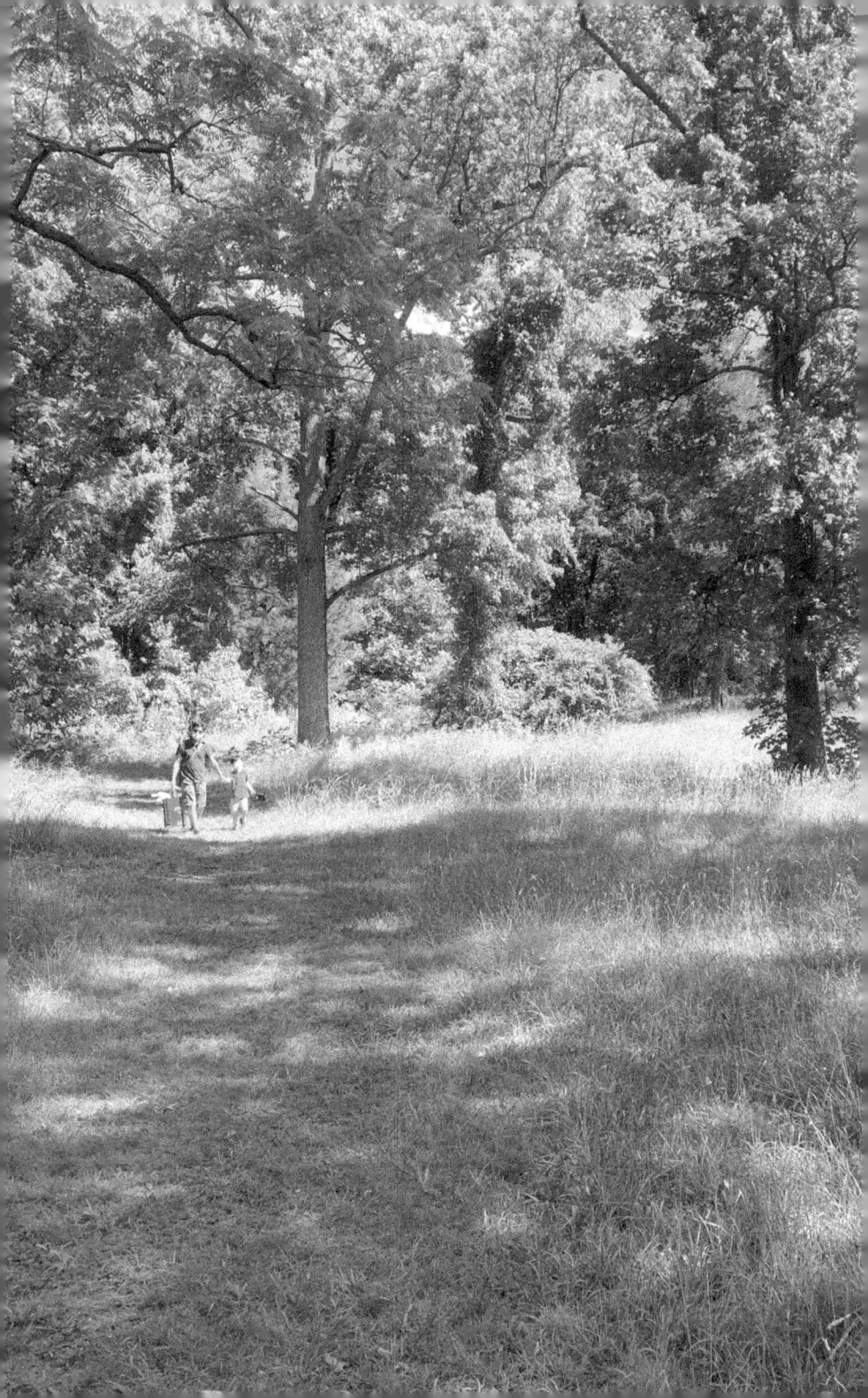

Walk 13

Hooking Sea Monsters at South River Farm Park

I was pleasantly surprised by my visit in late June 2020 to South River Farm Park in Mayo. I'd never been past the county's greenhouse located there, set at the end of a long, open field, and I wasn't expecting much in the way of a walk. Imagine my delight when I stepped into the woods beyond and strolled down a quiet gravel lane, surrounded by towering yellow poplars and oaks.

The road narrowed as it crossed a causeway over a marsh, and then the forest opened up on a park-like meadow on a bluff overlooking the river. I picked out a landmark on the far shore and realized I was directly across from my own Quiet Waters Park, just about three quarters of a mile away as the osprey flies, but 10 miles away by car.

South River Farm Park opened to the public just five years ago. It had long been a storage site for Anne Arundel County's public works equipment as well as the greenhouse where county agronomists grow marsh grasses to replenish shoreline projects. In 1995, a renowned local environmental activist named John Flood created 300 yards of living shoreline to protect the 170-acre peninsula. The low rock breakwaters he built then are still there, doing their job well.

That peninsula is surrounded by Limestone Cove on the upstream side, Brickworks Creek and Selby Bay on the downstream side, and the South River. The meadow on the bluff at Mayo Point overlooks the inlet to a salt pond, with a sandy spit that's begging for a barefoot wade.

On the way in, I met a young man and his little boy, walking along the lane hand-in-hand. He was carrying a bundle with the end of a fishing rod sticking out the top. Visions of Sheriff Andy Taylor and Opie came wafting up from my televised past. I struck up a conversation and learned that he was Jin Park from South Korea, working as a guest researcher at the National Institutes of Health in Rockville. He was meeting some friends at the park's beach. His son, Jeongwon, was a shy first-grader.

From the meadow, a narrow trail leads along the bluff, through a paw-paw patch and down to the shore, where there's a series of small beaches separated by reeds and protected by John Flood's low rock breakwaters. A huge fallen tree blocks access to part of the shoreline, but you can scooch under it, even with creaky old knees like mine.

There I met Jin's other friends, one of whom had an even younger son along. I chatted with them as little Jeongwon cast a line from atop the rocks. "We're giving their moms a break today," Jin grinned. He had learned from his friends that South River Farm Park was a secluded spot where they could enjoy a quiet afternoon on the water with their kids. He noted that Ocean City was far too crowded, and too far away from his home in Potomac, Maryland.

One of the adult friends, fishing as well, suddenly snagged something big, his rod arcing almost 180 degrees. General debate ensued as to what kind of fish might be giving the guy such a fight. Too big for a white perch, certainly. Unlikely that it's a rockfish, even this close to the mouth of the river and the open Chesapeake Bay. Could be a big blue catfish, an invasive beast that can grow up to 100 pounds, but this water's too shallow for them. The mystery was solved when twin fins popped up from the water a couple hundred feet offshore. That marked the critter as a cownose ray. Its wingtips break the surface, looking like shark fins, a sight that often alarms observers unfamiliar with the species. They fooled me the first time, too.

My friend, Dr. Matt Ogburn, a senior scientist at the Smithsonian Environmental Research Center on the Rhode River, just three miles south of this very spot, has studied cownose rays extensively. These beautiful and gentle creatures can have a wingspan three feet across and can weigh up to 50 pounds. They're native to the Chesapeake Bay, but migrate between here and Florida. Matt likens the migrating schools of majestic rays to the herds of wildebeests sweeping across the Serengeti Plains in Africa.

In one study in 2014, SERC scientists worked with local watermen who commonly find stray rays trapped in their pound nets. Matt and his crew implanted rays with acoustic transmitters, then tracked their migration, using hydrophones at receiver stations to pick up the signals from the transmitters. There are more than 200 receiver stations up and down the Chesapeake Bay, and more receiver arrays along the Atlantic coast between the Carolina capes and Florida.

The rays mate in July then leave the Bay by October to return to their wintering grounds. One individual female cownose ray was tracked from the Bay to Cape Canaveral and back. You can read about Dr. Ogburn's research on the SERC.SI.EDU web site.

I left the gang with the fisherman still hanging on to the ray. On my way back to the car, I met up with just a small handful of other visitors, several of whom were accompanied by their dogs on leashes. I've heard that some residents on the Mayo peninsula are leery of the county's plan to develop this and other nearby parks, but at least on this mid-week summer afternoon, this park did not appear to be a threat to anyone's tranquility.

I met two women who lived nearby, one with a chocolate Labrador retriever, the other with a matching light-blonde Lab, and I had to stop and say hello. As I shared the dog biscuits I always carry in my pocket, I told the tale of one time when I was walking my old chocolate Lab, Joe, in Quiet Waters Park. I had met an older man with a cane just as another walker came along with a light-blonde Lab. The old man asked me what kind of dog Joe was, and I said, "Well, sir, this is a chocolate Lab." He pointed to the other dog and asked, "So what's that, a vanilla?"

Overall, I walked a little more than 3.5 miles in just over two hours, and didn't explore all of the park's trails. I'll be back, but next time I'll bring my fishing rod along.

South River Farm Park
3553 Loch Haven Drive
Edgewater, MD 21037
410-222-7317
aacounty.org/locations-and-directions/south-river-farms-park
Open dawn to dusk daily
Plenty of parking on site
Free admission
Portable toilets on site
Well-disposed dogs on leash are welcome; bring your own doggy bags
Easy going

Walk 14

Discovering Sources at Severn Run Natural Environmental Area

We were on a mission, my friend Tom Guay and I, that hot day in July 2020. At the time, Tom served as the program officer for the Severn River Association, known as the oldest river group in America. For more than 110 years, the organization has been promoting the health of the Severn through monitoring, advocacy, and education. Tom runs the day-to-day operations, training, and managing volunteers who check for water quality, discover beds of aquatic grasses, and plant oysters on several sanctuary reefs up and down the river.

I had joined Tom and two of his volunteers the week before aboard his center-console patrol boat, monitoring the water quality on several sites up Whitehall Bay. The water seemed to be doing okay along Mill Creek and Rideout Creek, which was encouraging after several weeks of algae bloom. But Tom expressed some frustration about another source of pollution way up at the head of the river.

He has another boat, a smaller skiff that can get into really skinny water, but even that got stuck in the mud the one time he tried to poke up into Severn Run. He said he suspected that something was making that creek muddier than it should be, and whatever it was, it was contributing to the abundance of sediment in the river it flows into, but he needed to see it first-hand to confirm his suspicions.

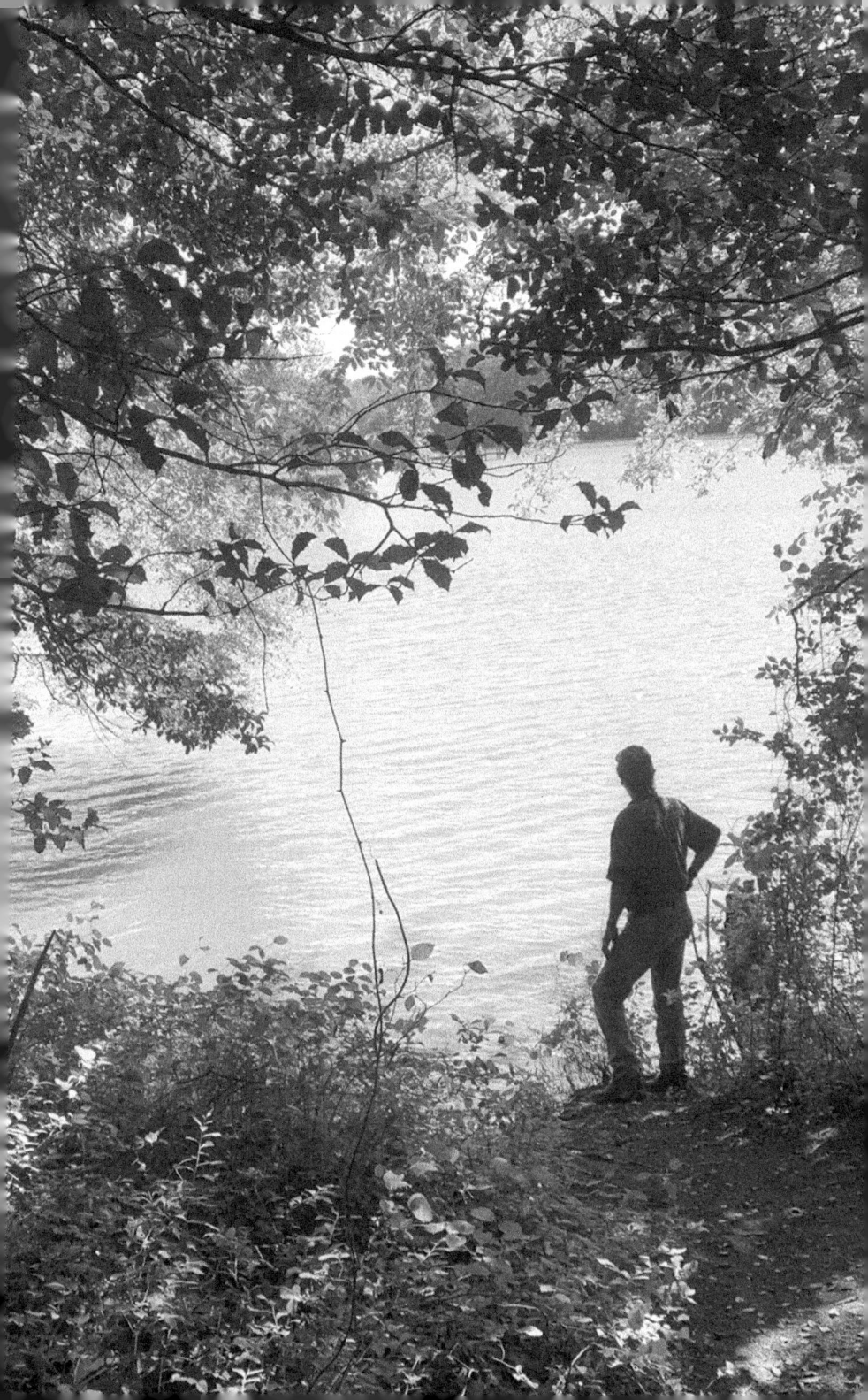

Later, I happened to find a trail on the AllTrails app that encompassed the mouth of Severn Run, so I invited Tom to join me on an exploratory jaunt. We met one sunny mid-week day by the Baldwin Memorial United Methodist Church on General's Highway in Crownsville. The app showed one of two trailheads toward the end of Indian Landing Road. We found it on the left. It's a little hard to see, since the sign sits back behind the tree line. The berm is wide enough to park, but there's a "No Parking" sign. A couple of neighbors walking their terrier suggested that we park around the corner on Larue Road. If you see the entrance to Arlington Echo Outdoor Education Center, you've gone too far.

The sign at the trailhead informed us that we were about to enter the Severn Run Natural Environmental Area, a name made up, no doubt, in some windowless conference room by a committee eager to move on to other agenda items before all the bars closed.

The site does, indeed, encompass the watershed of Severn Run, the headwaters of the Severn River. It has remarkably retained its natural character, thanks to the aegis of the Maryland Park Service. It's certainly environmental, as Tom Guay could attest to in his official capacity as the head of such an organization. And it covers an area of more than 1,400 acres. It's a title that's descriptive enough; it just doesn't sing.

I should mention here that before we both got into the business of protecting the environment, Tom and I played music together for years as members of the Eastport Oyster Boys band. So we're sensitive to these artistic nuances.

Fortunately, the trail we followed took us through forest and marsh, providing scenes of inspirational beauty. We even found a rustic amphitheater on a bluff overlooking the river where we could have performed an impromptu concert had we only known to bring our instruments along with our binoculars.

We followed the packed-earth trail single-file through a forest of white oaks and tulip poplar, with holly trees here and there. At its highest point, an elevation of about 100 feet above the river, the trail wove around several large pines, but I'm still trying to learn how to tell my pitch pines from the shortleaf and Virginia.

At one time, there were wooden signs identifying some of these trees, but they've rotted away over the years and nobody seems interested in replacing them. We picked up several bits and pieced together a sign that read Chinkapin Oak, and there it was, only the second one of its species that I'd ever spotted, a realization which gave me a pleasant reminder that I've still got a lot to learn. Other than this sign of neglect, the trails seem well used and free of litter.

The path dipped down to the water's edge, and we got a good view of the bight at the very end of the Severn River proper. Like the South River and the Magothy, the Severn is not so much a flowing river as it is a tidal estuary. It's named after the river separating England from Wales. Severn Run, on the other hand, is an actual fresh-water stream fed by no fewer than nine smaller streams, most notably the Jabez Branch.

We crossed over one of those smaller tributaries called the Sewell Spring Branch. It's a crystal-clear rivulet that slips underneath a quaint footbridge, its banks fringed with ferns. I learned a lot of this information from a reference book Tom gave me later called *Gems of the Severn*. Published by the Severn River Commission in 1988, it lists the findings of Todd Davison and Colby Rucker, who cataloged more than 500 natural, historical, and cultural "gem" sites along the river. It's out of print, but you can find it in the county library.

It turns out that this creek was named after a Methodist preacher named John Sewell, who hosted meetings of the Methodist Society in his nearby home in 1777, years before the Methodist Episcopal Church was formed in 1784. Sewell's home, Brooksby Point, is still standing and privately owned. It's just upstream of the bridge, outside the limits of the natural area. Bishop Francis Asbury himself preached there several times. Asbury was the first bishop of the Methodist Episcopal Church consecrated in the United States. I mused at the contrast between Sewell's humble frame house up the creek and the Gothic Revival elegance of the granite Methodist church built at the far end of the road in 1894.

The trail led us up another steep hill and down again onto the spit of land that marks the confluence of Severn Run and the Severn River. There, Tom could plainly see that the water in Severn Run was the color of a Starbuck's grande mocha latte.

"We've been tracking the water quality at Indian Landing, and we always have the worst readings there," he said, shaking his head. "We haven't been able to get the boat up here; it's too shallow. But this is exactly what I expected." The next step, he explained, was to determine that the excess sediment has something to do with stormwater runoff from Route 32 and I-97. Then to fix it.

The good news is that the marsh vegetation at the mouth of Severn Run seems to be uncontaminated by invasive phragmites reeds. We wound through the native cattails, rose mallows and cordgrass to the very tip of the spit where the freshwater meets the tide. As if on cue, a majestic great blue heron swept right overhead.

When we got back to our cars, we were surprised to learn that this portion of the trail was only about a mile out and back. Another leg of the trail parallels Severn Run and ends up at Veterans Highway. You can start at that end by driving to the end of General's Highway, turning north onto Veterans Highway and keeping a lookout for a gravel drive on the right with a mailbox marked "8737." You'll find a parking area and the second trailhead at the top of the drive.

Severn Run Natural Environmental Area
8737 Veterans Highway
Crownsville, MD 21108

aacounty.org/boards-and-commissions/severn-river-commission/severn-watershed/severn-run-and-jabez-branch/

Parking for the Indian Landing Road trailhead is in the neighborhood on Larue Drive; please be respectful of neighbors

Parking for the Veterans Highway trailhead is limited, located at the end of the driveway of 8737 Veterans Highway

Open dawn to dusk

Free admission

No toilets

Docile dogs on leash are welcome; bring your own doggy bags

Moderate, some topography

Walk 15

Spritely Whimsy of Spriggs Farm Park

I've always been curious about the origin of the name of the Magothy River. According to the U.S. Geological Survey, the river was labeled Maggotty River on a map drawn in 1690. The USGS web site speculates as to whether the name refers to mosquito larvae or an Algonquian phrase meaning small plain devoid of timber.

My impish nature leads me to think that the name actually stems from English word "maggot," but not in the way you're thinking. In the mid-1600s, when this area was first settled by English persons, they used the word maggot to mean a "whim" or "fancy," as if one had a maggot wiggling about in his brain. "Maggoty" meant full of whimsy.

I'd like to think of the whimsical nature of the name because of my excursion to Spriggs Farm Park on the Magothy in late July 2020, where I met my old friend Jack Neil, a lobbyist for the geo-thermal industry who lives nearby with his family. Jack showed me a black-and-white photograph of a grinning Mrs. Spriggs proudly cradling a watermelon the size of a pot-bellied pig in her arms. At her side, perched upon another colossal gourd, sits a cat, looking about as if he's trying to detect lurking watermelon rustlers.

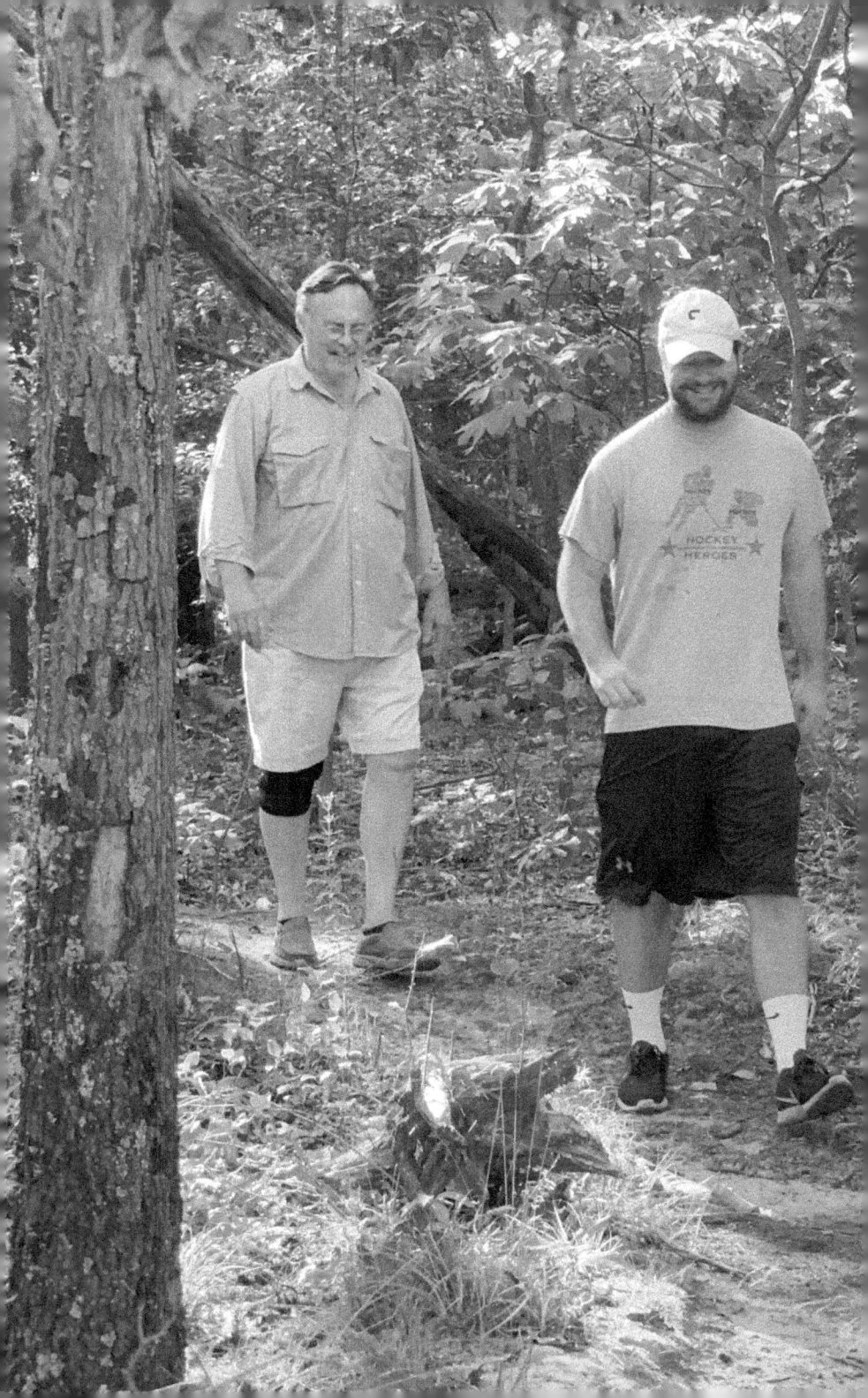

The farm, located on the banks of the Magothy River between the modern suburban communities of Ulmstead Estates and Bayberry, was actively cultivating watermelon, peaches, and tomatoes for about 100 years before Mrs. Spriggs' husband, Frank, died in 1982.

Frank Spriggs was the Arnold postmaster. He wrote a letter in 1967 about life on the farm. They would ship the produce to market in Baltimore aboard a bugeye schooner. "Some of these watermelons grew so large one year," he wrote, "that the captain of the Bug-eye refused to handle them as they weighed 70 to 90 pounds apiece." To me, that's whimsical. Downright maggoty.

According to Jack, Mrs. Spriggs lived to the venerable age of 100 and a half. When she died in 2008, the 54-acre farm passed on to her friends and caretakers, Bill and Lynn Hatch, who could easily have sold the property to developers. Instead, Jack Neil and other concerned citizens formed the Spriggs Farm Preservation Foundation and spearheaded the transformation of the farm into a county park.

Under their aegis, Anne Arundel County purchased the site in 2011 for about $3 million, including $1.3 million from Maryland's Program Open Space and $700,000 from the federal Land and Water Conservation Fund, matched by $1 million from the county Forest Conservation Fund. This is the fund that developers contribute to when they cut down too many trees.

I met Jack and his son, Devin, a recent environmental studies graduate of Salisbury State, on one of those hot-and-muggy mornings typical of July. Jack opened the gate—you need to log onto the web site to get the combination to the lock—and we drove up the hill to park by the Spriggs' old farmhouse.

Jack was eager to show me around the property and talk about the success of the foundation to preserve the farm from development and make it accessible to the public. He told me about the Spriggs family and the history of the place as we walked down the gravel road to the river's edge. As the road opened up onto the former watermelon patch, now a meadow, a large doe emerged from the brush and gave us a long, studious look before sauntering across the road and disappearing into the woods.

"We see deer all the time," Jack grinned. "They spend the night carousing around the neighborhood, then in the morning we see them sneaking back into the park."

We stopped at the picnic area overlooking the river. You can see Gibson Island and Dobbins Island and catch a glimpse of where the Magothy estuary meets the Chesapeake Bay. Baltimore Lighthouse would be there at the mouth, just out of sight.

The water here is pretty shallow, Jack noted. "When the north wind blows all the water out of the Bay in the winter, you can walk all the way out to the end of that pier," he said, pointing to a neighboring dock that extends at least 100 yards out into the river. The park property has more than 600 feet of shoreline. We walked down the bank along a narrow path through the towering phragmites, the invasive reeds from Eurasia. There was a narrow beach along the shore that would be walkable at low tide. You can launch a canoe or kayak here, but if you do, take care, as the trail down the bank is quite steep.

"We're working on plans to eradicate these phragmites," he noted. "We'll also build a living shoreline to protect this bluff from erosion." The path led through the reeds to an inlet where a trickle of water feeds a three-acre tidal pond.

I followed Jack and Devin back up the bank and into the oak and holly forest. A sandy path led us through the woods to emerge on a hilltop overlooking the pond. As we talked, we watched an industrious muskrat swim across from the far bank with a thatch of reeds in its mouth to feather its nest. An eastern kingbird swooped to snatch a bug from just above the surface. A great blue heron scrawked across the pond, gliding pterodactylly.

"There's an eagle's nest over there somewhere," Jack said, gesturing to the woods on the other side of the pond. Neighbors on that side of the park have their own access at the end of Stonington Way.

"When you're here early in the morning, the bird songs are like a symphony," Jack said. "The slopes around the pond act like an amphitheater, so if you stand here on this bluff, it's an amazing sound. Then the mockingbird starts to sing and everybody else shuts up."

The path led us along the rim of a ravine back to the farmhouse near the entrance to the park. The old house looks run down, but Jack reported that there are no definite plans to renovate it any time soon. He hopes the foundation can use the site to develop environmental education programs for county schools as well as the community college.

I noted earlier that the name Magothy might be Algonquian in origin. We ran across lots of ancient oyster shells on the path high up on the bluff overlooking the pond, indicating that people were there feasting on the luscious bivalves perhaps thousands of years ago. Jack also mentioned that prehistoric arrowheads and tool points have been found in the eroding river shoreline.

Still, this site seems more significant in its preservation of the history of the truck farms that once made northern Anne Arundel County famous for its produce. Even more than that, Spriggs Farm Park is a prime example of how local citizens can band together to preserve places like this for the rest of us to enjoy.

Spriggs Farm Park is a gated park with a combination lock. Access to the park is limited due to site conditions and capacity. Secure the gate on entering and leaving the park.

Spriggs Farm Park
965 Bayberry Drive
Arnold, MD 21012

410-222-7317

aacounty.org/locations-and-directions/spriggs-farm-park-on-the-magothy

Parking is limited; park only in fenced parking lot and not on the road

Open dawn to dusk daily

Free admission

No toilets

Attentive dogs on leash are welcome; bring your own doggie bags

Easy going

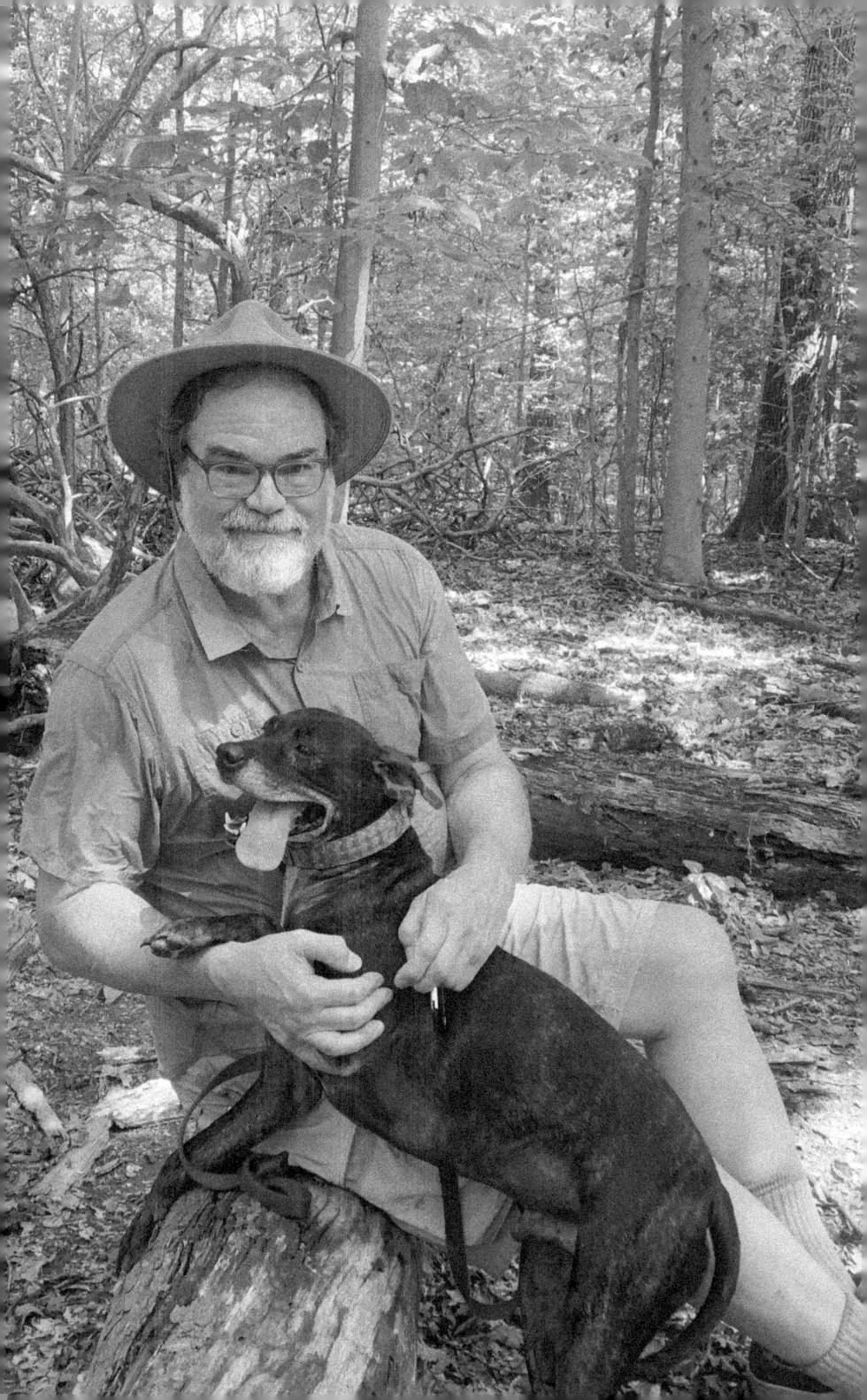

Walk 16

Keeping Broad Creek Trail Safe from Bears

I'm still trying to learn my trees, so I was a little shaken when an alert reader wrote in questioning my calling a certain tree by the name "tulip poplar." I dropped my newspaper and grabbed my laptop to see if I've been doling out inaccurate information, as has been known to occur from time to time, much to my embarrassment.

To my relief, according to the U.S. Department of Agriculture Natural Resources Conservation Service web site, what I call a "tulip poplar" is also known as yellow poplar, tulip magnolia or whitewood as well as the name the reader knew it by, "tulip tree."

Whatever you call them, these trees are truly magnificent. They are actually not poplars at all, but members of the magnolia family, which accounts for their yellowy flowers, as big as your fist, that bloom between April and June.

Tulip poplars are the tallest, straightest trees in any forest on the East Coast. Indians in this region used their trunks to build dugout canoes. They would fell a tree and lay burning coals along the top, then scrape out the charred wood with stones or oyster shells. They would repeat the process laboriously until the log was hollowed out in the shape of a canoe. Some of these canoes were 40 or 50 feet long.

Captain John Smith was impressed by their speed. "Instead of Oares, they use Paddles and sticks, with which they will row faster than our Barges," he wrote in his journal. They "row faster with three oares in their canoes than we with eight."

The English quickly adopted the concept of shaping a log to turn it into a boat and refined it by fastening several sculpted logs together to form a single hull. Eventually, boatwrights whittled our local forests into the traditional Chesapeake Bay brogans, bugeyes, and pungy schooners you can still see at maritime museums as well as the smaller, sleeker log canoes that are actively raced on the Eastern Shore today, even though some of them are more than a century old.

I found a lot of tall tulip poplars at Broad Creek Park, along with some truly remarkably large specimens of gray beech. I checked out the trail on one hot and muggy afternoon in mid-August 2020 with a new companion.

The park surrounds the headwaters of the creek, which opens up onto the upper reaches of the South River. It's nestled in between Annapolis High School on Riva Road and the Anne Arundel County offices on Harry S Truman Parkway. There are several trail loops on either side of the creek running a total of about four and a half miles.

The trail head is a little hard to find—it's not marked—but I followed the AllTrails app to the parking lot of the county health department on Truman Parkway, across the road from the department of agriculture offices, where the statue of the cow is whimsically decorated in a fashion to celebrate various holidays throughout the year. At that time, it was wearing an appropriately sized surgical mask over its muzzle. The trailhead is in the corner of the parking lot nearest the dumpsters.

🐾

But before we head down the trail, I have to tell you about my new hiking companion. I received many kind notes and comments about the passing of my sweet Irish setter, Bonnie, last spring. Since then, I've been trying to get my "doggie fix" by accosting passing dog-walkers and begging for a chance to say hello to their pooches. This has been met with varying degrees of success—and suspicion.

Eventually, I got the idea to call the SPCA of Anne Arundel County and see if I could borrow a dog to take for a walk. To my surprise and delight, I got invited to take some special training and earned the privilege of taking one of their charges off the premises for a few hours.

I showed up at the adoption center in Eastport, ready with my own leash, pockets stuffed with doggie bags and biscuits, my mask responsibly in place. The first candidate the volunteers brought out for me was a nice little shepherd mix. We got along fine as we trotted down the sidewalk toward the parking lot, but then he balked at getting into the back of my car. He simply would not get in. Maybe it was because of what happened to him the last time he got in a car. Obviously, this one just wouldn't do.

The second candidate was a nice little female pit bull mix who took one look at me and shrank back in horror. "Maybe it's your mask," the volunteer offered. And truly, what dog wouldn't wonder why all the humans are going around muzzled all the time? I lowered my mask and the poor pup reared back even more sharply. Perhaps it was my full beard. I was certainly furrier than she was. On the other hand, I frequently get the same reaction from other females, no matter what species. So this one wouldn't do, either.

Next came the Duchess Ripley, an elderly, dignified Lhasa apso. At first I admit that I was a little disappointed, since larger dogs have been my main companions over the years, but I'm not a specieist, and I determined to give this little one a chance. I picked her up and placed her in the back of my Forester, where she sat down. I think. Between her short legs and long fur, it was hard to tell.

I took the Duchess for a test walk at the Homeport Farm Park off Solomons Island Road. It's a long drive to the parking lot, then a short walk down the hill to the kayak launch on Church Creek. The Duchess made it down the hill all right, took a sniff or two at the sand on the beach, then headed back up the hill.

Since I was attached by the leash, I followed. She was pretty tired by the time we got back to the car, and I realized that my legs are 36 inches long compared to hers at six inches, which meant that my quarter-mile walk was a mile and a half for her, a pretty good haul for an old gal on a hot day. She enjoyed the pan of water I had waiting for her in the back of the car as we drove back to the SPCA

Finally, the volunteer brought out Loki Loc, a medium-sized, short-haired breed called the Plott hound. I had never heard of such an animal. According to the American Kennel Club web site, Plott hounds are descended not from English foxhounds but from German Hanover hounds. In 1750, Johannes Plott arrived in North Carolina from Germany with five Hanover hounds. Plott settled in the mountains, where he raised a family and hunted bears with his hounds. His son, Henry, bred the family pack to local hounds and produced a big-game hunter originally known as "Plott's hound." It is now North Carolina's state dog.

True to his nature, Loki was bright and curious and eager to get out on a walk. He jumped into the car and then behaved well on the leash once we arrived at the park. As we walked along the trail, Loki would stop at regular intervals, sniffing to check for messages, then hike a knee to leave a reply. This occurred so frequently that after a while, it was obvious that the reply part was strictly out of habit, like a printer that keeps chugging out sheets of paper even when the ink cartridge had long run out of toner.

Since it was hot and we were running a bit late, we stuck to the nearest loop of trails, hiking only about two miles in a little over an hour. The trail is a good one, with plenty of topography and a variety of trees to learn about. By the time we got back to the car, we were fairly well bonded.

This was a happy dog, even though we found no bears to hunt, and I was happy to have had some time together. I got Loki Loc back to the SPCA in time for his 3 o'clock curfew. Now that we know the system works, I'm looking forward to meeting other new friends to hike around with.

The SPCA of Anne Arundel County is the largest and oldest animal welfare organization in the county. They provide shelter and humane care for homeless animals in need and serve as advocates for animal welfare in our community. Unlike other shelters in the region, the local organization does not set a time limit on how long an animal is available for adoption.

The SPCA shelter in Eastport takes in homeless animals regardless of age, breed, or physical condition, and provides them with the care they deserve for as long as it takes to find the critters a home. They have maintained a record high life-saving rate of 98 percent every year since 2014—one of the highest in this country—a remarkable achievement as they accept animals that other shelters turn away.

The SPCA is located at 1815 Bay Ridge Avenue in the Eastport neighborhood of Annapolis. You can make an appointment by calling 410-268-4388. For more information, log on to www.aaspca.org.

Broad Creek Park
1A Harry S Truman Parkway
Annapolis, MD 21401

410-222-7317

aacounty.org/locations-and-directions/broad-creek-park

Plenty of parking in the Anne Arundel County Health Department lot

Open dawn to dusk daily

Free admission

No toilets

Well-trained dogs on leash are welcome; bring your own doggie bags

Moderate, some topography

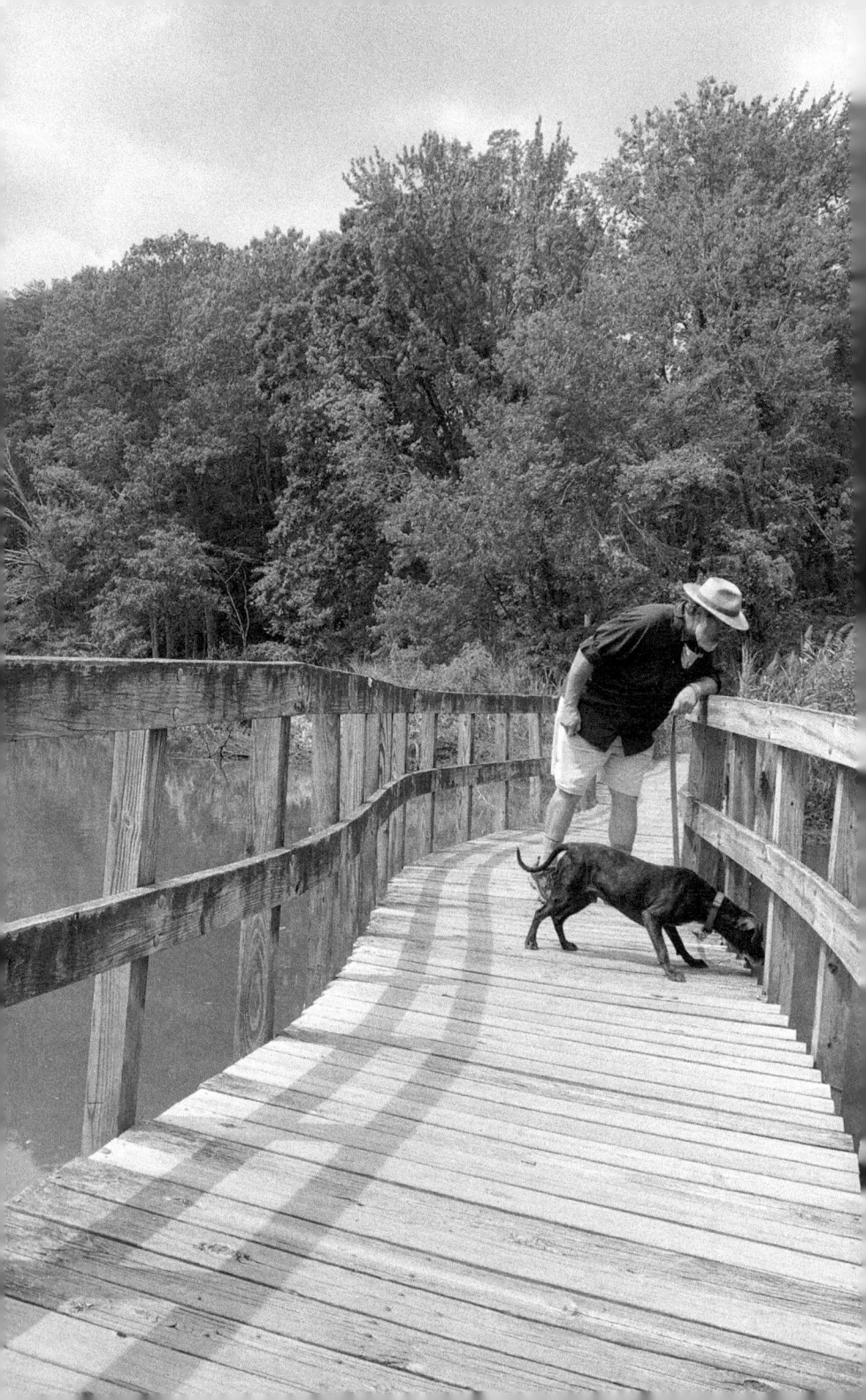

Walk 17

Trekking Through Truxtun Park

People ask me if I've lived in Annapolis my entire life, and I never tire of answering, "Not yet."

I explain that I'm a newcomer. I've only lived here 40 years. Still, in all that time, I had never bothered to explore the city's Truxtun Park until one hot and muggy afternoon in late August 2020.

Truxtun Park covers more than 70 acres between Hilltop Road and Spa Creek. The centerpiece of the park is the Roger W. "Pip" Moyer Recreation Center with its many recreational amenities. Other features of the park include a newly renovated swimming pool, a skateboard park, several well-manicured baseball fields, basketball courts, recently renovated tennis courts, a picnic pavilion overlooking the creek, and playgrounds for kids.

Down at the end of Truxtun Park Road off Primrose Road, you'll find a small beach that's a happy place to launch a canoe or a kayak, and a public boat ramp, one of the few near Annapolis besides the small ramp at the end of Tucker Street in West Annapolis and the huge ramp complex at Sandy Point State Park.

I knew that the park was named after Thomas Truxtun, one of the first six commanders of the United States Navy appointed by President George Washington. Truxtun was born in 1755 in Hampstead, New York, on February 17, which also happens to be my birthday. He served aboard the newly commissioned frigates USS *Constellation* and then the USS *President* during the Quasi-War with France from 1798 to 1800. But I couldn't figure out Truxtun's connection with Annapolis.

It turns out that the park was named by the commander's grandson, Truxtun Beale, who donated the property to the city in 1931, just a few years before his death. According to several web sites, Beale died in 1936 "in his country home near Annapolis." This was a place called Laurel Banks Farm, which turns out to be the site of what is now Quiet Waters Park.

Truxtun Beale was a fascinating character. He was born in San Francisco in 1854 and became a diplomat who served as our ambassador to Persia, Greece, Romania, and Serbia. When he wasn't staying at his country home near Annapolis, he lived in his townhouse in Washington, D.C. That townhouse is still there. It's known as the historic Decatur House. Beale's widow, Marie Oge Beale, bequeathed the house to the National Trust for Historic Preservation just before she died in 1956.

On my way to explore Truxtun's park, I stopped by the SPCA shelter in Eastport and sprang my old buddy Loki Loc out on parole for the afternoon. If you recall from my last outing, I've undergone special training and have earned the privilege to take adoptable dogs off campus for walks. I was surprised to see that Loki Loc, the dog I took out last time, was still there and had not yet been adopted, as he's such a wonderful pup. Sure, he's a bit gray around the muzzle, but so am I. He's still lovable, and so am I, as my emotional-support spouse will attest to. Sometimes.

Loki was happy to see me waiting for him on the bench outside the shelter. He politely plopped his front paws up onto my knees, wagged his skinny tail, and gave my nose a friendly lick. Loki Loc is a Plott hound at heart, a medium-sized dog bred to hunt mammoth-sized bears in the Appalachian Mountains of North Carolina. His sleek, brown-and-black brindle fur and bright eyes give him charm, but those perky ears are his mainstream medium of communication. They're jerked upright most of the time as he sniffs the shrubs and tree trunks, searching for evidence of anything that might be of interest, like signs of grizzlies.

We parked in the lot off Primrose Road. It's usually packed with boat trailers on any weekend, but on this mid-week day in late August 2020 it was nearly empty. With leash in hand and doggie bag in pocket, I led Loki up the hill to take a look at the back reaches of Spa Creek below us through the woods dominated by mature chestnut oaks.

On the right, you can see a deep gully cutting through the hill. This is all that remains of the Bay Ridge and Annapolis Railroad, built in 1886. As Jane McWilliams and Carol Patterson wrote in *Bay Ridge on the Chesapeake,* (1986) "the Bay Ridge and Annapolis Railroad Company built a line from Annapolis to Bay Ridge, the Victorian resort on Tolly Point then in full summer swing.

"Track ran from what is now Amos Garrett Boulevard across Spa Creek and across Primrose Hills toward what is now Bay Ridge Avenue, across the land that was later the Annapolis Airport (where the Giant shopping center on Bay Ridge Road is located today), the entrance to what is now Annapolis Roads, and on to Bay Ridge. Trains ran until the resort closed in 1903, although there was still some informal use of the track after that. Parts of the line are still visible, but the actual track was torn up for metal in WWI."

Loki and I enjoyed the cool breeze at the top of the bluff. We followed the hard-packed trail as it paralleled the creek. There's a good amount of bare earth crisscrossed by exposed tree roots that could trip you up. Some of the steps up steep slopes have eroded away over time, so it would be wise to exercise caution. If you have any mobility issues, you might consider sticking to the paved walkways elsewhere in the park. Still, this is a lovely trail, refreshingly free of litter and, on this day, free of other people, too. We only met two other walkers, one dogless and one with an aged poodle.

We heard the piercing whistle of the osprey whose nest I've seen nearby from the water. They'll be heading down to South and Central America in just a few weeks. We also heard the maniacal cackle of a pileated woodpecker, but as hard as Loki searched, we did not see any other wildlife.

A fork in the trail led across an old wooden bridge to the Truxton Heights neighborhood, spelled with an "o" in lieu of the second "u" for some unknown reason. From there, it connects with the Spa Creek Trail that winds up behind the Wiley H. Bates Legacy Center on Smithfield Street.

We stayed on the main trail and came out of the woods behind the Pip Moyer Recreation Center. We dove back into the trees and wound up at the old tennis courts. The trail roughly circumnavigates the public swimming pool, and no matter where you are, you can hear the high-pitched squeals of delighted little swimmers through the treetops.

We got back to the car after walking about two miles in about an hour. Loki lapped at the pan of water in the back of the Forester, and I turned the AC up full blast on the way back to the SPCA. Once there, Loki hopped out of the car and trotted cheerfully up the walkway to the shelter, where a staffer took him in. He slipped through the door without even saying goodbye.

The SPCA is located at 1815 Bay Ridge Avenue in the Eastport neighborhood of Annapolis. You can make an appointment by calling 410-268-4388. For more information, log on to www.aaspca.org.

Truxtun Park

Off Primrose Road at Roger W. "Pip" Moyer
Recreation Center
Annapolis, MD 21403

410-263-7958

Open dawn to dusk daily

Plenty of parking on site

Free admission

Toilets in the Rec Center

Cheerful dogs on leash are welcome; doggie bag dispenser available

Moderate, some topography

Walk 18

Waterworks Park Redux

There are some places you just can't get enough of, and the City of Annapolis Waterworks Park is one of them. I hiked part of the trail earlier in the year from the trailhead on Housley Road and wound up at the reservoir of the old waterworks on Defense Highway. This time, in early September 2020, Louise, my emotional-support spouse, and I started at the dam and took a short walk along the lake.

Waterworks Park is a little hard to describe. There are 11 miles of trails winding through 600 acres of dense hardwood forest in an area tucked between General's Highway and Defense Highway. All of that is open to the public with no admission fee.

The Reservoir Trail is a flat, hard-surfaced trail that winds along the eastern bank of the main reservoir and two small ponds. This is the only handicap-accessible trail in the park.

The Overlook Loop Trail is marked with blue blazes and runs about a half-mile from the northern edge of the earthen dam that separates the two small ponds to the east. This one climbs to the top of the hill overlooking the reservoirs and ends up by the Reservoir Trail picnic area. The Woodland Loop Trail, marked with white blazes, extends the Overlook Trail by another mile.

We parked at the foot of the concrete dam. The Annapolis Water Works facility dates back to 1866, when it pumped clean, potable water from this reservoir about three miles to Annapolis through what at the time were innovative concrete pipes. The city augmented the drinking water from the reservoir with well water beginning in the early 20th century. Today, the city pumps all of its water—1.5 billion gallons every year—from eight wells ranging from 250 to 1,000 feet deep. The reservoir is now just for catch-and-release fishing.

The only other folks we met that day comprised a family group watching one kid fish in the stream that stemmed from the dam's outflow. The boy grinned as he pulled out a good-sized smallmouth bass. I got to chatting with Chris Breece of Ellicott City, who was there with his eight-year-old twins Christopher and Autumn. Chris' friend Meaghan Masella of Severna Park was there with her four-year-old daughter, Shelby Massella Walker, and seven-year-old son Guy Massella Walker, the fisherman.

"We love it here," Chris told me. "We've been here four or five times this summer. We park over on Housley Road and walk about two miles to get here. The kids enjoy the hike." He said the kids hooked at least 20 fish in this spot, which rankled me a bit because the last time I was here with my fly rod, I got skunked. Apparently, these bass like to entertain kids more than us old guys.

Louise and I strolled across the footbridge over the stream, which is one of the tributaries to Broad Creek on

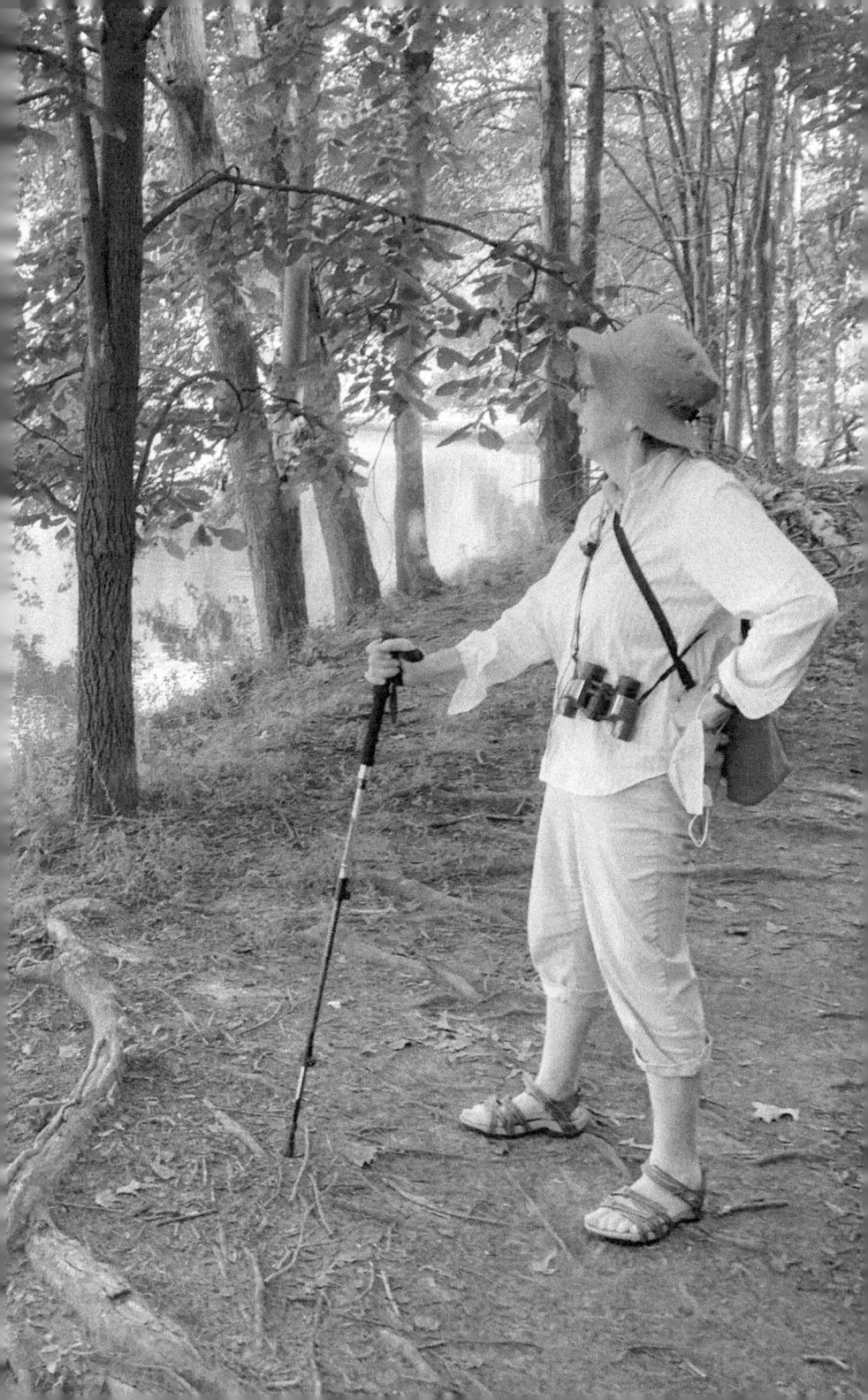

the South River. We were up for just a short walk, so we chose the one-mile Housley Loop. This is a hard-packed earthen trail that leads along the western edge of the reservoir underneath the locust trees and cottonwoods.

One leg of the trail stops at the end of the earthen dam that separates the main reservoir from a smaller holding pond. Another leads up the hill into the hardwood forest of beeches, oaks, and holly trees. It rises about 100 feet to the top, where the old landfill is now covered by an 80-acre field of solar panels.

We admired the view of the lake below and a glen covered with bright yellow coreopsis blossoms, looking like a field full of little black-eyed Susans shining in the sun. We looped back from there, but you can hike about four or five miles farther, all the way up to Honeysuckle Lane in Crownsville.

Somewhere in this park lies the grave of one of my favorite dogs of all time. My father, Bill Holland, served as the director of Public Works for the city of Annapolis under the Hillman and Callahan administrations. Louise and I lived in Eastport when we were first married way back in the last century, and Mikey, a Brittany spaniel who'd been my dog since he was a pup back in Pittsburgh, lived with us.

Mikey was the smartest dog in the world, and the sweetest. I remember one spring I was recovering from a nasty car wreck that should have killed me. I was convalescing at my mother's house in Sewickley, a small town down the Ohio River from Pittsburgh. The public elementary school was right across the street. Mikey and I would be sitting on Mom's front porch enjoying the morning air, when the school bell would ring and all the kids would come pouring out onto the playground for recess.

Mikey would get up, stretch his back with a yoga-esque "down dog," take a deep breath, and trot across the street. I would hear the kids calling, "Mikey! Mikey!" I would watch him romp with the kids on the playground and 15 minutes later, the bell would ring and the children would line up and file back into the school building. Mikey would trot back across the street, find his place on the porch and curl up with a sigh. I likened the scene to the one in the classic Warner Brothers cartoon where the sheep dog punches his timecard after a long day of guarding the flock.

Not long ago, I signed up for a Growing up in Sewickley group on Facebook, and several of its members recalled playing with good old Mikey at that school.

Mikey was pretty old when Louise and I went on our honeymoon tour around the country. We left him with my dad, and when we got back, Mikey was gone. Dad perhaps took advantage of his position when he chose one of the hilltops overlooking the reservoir as Mikey's resting place, but that was long ago, and Dad's not around any more, either, so I have no way of knowing where Dad left the bronze plaque.

Knowing my dad, I'm sure he left one to commemorate the spot. Let me know if you find it.

Annapolis Waterworks Park
260 Defense Highway
Annapolis, MD 21401

410.263.7958

annapolis.gov/DocumentCenter/View/449/Waterworks-Park-Brochure-PDF?bidId=

Open dawn to dusk daily

Plenty of parking on site

Free admission

No toilets on site

Amiable dogs on leash are welcome; bring your own doggie bags

Moderate, some topography

Walk 19

Chillin' Out with Max at Bacon Ridge

This old adage used to be my motto: "I want to be the guy my dog thinks I am."

Now, I just want to be like Max.

Max is my latest parolee from the SPCA in Eastport. We went for a walk in the Bacon Ridge Natural Area in mid-September 2020 and had a wonderful time together. Max is mostly bulldog, a beefy 90-pound bundle of laid-back sweetness with a massive head, big brown eyes, and teeny little ears. He's bright and curious yet unfettered by any need to exert his male ego. At nearly eight years old, he's a gentle being all around.

I stopped by the shelter that afternoon with blind-date nerves, not knowing who they'd match me with this week or if we'd get along. Then one of the staffers brought Max out to meet me in the lobby, and it was instant bonding. We exchanged introductory sniffs and very quickly, Max was pressing against me and then, in the ultimate compliment, sat on my foot. He had claimed me then and there.

We got out to the car, where I had carefully piled all of my stuff—duffle bags of foul-weather gear, fishing paraphernalia, other detritus—in the front end of the rear compartment, clearing a large space in the back for Max. I helped him up and carefully closed the rear hatch. By the time I opened the driver's door, Max had already made

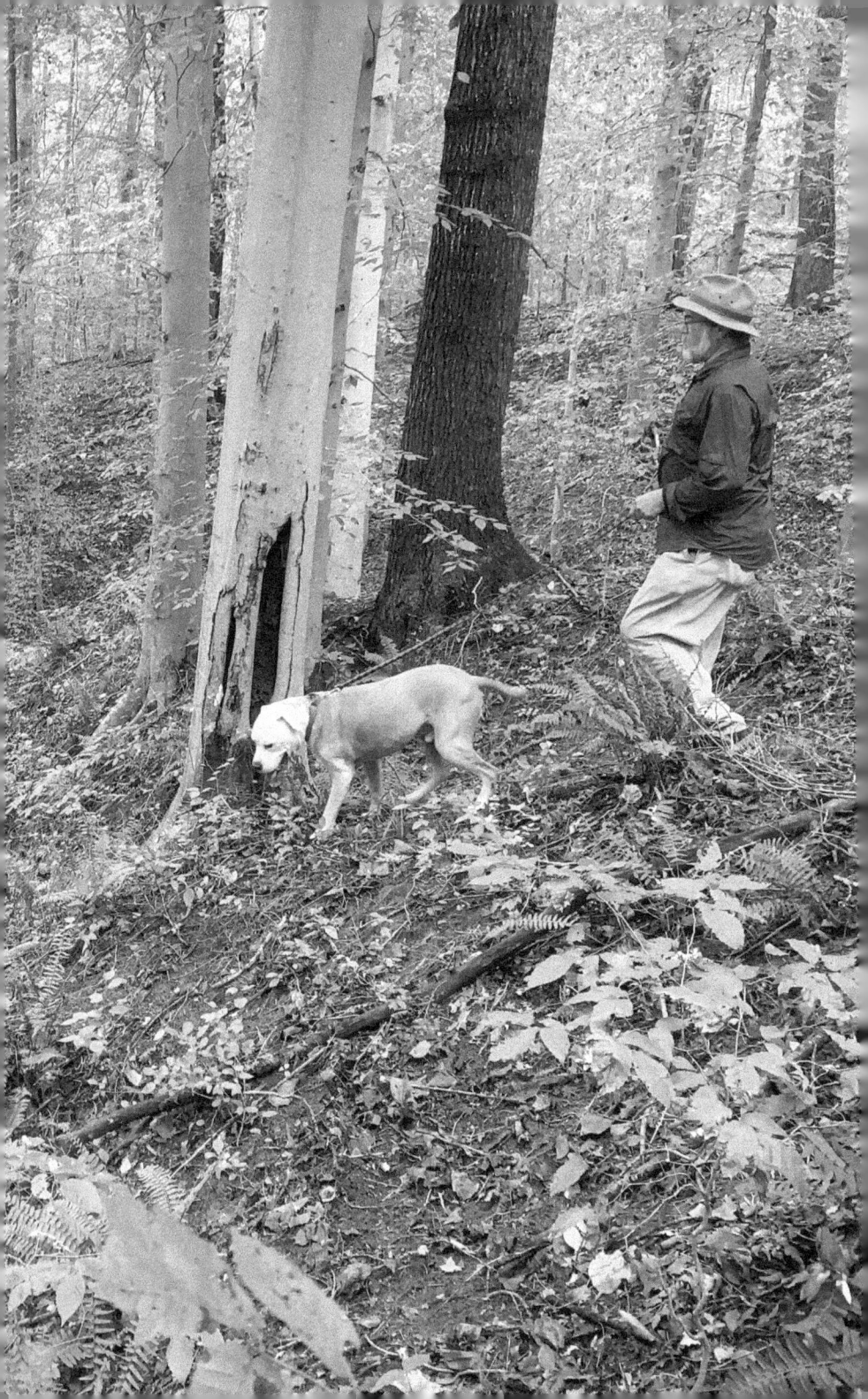

himself a comfy nest on top of my pile. Fortunately, I had moved the ukulele and the fly rods to the front seat.

🐾

We drove up General's Highway to Crownsville Road and crossed over I-97 on Hawkins Road, where the trailhead for Bacon Ridge can be found on the right. Bacon Ridge Natural Area is 630 acres of permanently protected land through a conservation easement between Anne Arundel County, Maryland Environmental Trust, and Scenic Rivers Land Trust.

Bacon Ridge Natural Area comprises tracts of marsh and mature forest nestled between I-97 and St. Stephens Church Road in Crownsville. The creek called Bacon Ridge Branch flows into the headwaters of the South River.

The property is owned by Anne Arundel County and managed by the County Department of Recreation and Parks. Since 2010, the natural area has been protected by a conservation easement held jointly by Scenic Rivers Land Trust and the Maryland Environmental Trust.

According to the Scenic Rivers web site, "a conservation easement is a voluntary legal agreement between a landowner and a land trust that limits future development on a property in order to protect its environmental features. The easement states what will be allowed on the property and how it will be managed. These requirements are permanent; the restrictions travel with the deed if the property is sold or transferred."

The terms of this easement allow for the land to be open to the public as a park for passive recreational activities like hiking and biking. The trust approved the county's request to create about 5.5 miles of hiking and biking trails in 2015 and 2016. Scenic Rivers also hosts the annual Walk for the Woods every spring to encourage families to explore the outdoors in general and the beauty of Bacon Ridge in specific.

Max and I parked and set off into the woods. Max was as gentlemanly on the other end of a leash as he is in all other respects. He didn't pull, he didn't yank, and he didn't stop at every rock, tree, post, or protuberance to mark his presence like some male dogs do. He was simply happy to be out on this trail on one of those cool days at the tail end of summer, and I was happy to be there with him.

There were nine other cars in the parking area, but we only encountered two other people the whole two hours we were there. We stepped aside to allow a mountain biker to pass us, and Max never flinched.

We walked the southernmost of the two loops. It's a well-packed dirt trail that follows the top of the ridge for the most part, so there are just a few steepish bits, which is remarkable considering how hilly the area is. The hollows drop nearly straight down almost 100 feet in places. It would seem that this trail was blazed artistically to let both hikers and bikers enjoy this beautiful forest.

A portion of the Bacon Ridge area was once part of the Crownsville Psychiatric Hospital, which opened in 1911 to serve African American patients needing psychiatric care. Somewhere near here, there's a cemetery where the bodies of 1,800 Black patients lie in graves marked only by numbers. County archaeologists have also documented 16 sites where they have discovered intact evidence of prehistoric or Native American campgrounds.

Near here, the Arundel Rivers Federation completed a stream restoration project on the Bacon Ridge Branch. The Federation received grants from Maryland Department of Natural Resources and the Chesapeake Bay Trust to restore a stretch of this stream using innovative techniques.

But before I tell you about that, let's take a walk back through history. The first Europeans to settle in this area were fur trappers. The first thing they did was trap all the beavers and send their hides back to England so gentlemen could wear fine hats.

Until then, the North American continent was teaming with beavers building dams and creating what essentially served as holding ponds for excess stormwater. The water was trapped so it could slowly filter into the ground.

With the beavers all gone, the ponds dried out, filled up and became more forest. And with no more furs to trap, the trappers moved on west. The next wave of immigrants cut down all the trees to grow corn and tobacco. With all the trees gone, the stormwater washed all the soil into the rivers and creeks and then on into the Chesapeake Bay.

One creek off the West River was 26 feet deep in the Colonial era, deep enough to launch ocean-going ships. Today, that same creek is just three feet deep.

As the stormwater flushes down narrow creeks, the force of the flow cuts a deep channel, eroding the sides of the creek bed and sending the sediment downstream. In some places along Bacon Ridge Branch, you can stand in the bottom and not be able to see over the top. This heavy erosion is known as a "headcut."

The traditional way to solve this problem is to haul in truckloads of rock and build small dams, or weirs, to eventually raise the level of the stream bed so that it reconnects with the surrounding flood plain. This is a very costly method and requires building temporary roads through the forest to allow trucks and other heavy construction equipment to reach the site.

With the available funds, the Federation and its environmental consultants at BioHabitats could have restored about 700 feet of stream with a traditional rock-based approach. Instead, they imitated beavers and built dams made from wood harvested on site. Impact on the surrounding habitat was minimal, and they were able to stretch their funds to restore 4,300 linear feet of stream. That's six times the length of stream restored for the same amount of money, with far less negative residual impact on the surrounding habitat. This project was the first stream restoration in Maryland to use all-wood grade-control structures, just like the beavers used to do.

We had a lot to contemplate, Max and me. To top it off, just before we reached the end of the loop, we came across an old automobile dumpsite with a curious beauty to it. It's not a dump so much as it is unintentionally artistic sculpture comprised three or four 1940s and '50s vintage wrecks teetering over the edge of a ravine. Max was particularly interested in one wreck that has been squeezed like an accordion between two trees that have grown up on either side of it. One hiker later identified it as a 1956 Mercury Monterey.

Our walk completed, I reluctantly escorted Max back to the SPCA.

The SPCA is located at 1815 Bay Ridge Avenue in the Eastport neighborhood of Annapolis. I was pleased to learn later that a family read about Max when this column was printed and they came in and took him home with them. SPCA volunteers sent him off with a clipping from the newspaper. If you'd like to find your own wonderful dog to adopt, you can make an appointment by calling 410-268-4388. For more information, log on to www.aaspca.org.

The Bacon Ridge Natural Area Stewardship Committee makes recommendations to the county on how the parkland can be best managed to provide public access in a way that promotes preservation of the area. The committee welcomes suggestions on how this public asset should be used.

Bacon Ridge Natural Area
1700 Hawkins Road
Crownsville, MD 21032
410-222-7317
aacounty.org/locations-and-directions/bacon-ridge-natural-area
Open dawn to dusk daily
Limited parking available at the Hawkins Road trailhead
Free admission
Portable toilet in the parking area
Mellow dogs on leash are welcome; bring your own doggie bags
Moderate, some topography

Walk 20

The Goddess of Glendening Nature Preserve at Jug Bay

We took a goddess for a walk along the Patuxent River at Jug Bay on one of those spectacular autumn days in October 2020.

Athena is the latest of the string of adoptable dogs I've had the privilege of borrowing from the SPCA of Anne Arundel County's shelter in Eastport.

The "we" in this case, was me and my emotional-support spouse, Louise. While we were all together for the walk, I took care to keep Athena apart from Louise as part of my SPCA training protocol. The training stipulated that the adoptive dogs must be kept isolated from other people and animals because the dog might have unknown issues that could emerge as aggression. Still, we all had a splendid afternoon.

Athena is tall for her age, just a little over a year old. She's part hound of some sort, which accounts for her floppy ears and short, smooth pelt; and part German shepherd, which accounts for her black-and-buff coloration. But her most distinguishing feature—beyond her expressive brown eyes—is that long snout—all the better to sniff with, my dear.

And sniff she did. In Athena, the phenomenal olfactory fortitude of the hound has been compounded by that of the shepherd, resulting in a creature who lives through

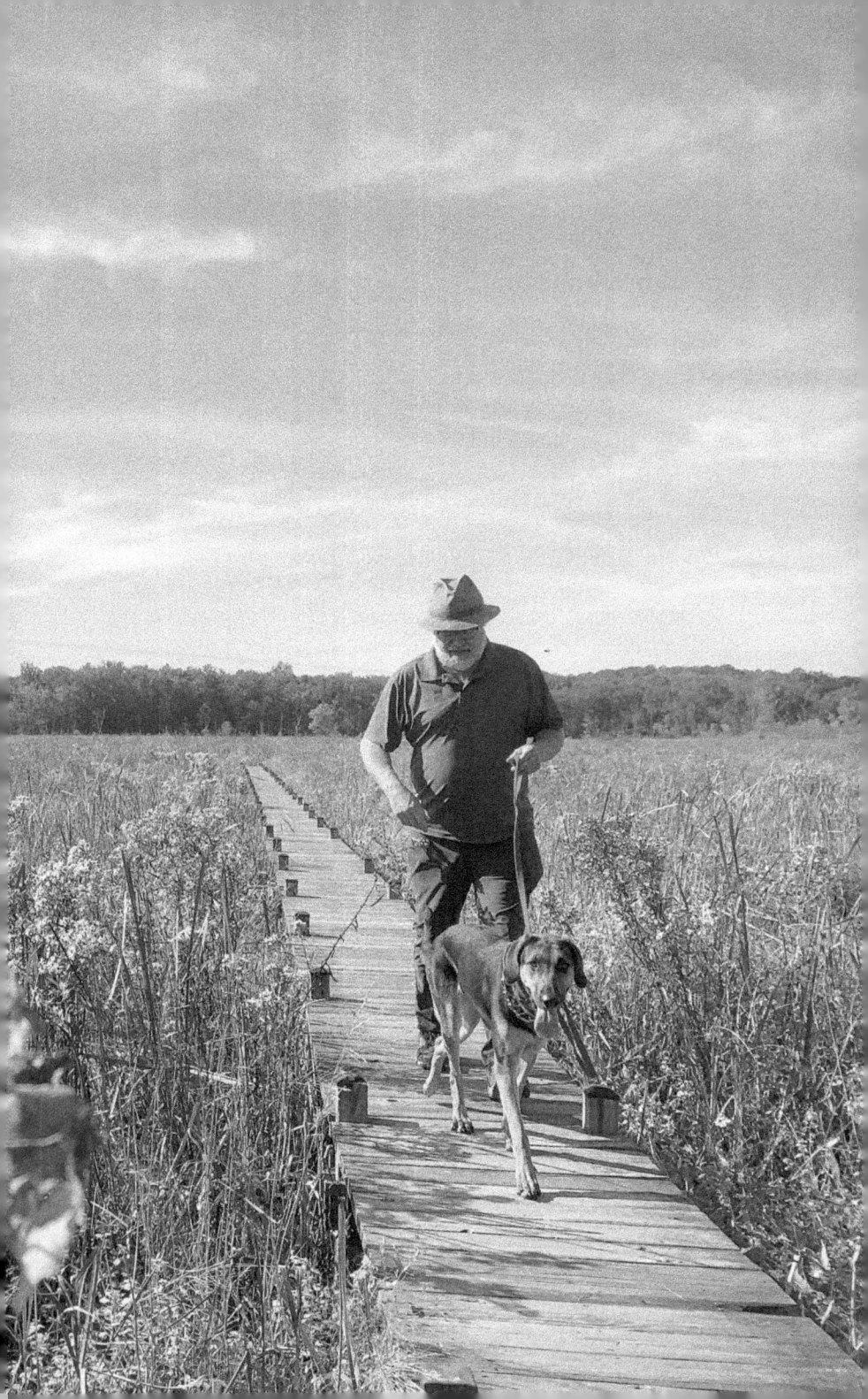

her nostrils. The minute I took hold of her leash at the door of the shelter, she bounded for the nearest fence post, nearly yanking my wrist into something that felt like an exhausted accordion. She quickly inhaled every loose atom of information from that spot, then lurched for the next one, and the next, on down the very long sidewalk to our car. Athena continued this impulsive mode of investigation after we reached our destination.

Jug Bay Wetlands Sanctuary comprises about 1,700 acres of tidal and freshwater marshes, forests, creeks, meadows, pine barrens, and fields along the Patuxent River in the southwest corner of Anne Arundel County. Since it was established in 1985, Jug Bay has secured its stature as one of the most spectacular natural sites in the realm of the Anne Arundel County Department of Recreation and Parks.

Note that the Jug Bay site includes not only the actual wetlands sanctuary but also the Glendening Nature Preserve, Patuxent Wetlands Park, and the Nature Preserve at Waysons Corner. You'll find an excellent visitor center at the sanctuary proper near the end of Wrighton Road. There is an admission fee of $6 per vehicle, but pets are not permitted. So we chose to ramble around the Glendening Preserve, where there is no admission and dogs on leashes are welcome.

There are two entrances to this section of the park, the southernmost one on Wrighton Road before you get to the entrance of the sanctuary, and the main entrance on the north side where Plummer Lane meets Maryland Route 4. We parked at the southern entrance.

In between the Glendening Preserve and the Jug Bay Sanctuary, at the very end of Wrighton Road, there's a bend of the river called Pig Point. Archaeologists from the county's Lost Towns Project have been studying this site since 2009, and they've discovered evidence of thousands of people living there for thousands of years. They've uncovered no fewer than 14 sites within a mile of the original Pig Point dig site, unearthing arrowheads and other projectile points that date back 6,500 years and older.

As we walked along the paths crisscrossing the preserve, underneath the canopy of oak and other hardwood trees still in full leaf, it reinforced my long-standing impression that these ancient people had exceedingly excellent instincts for finding delightful places to live. We crossed a freshwater stream cut deep into a hillside and stopped for a breather on a bluff overlooking the river, where the wild rice is still plentiful. Back when these ancient people lived here, the abundance of waterfowl and fish, deer and other wildlife must have made this a true land of pleasant living.

Athena was certainly delighted to be there. She plunged from tree to tree, quickly but carefully researching every trace of anything discernible from every square centimeter of bark. Like other dogs of her particular blend of breeds, Athena's schnozola has more than 200 million scent-gathering receptors, while we two-legged types have a measly five million. I've read that a dog's nose is 100,000 to 100 million times more sensitive than those of us mere humans.

Unlike humans, dogs have something called the Jacobsen's organ inside their nasal cavities. It opens onto the roof of the dog's mouth behind the incisors. The nerves from this organ lead directly to the brain and respond to a range of invisible substances that often have no odor at all, like pheromones.

This is what makes dogs like German shepherds so effective when trained in search-and-rescue operations. They can detect survivors buried under earthquake rubble, drowning victims at the bottom of a river, or explosives and drugs hidden in baggage at airports. Some can even discern the presence of cancer or detect oncoming epileptic seizures.

We walked along the Cliff Trail that follows a creek as it cuts into the terrain on its way to meet the river. Once there, it turns to run along the bluff overlooking the Patuxent. The farther along we walked, the less impulsive Athena's lunges became. Instead of pouncing on every single tree, she selected every third or fourth tree to inspect, and eventually calmed down to only having to pounce on every fourth or fifth tree.

What she was finding so interesting is still a mystery. But it occurred to me that here we have an opportunity to advance the Lost Towns Project's mission. Why not train dogs like Athena to track down ancient artifacts? Human bones, no matter how old or no matter how deep they're buried, must still have some detectable scent. Athena might have discovered the remains of several thousand ancient souls that one afternoon alone; she just didn't have the training to tell anybody about them.

One thing is worth noting: One of the first SPCA dogs I took out was a male who also had hunting genes, and like Athena, spent a lot of time in nostrilized investigation; but unlike Athena, he felt impelled to leave a mark at every spot he checked out. This left him pretty well drained before very long, but that didn't keep him from going through the motions every time. Athena, the goddess she is, never deigned to leave evidence of her having been present.

We found a boardwalk that extended way out across the marsh to where it met Galloway Creek, an offshoot of the main channel of the Patuxent. It's astonishing to be out in the middle of a pristine tidal marsh, surrounded by native wild rice and cattails, untainted by the presence of invasive phragmites reeds.

We took the Blueberry Trail back and logged more than three miles without covering anywhere near half of the trails in the Glendening Preserve. On that last mile down the grassy lane, Athena had calmed to the point of downright daintiness at her end of her leash. Until we got back to the SPCA. Once on her home turf, Athena again lurched at every post and pole along that long sidewalk to the shelter like the pup she still is.

Ending on an upbeat note, I was pleased to learn that my buddy Max, the last dog I borrowed from the shelter, has found a new home. I'm sure he'll make his new family very happy.

The SPCA is located at 1815 Bay Ridge Avenue in the Eastport neighborhood of Annapolis. Call 410-268-4388 for an appointment to see who's available for adoption. For more information, log on to www.aaspca.org.

Jug Bay Wetlands Sanctuary, Glendening Nature Preserve
1361 Wrighton Road (southern entrance)
Lothian, MD 20711 410-222-8006

jugbay.org

Free admission to Glendening Nature Preserve

Parking available on site

Amiable dogs on leash are welcome at Glendening Nature Preserve, but not at the main section of Jug Bay.

Bring your own doggie bags

No toilets

Open dawn to dusk

Easy going

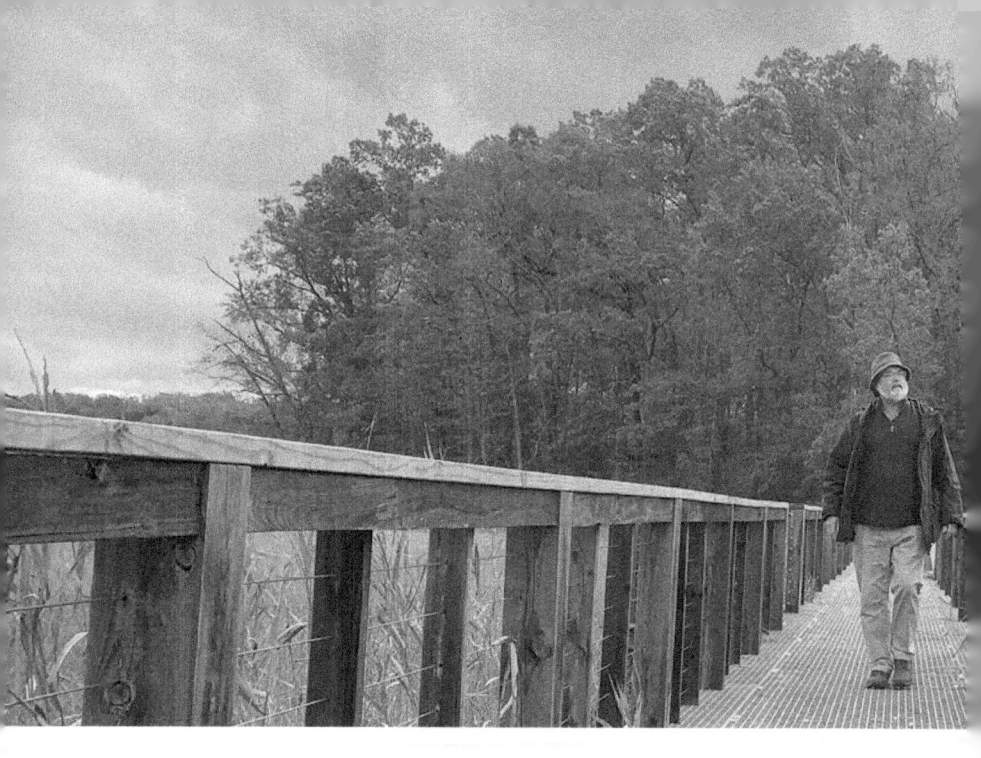

Walk 21

Dogless on the Hog Island Trail at Smithsonian Environmental Research Center

How did Hog Island get its name? It's not technically an island at all, more like an isolated bump of oak trees, holly and mountain laurel set between a salt marsh and Muddy Creek, where it opens up to meet the Rhode River.

You'd think that perhaps somebody found it a safe place to keep a herd of pigs, but that doesn't hold up to logic. I don't know of any local families named Hog with only one "G." Still, Hog Island is a delightful microhabitat to explore.

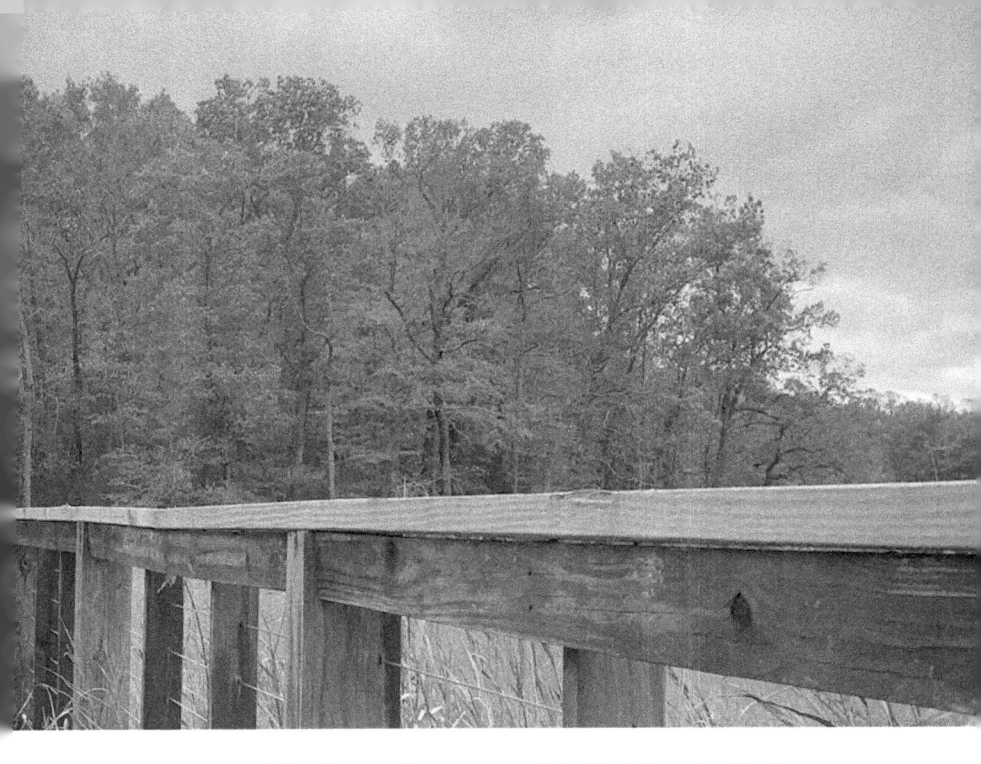

Hog Island is on the campus of the Smithsonian Environmental Research Center (SERC) in Edgewater. The Center is one of my favorite places on the planet. Just 10 miles south of Annapolis, it covers 2,660 acres of forest, field, and marsh nestled along the 15 miles of the Rhode River shoreline. It was founded in 1965, and some of the scientists' studies on water quality, land use, and global warming have been ongoing since that time.

On top of providing long-term, cutting-edge ecological research on the issues impacting anywhere on Earth where land meets water, this Smithsonian Center also offers public education programs and access to trails that crisscross the landscape and Bayscape.

So I was pleased to learn in November 2020 that the campus had recently reopened to the public. Downtime had been used wisely, and the main trails and boardwalks were almost completely refurbished. Several legs of the trail were still undergoing renovation, but the main route from the Reed Education Center to Hog Island has been completed.

I picked that particular day midweek, just after the dregs of the most recent hurricane had slogged through. I went reluctantly dogless this time, since pets are not allowed on the campus, which is not only an active research center but also a wildlife sanctuary.

The Smithsonian Environmental Research Center is located on Contees Wharf Road off Muddy Creek Road. You first check in with the guard at the gate. Bring along a photo ID, which is sometimes required. Follow the signs to the Reed Education Center.

It's open to the public Monday through Saturday, 8:30 a.m. to 4:30 p.m. except for federal holidays.

The Reed Center is open during those days and times, so you can see the exhibits as well as use the restrooms. Paddlers can launch a canoe or kayak at the boat ramp and explore the creeks and islands that make the Rhode River such a treasure. Since the Center occupies most of the shoreline, it's one of the least developed rivers in Anne Arundel County. You can find creeks with a 180-degree viewshed that hasn't changed much since Capt. John Smith sailed by 400 years ago.

Follow the trail behind the Reed Center, along the river's shore. You'll find a sandy beach where educators get kids to drag seines so they can study all the crabs, fish, eels, and other squiggly critters that live in the brackish water. The Center educates thousands of school children every year on the environmental issues impacting the Chesapeake Bay.

The trail has a new gravel surface, and all of the steps and boardwalks have been rebuilt. Keep an eye out for deer, foxes, and other wildlife. River otters have been spotted along here as well. The trail runs along the appropriately name Fox Creek, then rises through a forest of mostly large beech trees. While the leaves on the hickory trees had turned yellow-gold, the leaves on the beeches were still green when I walked through here.

The trail meets Fox Point Road. If you turned right and walked up the road, you'd eventually come out with a view of the Charles McC. Mathias Laboratory building. Turn left and you'd wind up at Fox Point with an overlook through the trees of the mouth of Muddy Creek. The main trail, however, dives back into the woods on the other side of the road.

You'll wind up at the boardwalk that crosses the marsh. Hog Island is the oak-covered hill at the far end of the boardwalk. You'll pass along a stand of Atlantic white cedars, then cross a meadow of salt marsh cordgrass and notice how the knee-high native grasses are being overtaken by the taller invasive phragmites reeds.

I've seen eagles overhead along here after the osprey have gone for the season, but on this particular day there were only turkey vultures playing in the after-hurricane currents that were blowing the clouds away.

Once you've climbed up the slope to the top of the island, it's almost like you've entered a different world. The mountain laurel, the massive white oaks, the holly, all make the setting seem fit for a fairy-tale. In fact, I came across evidence of such spirits: Some sprite had decorated the path with a colorful mandala, an elaborate mosaic carefully crafted of yellow and red leaves laid out in a circular pattern about the size of a dinner platter.

While I was admiring the mysterious organic art on the trail, a couple of walkers came over the crest of the hill. We all put on our masks and struck up a coronavirus-era conversation from a respectful distance. They were Beth Elzer and her teenage son, Rowen Green, both from Silver Spring.

"This is the first time here for us," Beth told me. She searches for nearby walkable trails on the internet. "I look for big, green blobs on Google Maps, then I look to see if it's a place that it's legal to visit."

Both of them had cameras with zoom lenses strapped around their necks.

"It's so wonderful to get out and see new places where we can go on different hikes. When you go on a weekday, you have it all to yourself."

Rowen, a seventh grader at the time at a Silver Spring Catholic middle school, admitted that he doesn't mind tagging along with his mom on these field trips. "It gets me off the video games," he said. I took their picture and headed back to the Reed Center.

Later, when I reviewed all the photos I had taken that day, I stared at one of me walking down the boardwalk, away from Hog Island. There, behind me, was the answer to my question. The wooded hump in the middle of the marsh made the shape of a giant sleeping hog.

Smithsonian Environmental Research Center
647 Contees Wharf Road
Edgewater, MD 21037 443-482-2200
SERC.SI.edu
Open Mon.–Sat. 8:30 a.m.–4:30 p.m., except federal holidays
Free admission, but be prepared to show photo ID at gate
Plenty of parking on site
Dogs are not allowed (this is a designated wildlife refuge)
Toilets available at the Reed Center
Easy going

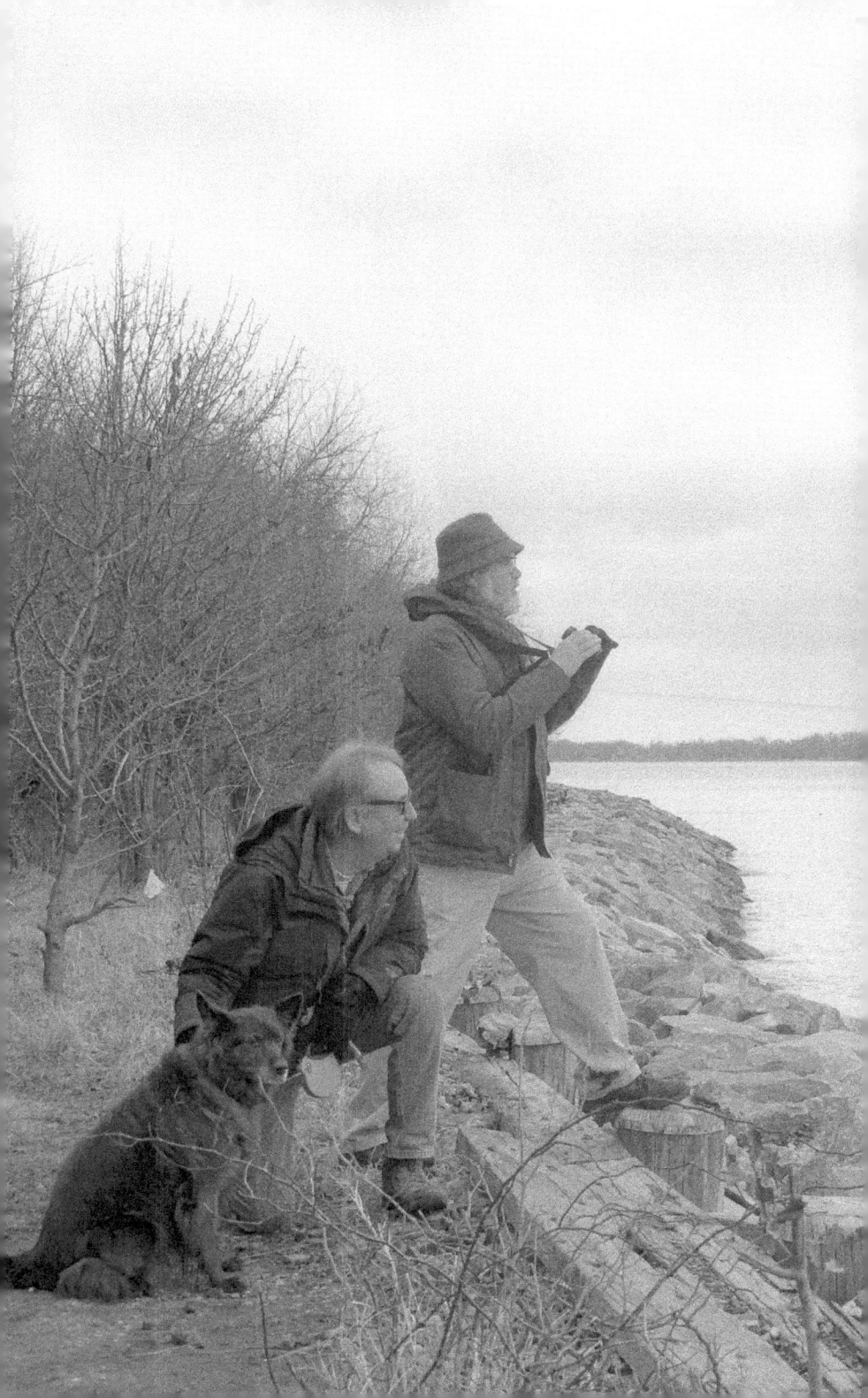

Walk 22

What's Towering over Greenbury Point

You can see them from just about anywhere around Annapolis: the three Eiffel-shaped towers on the far side of the Severn River. As ubiquitous as they are, they have an astonishing story to tell.

A while back, I explored the head of the Severn River with my friend Tom Guay, who at that time served as the executive director of the Severn River Association, so it seemed right that we should check out the other end of the river together. Then one frigid January day early in 2021, we hiked some of the trails at Greenbury Point that wander around the base of those towers.

We met at the nature center on Bullard Boulevard, just past the Naval Academy golf course. Tom's family dog, Mahki, joined us on that chilly, overcast day. She's a fairly spry 11-year-old rescue mix of retriever and Australian shepherd "with a tiny dash of chow mixed in," Tom explained. Dogs are permitted as long as their human is at the other end of a leash. Mahki gave me an introductory sniff and we were off on the trail.

I always enjoy spending time with Tom. We talk about history and books, music, birds, and more history. As we rambled around the 231-acre peninsula, we wondered what it must have been like when the first English settlers

JEFFERSON HOLLAND | 143

showed up here in 1649 and established a gathering of tobacco plantations they would call Providence.

Part of this peninsula was once owned by Col. Nicholas Greenberry (1627–1697), who became one of Gov. Francis Nicholson's commissioners of the new city of Annapolis in 1696. His tombstone was moved in 1925 to the St. Anne's churchyard, where you can see it today. How or why "Greenberry" became "Greenbury" is a piece of history that's a mystery to both of us.

The trail took us along the banks of Carr's Creek that separates this part of the peninsula from the old North Severn Naval Station. The Naval Academy's firing range is on the far side of the creek, and when the Mids are using it, the trails on this side are closed to the public. You can log onto the Academy's X (formerly Twitter) account to check the current status.

The far side of the creek was also once the site of the first Naval Air Station. This is where naval aviation was born. In 1911, Lt. John Rogers flew the Navy's first biplane, a Wright Brothers B-1, fresh out of the crate from Dayton, Ohio, and assembled in the Academy's armory. Over the next few years, pilots and mechanics tested early versions of floatplanes as well as the first catapult-launched plane that would eventually lead to modern aircraft carriers. An exceptionally nasty winter in 1917 compelled the Navy to move the air station to Pensacola, Florida, where it remains to this day.

We got off a muddy side-track and onto a wide, hard-packed gravel road. I've been asked by volunteers who tend to our local trails to remind readers to avoid using muddy paths. Churning up the mud makes an even bigger mess when the mud dries. There are plenty of paved or hard-packed trails to choose when it's been raining, and the volunteers work hard enough without having to deal with the mess left by inconsiderate hikers and bikers.

The road came out to the bank at the mouth of Carr's Creek with an astonishing vista of the Naval Academy, Annapolis, and Eastport far across the river. I told Tom about a chart I have dating from 1846 that shows the domes and spires of the city skyline from different angles of approach. That skyline hasn't changed all that much since that time, with the exception of the St. Mary's church steeple and the Academy chapel dome. In the foreground, we saw large rafts of diving ducks: pintails, canvasbacks, buffleheads, and surf scoters.

At the end of the point, we had a panoramic view of the Bay, from Hackett's Point on the far side of the mouth of Whitehall Bay and the expanse of the Chesapeake Bay Bridge, all the way down to Thomas Point Light and Bay Ridge across the mouth of the Severn River.

This was Greenbury Point proper. Somewhere near here was the site of the first Greenbury Point lighthouse, built on shore in 1848. It proved to be not very useful, since ships sailing from the northern Bay couldn't distinguish the lighthouse light from the lights of the city in the background.

It was replaced by a screw-pile lighthouse, which looked very similar to the Thomas Point Light, a half-mile offshore in 1892. Like most of the other 42 screw-piles built around the Chesapeake, this one succumbed to ice damage in 1918. The cottage was demolished in 1934, leaving just the platform sitting on its pilings. For the next seven decades, this structure was known by local sailors as "the spider buoy." It, too, was demolished around 2002 and replaced with the bundle of pilings we could see out there now.

The road took us underneath the outermost tower. These towers have been part of the skyline since 1938, when they were added to a grid that the Navy had started building 20 years earlier. These three towers are all that remain of a complex of 19 towers that together formed one huge antenna capable of broadcasting radio waves to ships all around the globe. America learned of the armistice that ended the War to End All Wars from here.

In the 1960s, the system was enhanced to the point where it could communicate with nuclear subs operating 65 feet below the surface anywhere in the world. By 1994, satellites had made the radio-based system obsolete, and the other towers were blasted down in 1999, leaving these three as landmarks.

The USNA Museum produced a fascinating video series called "The History of the Navy in 100 Objects." You can learn more about the towers' history and watch dramatic footage of their demolition by searching for usna.edu/100objects on YouTube. It's Object #39.

We followed the road to the end of Bullard Boulevard and headed back to our cars at the nature center. We had logged about two and a half miles in about two and a half hours, which is about right for the amount of stopping we did to gawk at the birds, gape at the scenery, and talk with each other as well as some of the few other walkers we met up with.

We didn't follow any trail in particular, but you can take the Poet's Nature Trail, a one-and-a-third mile loop that meanders through scrubby woodland and meadows along Carr's Creek or the shorter Bobwhite Circuit Trail. The Pipsissewa Trail, presumably named after the flowering native herb, starts on the other side of Bullard Boulevard, then crosses Hooper High Road and connects with the Timberdoodle Trail.

Because this is a military installation, taking photographs of buildings is not permitted. Greenbury Point is a facility of the U.S. Navy and when you visit, you are a guest of the Navy. Please be on your best behavior.

It was a good workout for Mahki, and a good catch-up time for Tom and me. Since that visit, the Naval Academy Golf Association/Naval Academy Athletics Association stirred controversy by announcing plans to develop a portion of the conservation area into an exclusive golf course.

The Chesapeake Conservancy joined partnered with Severn River Association and Chesapeake Bay Foundation along with a grass-roots group called "Save Greenbury Point" in opposition to this ill-conceived proposal.

A statement on the Conservancy's web site reads, "Such a development would cause serious and irreparable damage to the environment and an area steeped in pre-Colonial and Colonial history." Recently, 25 nonprofits signed a joint letter in opposition. Senators Ben Cardin and Chris Van Hollen, along with Congressmen "Dutch" Ruppersberger and John Sarbanes also wrote a letter to Navy Secretary Carlos Del Toro voicing their concern. You can learn more about this issue at chesapeakeconservancy.org/greenbury-point-conservation-area.

Greenbury Point Nature Center
Bullard Boulevard at McLeans Road
Annapolis, MD 21402 410-293-1084

navymwrannapolis.com/programs/bedd477e-9ba4-49a2-9d91-8cd6f02dcd8f Open daily dawn to dusk except when the firing range is in use (closures announced on x.com/nsaannapolis)

Nature Center is open daily except holidays or when otherwise reserved

Free admission

Parking available on site

No toilets

This particular site is fanatic about keeping dogs on leash and staying on designated trails; bring your own doggie bags

Easy going

Walk 23

Thank Volunteers for Beachwood Park

There are dedicated volunteers in our community you'll probably never meet, people who work hard to make your life a better one. I had the privilege of meeting up with a bunch of them—old friends and new friends alike—to tour Beachwood Park in Pasadena, one of those pocket wildernesses perched on the upper reaches of the Magothy River. This group of volunteers has been working for the past six years, transforming the junked remnants of an abandoned beach resort into wooded waterfront access for us all.

My wife, Louise, and I drove up to Pasadena one chilly Sunday afternoon in late January 2021 to meet Paul Spadaro, president of the all-volunteer Magothy River Association, and his wife, Sandy, along with long-time volunteers David and Kathy Nolte and our long-time friends, David and Ginger Hildebrand. Of course, we were all masked up and carefully distanced.

The Noltes own the Suspender Store in Millersville, and the Hildebrands are renowned musicians and musical historians. Ginger teaches music and performs with the Ensemble Galilei, and David teaches at the Peabody Institute and recently co-wrote the definitive history, *Musical Maryland*, with Elizabeth Schaaf, published by Johns Hopkins Press. All these folks live

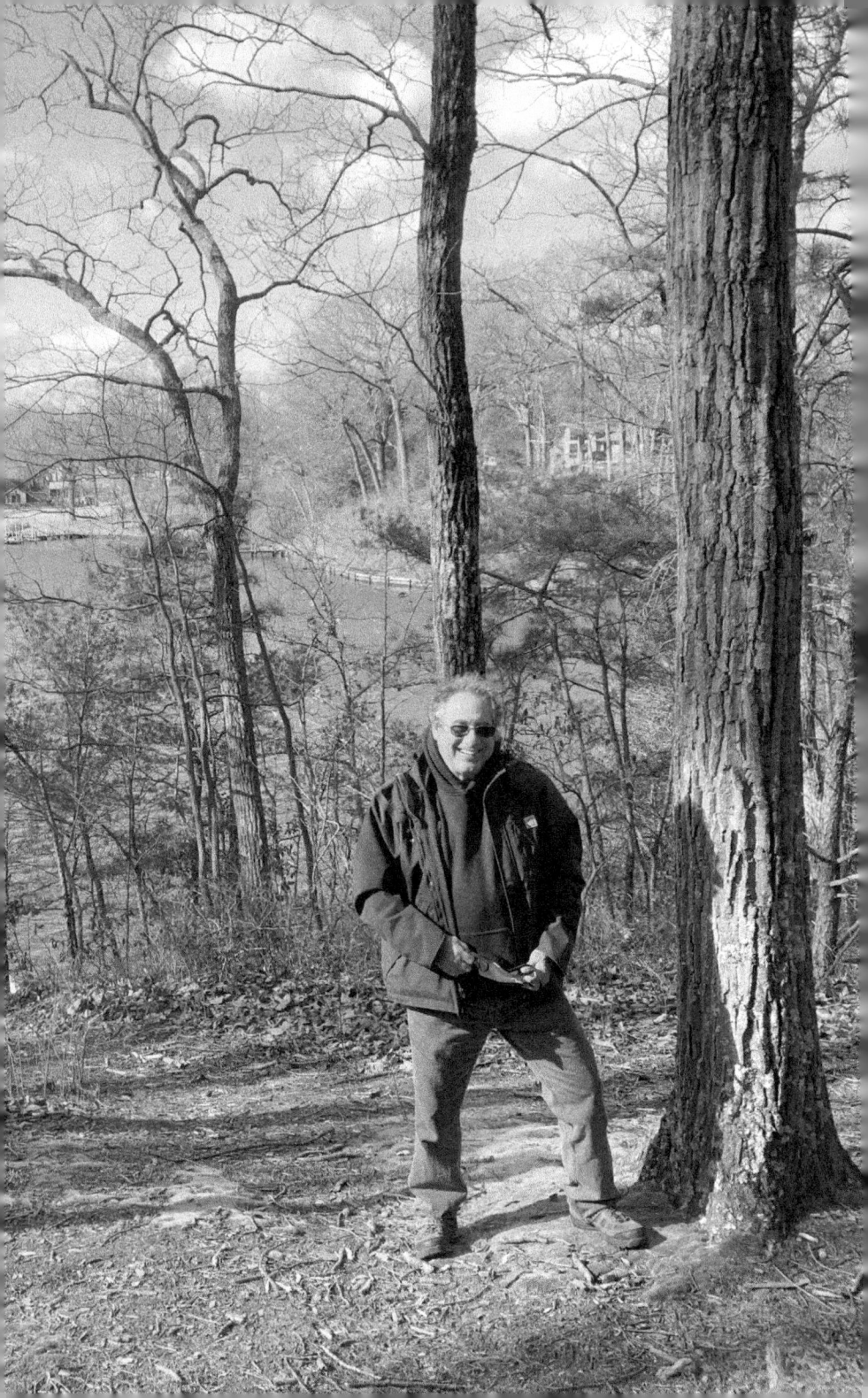

in and around Severna Park. For Louise and me, this was one of our rare excursions north from our home in Annapolis. It's not often that we venture all that way across the Severn River Bridge.

Paul gave us the background on the site. It had once been an interracial waterfront amusement park in the era when most such attractions were either all-white, like Beverley Beach in Mayo, or all-Black, like Carr's Beach and Sparrow's Beach in Annapolis.

It was owned by a Black Baptist minister and businessman named Hiram E. Smith, who managed to purchase the property in 1943 despite local restrictive covenants that barred the sale of land to anyone "of Negro, Chinese or Japanese descent," according to a 2002 article in *The Baltimore Sun*. In 1949, Hiram Smith bought the adjacent Beachwood Grove Park, enlarging his park by 16 acres.

In its heyday, Beechwood Park boasted a Ferris wheel, arcade games, and a dance pavilion where the likes of Ike and Tina Turner and James Brown performed for avid audiences. Busloads of church groups came down from Baltimore for weekend picnics. The Rev. Smith would even perform baptisms along the Magothy riverfront. Since it was one of the few integrated parks in the region, local businesses like Black & Decker and Westinghouse held their annual company picnics there.

Then the Bay Bridge opened, attracting audiences to other beach-front holiday venues "down the ocean," and by the early 1960s, most of the Chesapeake waterfront resorts like this one were on the decline. Smith lost Beechwood Park to foreclosure in 1963 owing to his failing health. He died the next year.

The property was slated for development when Anne Arundel County bought it for $1.3 million in 2002. But then it sat fallow, the structures crumbling and the trees becoming strangled by invasive vines, until the Magothy River Association came along in 2015 to reclaim it as a park. While they've made a lot of progress, there's still a lot work to do, Paul explained.

Paul led the group down one of the newly formed trails that leads from the 20-car parking lot through the mature red oak and pine forest to the riverfront. He and his volunteers had recently completed a project to protect the steep bank from erosion. Below, we found a small beach along a secluded cove. Despite the cold, a gaggle of guys was fishing for white perch, waist deep in their waders.

Paul pointed out vestiges of the old amusement park. There's a rusted streetlamp dangling from high up in a tree that indicated where the main entrance used to be. The walls of an old staircase had recently been painted by a local Girl Scout troop with a mural depicting kids fishing and crabbing.

He led us along a newly blazed trail that follows the crest of the ridge overlooking the river and pointed out strategically placed benches where you can relax and enjoy the vista through the trees. The path led to another beach where they had created a soft canoe and kayak launch.

A fisherman had just hauled his kayak out of the water and stood on a log, making a few last hopeful casts before calling it quits. I was pleased to note that he was wearing a dry suit appropriate for surviving a spill in the frigid water.

Paul explained that the county recently expanded the parking at the end of Beachwood Road so that paddlers could more easily access the boat launch. We watched the kayaker roll his rig up the path on a dolly with ease.

Dave and Kathy Nolte sat on a park bench by the beach and showed us the brass plaque dedicated to the memory David's father, Charlie Nolte, who was also a volunteer for the Magothy River Association. Charlie passed away in 2015 at the age of 79. "He used to play here when he was a kid," Dave recalled. Even as an adult, this was one of his favorite places. "The last time I saw him alive was right at this spot," he recalled.

Charlie grew up at his grandparents' home at the end of Lake Shore Drive and spent summer days exploring the river and creeks in his 14-foot Lyman outboard runabout. That love for the river motivated him as an adult to volunteer his time and energy to protect the water.

"He was always the first to volunteer to man educational displays or self-floating gardens," Paul told a reporter from the *Severna Park Voice* when the bench was dedicated. "He is greatly missed. He was a very kind, caring person."

JEFFERSON HOLLAND | 153

On our way back to the parking lot, Paul regaled us with fascinating stories of the history of the area, particularly of the Civil War era, like the Union gun emplacement at Mt. Misery in Severna Park, one of the highest points in the county and one with a view of both the Severn and Magothy riverfronts. In all, it was quite an educational afternoon. Louise and I agreed that we'd be back in the spring with our kayaks to explore the Magothy River water trail, and of course have a picnic by the water.

For more information on the Magothy River Association, and how you, too, can become a volunteer, check out their web site at www.magothyriver.org.

Beachwood Park
8320 Beachwood Park Road (off Magothy Bridge Road)
Pasadena, MD 21122

magothyriver.org

Open daily dawn to dusk

Limited parking along Beachwood Park Road

No toilets

Good-natured dogs on leash are welcome; bring your own doggie bags

Easy going

Walk 24

Mushing on Morning Choice Trail

I've been for a walk on a winter's day, even though I'm not particularly a winter person. But I do like a brisk midwinter's walk, so that's what I did on one of those clear, frigid days in early February 2021. And what better companion could I have had but Cody Boy, a purebred Alaskan husky borrowed from the SPCA for the afternoon.

Cody Boy was a spry nine-year-old at the time. He's got thick chestnut-and-white fur, a dark smudge on the tip of his tongue, one bright blue eye and one that's mostly brown but partly blue, too. The way he perked up his ears and swished his feather-boa tail assured that he was happy to see me and eager to hop in the back of the car for an adventure.

For no particular reason, other than I hadn't been there for a while, I chose to head for Patapsco Valley State Park. It starts just across the northwestern tip of Anne Arundel County and stretches along 32 miles of the Patapsco River. Eight developed recreational areas cover more than 16,000 acres crisscrossed by more than 200 miles of trails.

I picked out the nearest trail system, one that was new to me and less than 45 minutes away from my home in Annapolis. The Morning Choice and Ridge Trails cover the woods along the southern bank of the river between the Avalon Area and the Orange Grove Area. The trailhead is on Landing Road, off Montgomery Road in Elkridge. You can find it on the free AllTrails app or on the Maryland State Park web site.

The nice thing about winter trekking is that the trails are generally frozen solid, making for easy walking when they're dry and smooth, which these were for the most part. I really don't mind the cold, especially when the wind is calm, as it was that day. I've found that I don't need a lot of layers, since I build up a good amount of body heat when I get moving.

The bad thing, especially along some parts of this trail, is that lots of other people had been there over the past few days and they had left their boot prints deep in the slushy snow and mud. All of that was now frozen over, leaving the path in some stretches churned up in perma-chunks. It was like walking over an ancient lava field.

Still, breathing in that cold, still air while being out in these magnificent woods, mostly tall gray beech trees and towering columns of tulip poplar, with a few colossal white pines at the hilltops—all that more than made up for the uncomfortable spots in the trail.

And Cody Boy was in heaven. He behaved beautifully at the end of the leash—eager to move at a husky's pace, for sure, but responsive to the slightest tug if I wanted to turn onto a side path or urge him along when he'd spent a little too much time trying to figure out the origin of the particular odor on the trunk of a tree.

We followed the curiously named Morning Choice Trail through the woods, down a frozen hillside and

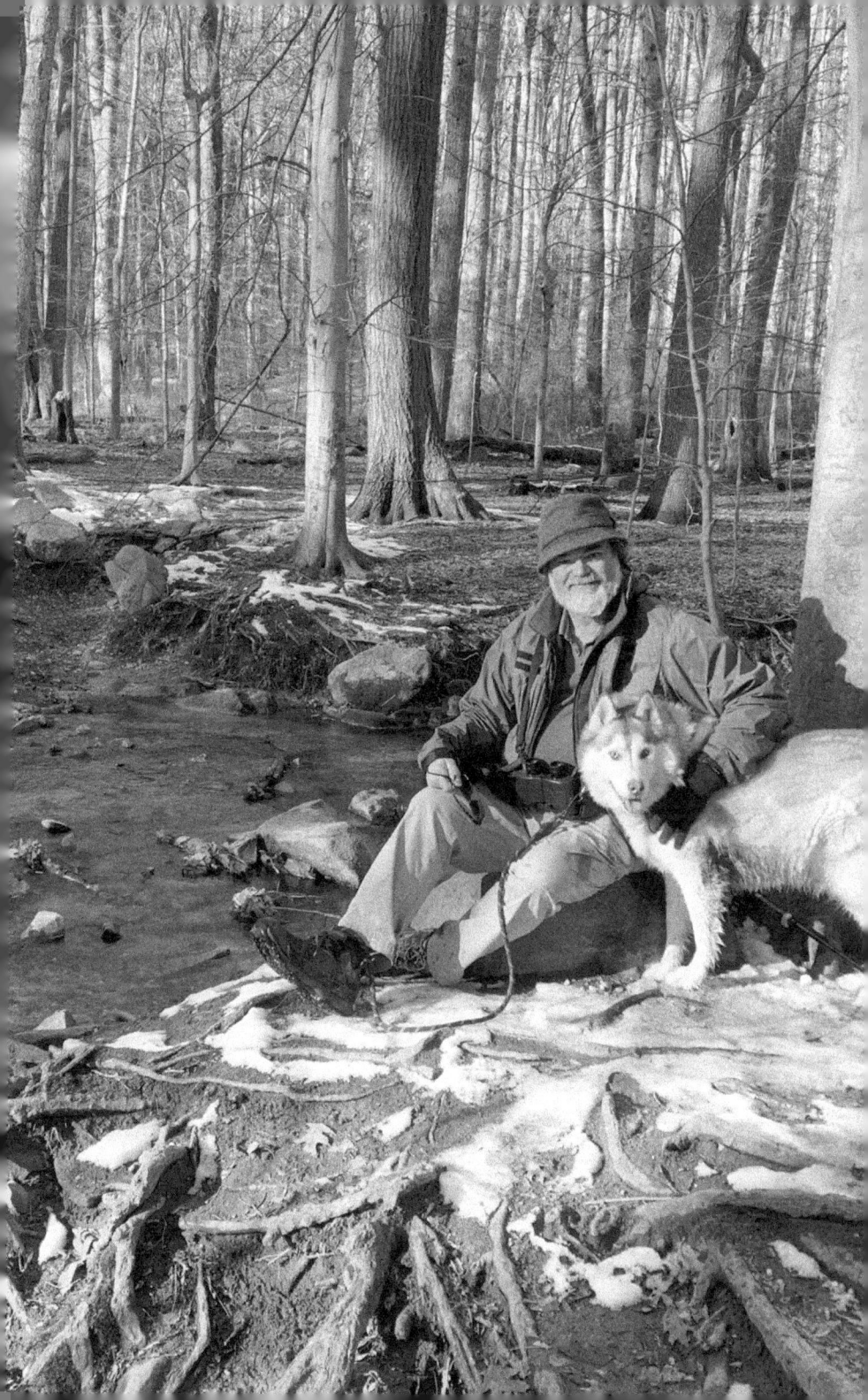

rock-hopped across the shallow Rockburn Branch creek. At the top of the next hill, the woods opened up onto a hillside field topped with what appeared to be a grand English manor house, a cream-colored Georgian mansion with outbuildings connected by hyphens and what looked like a walled garden to one side.

This turned out to be Belmont Manor, part of a 1,360-acre tract of land patented in 1695 by Mordecai Moore. According to the Maryland Historical Trust, Mordecai camped here "on the ridge of elk," and the next morning, he surveyed his newly acquired tract of land, with the mists rising up from the river below, and decided that this was an ideal place to build a home. He called the place Moore's Morning Choice, which accounts for the odd name of the trail.

Belmont is one of Howard County's oldest structures. I was surprised to find out that the land was acquired by Caleb Dorsey Sr. in 1732. He began building the mansion in 1738. This is the same Dorsey who owned Hockley-in-the-Hole, the estate that's now part of the Annapolis Waterworks Park. His wealth came from the Avalon Iron Works he operated in the valley below.

The property stayed in the Dorsey family for six generations, then was donated to the Smithsonian. The place is now owned by Howard County Recreation and Parks and appears to be a popular wedding venue.

The trail sidles up past an ancient graveyard sheltered by a sprawling poplar and surrounded by a wrought-iron fence. This reminded me of the time Louise and I visited Monticello. We had decided to park at the bottom of the hill and follow the path up the back way to the Jefferson family graveyard and on through the garden. And there was that magnificent mansion, so familiar in photographs and engraved on nickels, but in real life. A group of tourists had gathered on the back porch, so we joined them. Someone who appeared to be a tour guide counted heads, shrugged and led us inside.

The guide led us through the house and after a fascinating hour, we ended up at the front door. The guide opened the door and there we saw a line streaming down the hillside of hundreds of people waiting patiently for their turn to take the tour. We felt a little guilty about inadvertently cutting in line, but we got over it. We were sure that Mr. Jefferson would have let us in and shown us around, and he'd have offered us a glass of sherry, too.

The Morning Choice Trail connects with the Ridge Trail running parallel to the river, which seems to flow hundreds of feet below at the bottom of a steep hill. All of the trails are well marked with painted blaze marks on the trees and signposts at the intersections. Cody and I took a side trail marked Valley View that teetered across the face of the hillside, then made our way back to the Morning's Choice trail around the backside of the manor house.

While we didn't see a lot of birds, along the verge of the field we flushed an azure flurry of eastern bluebirds, then heard the lazy rap-rap-rap of a woodpecker high in the trees.

Considering that we were both about the same biological age, Cody Boy was way ahead of me by way of endurance. For the first few miles, we swung right along, Cody stopping only occasionally to sniff out an alluring aroma. But that last mile, I admit, had me winded, bewilderingly so until I realized I had been striding at a husky's pace up and down ice-packed tracks for the past couple of hours.

I sat down on a log to catch my breath and we had a little chat, Cody and me. I'm beat, I told him. We have to take it easy this last half a mile. He looked at me with that one blue eye and the one brown-and-blue eye, and he got it. He was an accommodating gentleman for the rest of the way. Almost downright condescending.

When we got back to the car, Cody Boy slurped up a bowlful of water and then gave me a big kiss. On our first date, too!

The SPCA is located at 1815 Bay Ridge Avenue in the Eastport neighborhood of Annapolis. Call 410-268-4388 for an appointment to see who's currently up for adoption. For more information, log on to www.aaspca.org.

Morning Choice Trail is just one of 200 amazing hikes in Patapsco State Park. Some of the areas require an admission, but there is none for Morning Choice and adjoining trails. From Annapolis, take I-97 North to MD-100 West, then US-1 North/Washington Boulevard.

Turn left onto Rowanberry Drive, then left onto Montgomery Road, then right onto Landing Road. The parking lot at the trailhead is about one mile up that road.

Patapsco State Park, Morning Choice Trail
5568 Landing Rd (off Montgomery Rd.)
Elkridge, MD 21075

410-461-5005

dnr.maryland.gov/publiclands/Pages/central/patapsco.aspx

Limited parking at trailhead on Landing Road

Open daily dawn to dusk

Free admission

No toilets

Neighborly dogs on leash are welcome; bring your own doggie bags

Moderate, some topography

Walk 25

Walking with Giants at Corcoran Woods

I always enjoy hanging out with people who are smarter than me. Now that I think about it, finding people who are smarter than me has never really been much of a challenge. I know a little bit about a lot of stuff, just enough to know I've still got a lot to learn. But I learn a little something new every day, which is a good thing for an old guy.

On one frigid day in February 2021, I learned a lot about trees from Dr. Geoffrey "Jess" Parker, who has served as the forest ecologist at the Smithsonian Environmental Research Center in Edgewater since 1987. Jess wanted to show me around the Corcoran Environmental Study Area or Corcoran Woods, a 215-acre tract of forest adjacent to Sandy Point State Park.

Corcoran Woods is not officially part of the park but is managed by the Maryland Park Service as a preserve where scientists can study forest diversity and where people can learn about trees—and where the human body and spirit can miraculously rejuvenate from just a couple of hours of goofing around in the woods.

I met Jess at the parking lot on Tydings Road off Log Inn Road. The weather was warm for this time of year, about 50 degrees, and all the ice and snow from the recent storm was melting, so we agreed that it was a good idea to don some serious bootage.

As a former Riverkeeper, I keep my car festooned with a variety of boots for any wet weather condition. I wear a pair of waterproof hiking boots and always keep a spare handy for when the first pair of waterproof boots inevitably gets waterlogged. Then there are the mid-shin white rubber waterman's boots for when I'm driving any boat. I've even got a pair of chest waders that have come in handy on occasion, especially when I happen to run across a promising fishing hole.

We suspected there would be a good amount of standing water on the trail, so both Jess and I chose our tall rubber boots. We headed down the main trail that runs through the middle of the tract, but after just a few hundred feet, there was so much water it wasn't so much a trail, more like a canal. I regretted not putting on the waders. In fact, I wished I'd brought along my kayak.

We backtracked and took a less soggy path off to the north toward the Magothy River. Sprouts of daffodils pushed up through the crunchy snow. We walked a plank that served as a bridge over the headwaters of Podickery Creek and through a thick stand of mature holly trees. As we trudged along, Jess told me about Colby Rucker, a legendary naturalist, historian, environmentalist, and tree expert who wrote a treatise on the Corcoran Woods in 2002.

To my surprise, I learned later that Rucker was a lifelong resident of Pines-on-the-Severn. He died at his home in 2004 at the age of 67. He wrote two authorita-

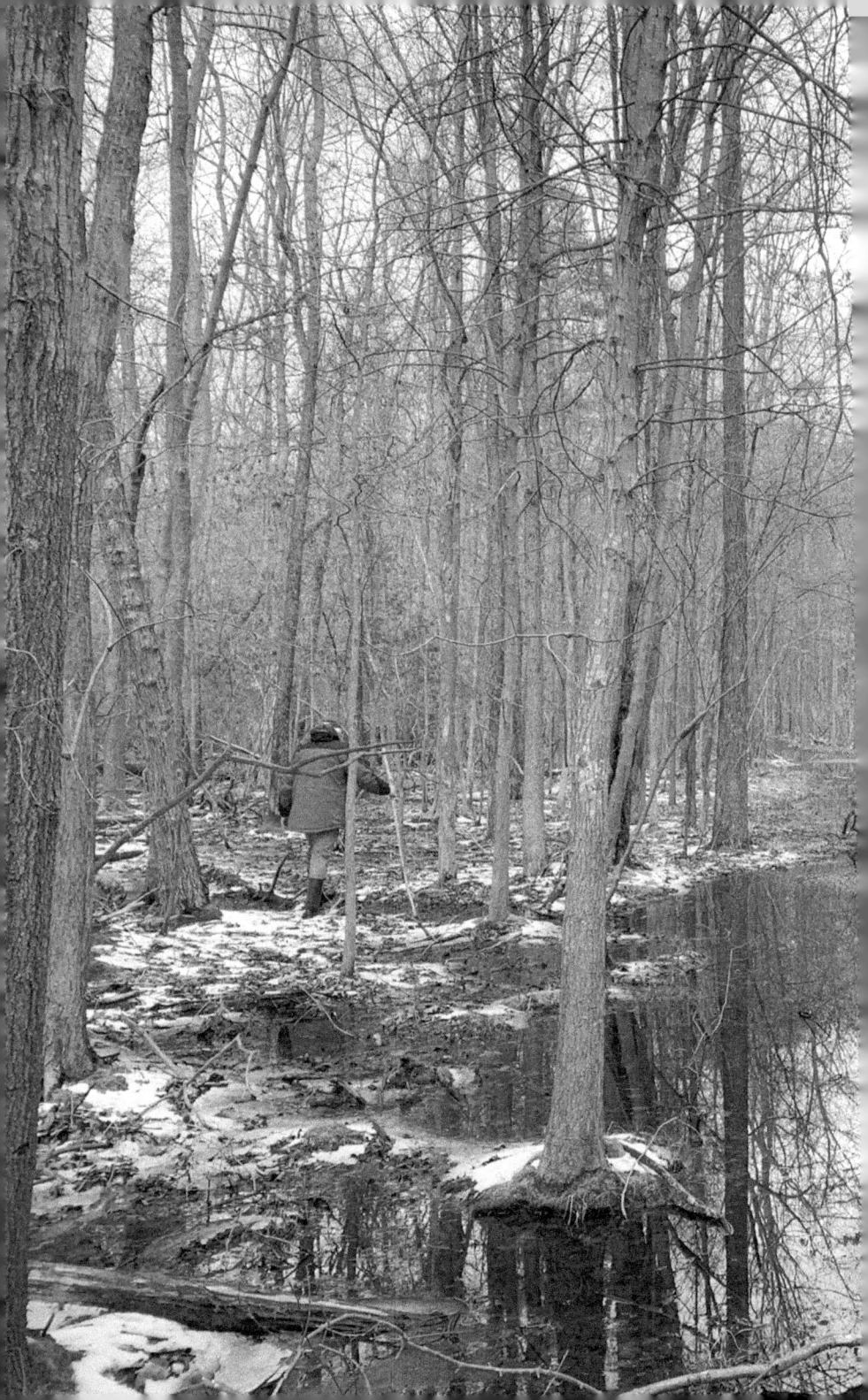

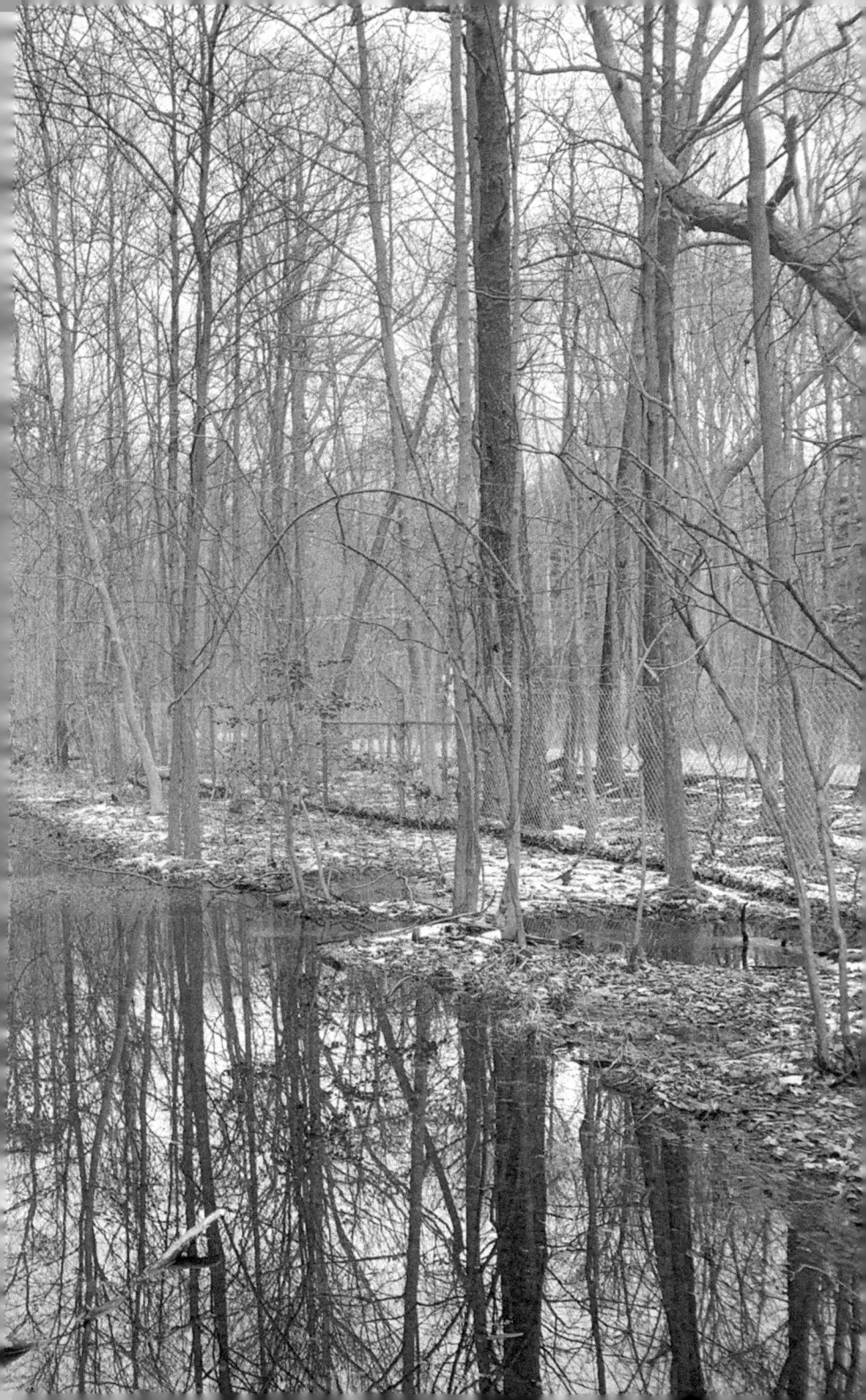

tive guides to the natural history of the Severn River: *Scenic Rivers: The Severn* (1983) and *Gems of the Severn* (1988). A man after my own heart, Rucker was also a poet. His obituary in *The Baltimore Sun* quoted a few lines from "Thoughts in a Maryland Woodland," which he wrote in the same year as his study of Corcoran Woods:

> This is the woods of home
> And I thought of things remembered
> And things before my time, some but yesterday
> To the ancient trees around me
> The measure of time is everywhere.

Rucker developed a scientific method of analyzing the character of a forest that has since become a standard in the forestry world. The Rucker Index lists the average height of the tallest examples of the 10 most prominent species of trees in the forest. In a list of 52 of the forests on the East Coast of the United States with the tallest trees, Corcoran Woods is right in there, ranked about halfway down with a Rucker Index value of 119.75 feet. By way of comparison, the top of the list, with a Rucker Index rating of 163.07 feet, is the Great Smoky Mountains National Park, where there's a white pine 185.5 feet tall.

Scientists like Rucker and Parker use state-of-the-art laser transits to accurately measure the height of individual trees. Rucker found that tulip poplar trees are the dominant species at Corcoran Woods, with the tallest measuring 142.1 feet tall with a circumference of nearly

12.5 feet. Curiously, the supposed official state champion tulip tree listed on the DNR web site is only 119 feet tall, located in Susquehanna State Park.

Rucker found seven other species at Corcoran Woods that set new state height records: sweetgum, mockernut, black locust, American holly, Hercules club, spicebush, and black highbush blueberry. One reason for the proclivity of such altitude lies in the fact that a good portion of the forest hasn't been touched by humans for many decades, likely because it's just too darn wet for agricultural pursuits.

It's named for Edward S. Corcoran, who once owned the 110-acre northwest portion noted for its ancient trees. Rucker identified a particular stand of tulip trees there, some of which were more than 150 years old.

The one bad thing about not being attended to by humans is that much of the forest has become heavily infested with vines, both native and invasive alien species. Rucker listed oriental bittersweet, multiflora rose, English ivy, and Japanese honeysuckle as common throughout. Bittersweet and grapevines as thick as your forearm have choked all but the tallest trees in some areas.

Jess showed me a 17-acre portion of the forest at the far end of the tract that had been cleared of vines and reforested with saplings of different species. Regimented rows of tall green plastic tubes spanned the cleared areas, each protecting a growing tree from becoming hors d'oeuvres for the deer. The saplings that seemed to be doing best were tulip trees, along with some black locust.

According to the DNR web site, "this is the first step in a multi-year effort to restore and reforest portions of Corcoran that have been overrun with numerous invasive and exotic vine species that have all but choked out the native forests." The project was funded by a grant from the Anne Arundel County Forestry and Greening Program administered by the Chesapeake Bay Trust, in partnership with the Alliance for the Chesapeake Bay and the Maryland Department of Natural Resources, Chesapeake & Coastal Service.

We managed to get back to our cars without stepping into water deeper than the tops of our boots. We'd pretty much circumnavigated the tract, logging about three miles all told.

I recommend visiting Corcoran Woods in the early spring or late fall, when the water should recede from the main trails and settle into the many vernal pools. But beware that the warmer the weather, the greater the risk of encountering ticks and mosquitos, both of which are apparently rampant there.

I learned a lot and had a lot of fun with Dr. Parker and his guided tour of Corcoran Woods. It was like visiting Joanie Mitchell's "Tree Museum," and I didn't have to pay a dollar-and-a-half just to see 'em.

Corcoran Woods
Tydings Road
Skidmore, Annapolis, MD 21409

410-974-2149

corcoranwoods.home.blog

Directions: Take Rt. 50 east toward the Bay Bridge. Take the exit to Sandy Point State Park. Cross over the highway on Oceanic Drive. Before you enter the park, turn left onto East College Parkway and take the first right onto Log Inn Road. At the next intersection, continue straight onto Tydings Road. The parking lot will be on your right. The trailhead is on the opposite side of the road.

Open daily dawn to dusk.

Free admission

Portable toilet in parking lot

Beneficent dogs on leash are welcome; bring your own doggie bags

Easy going

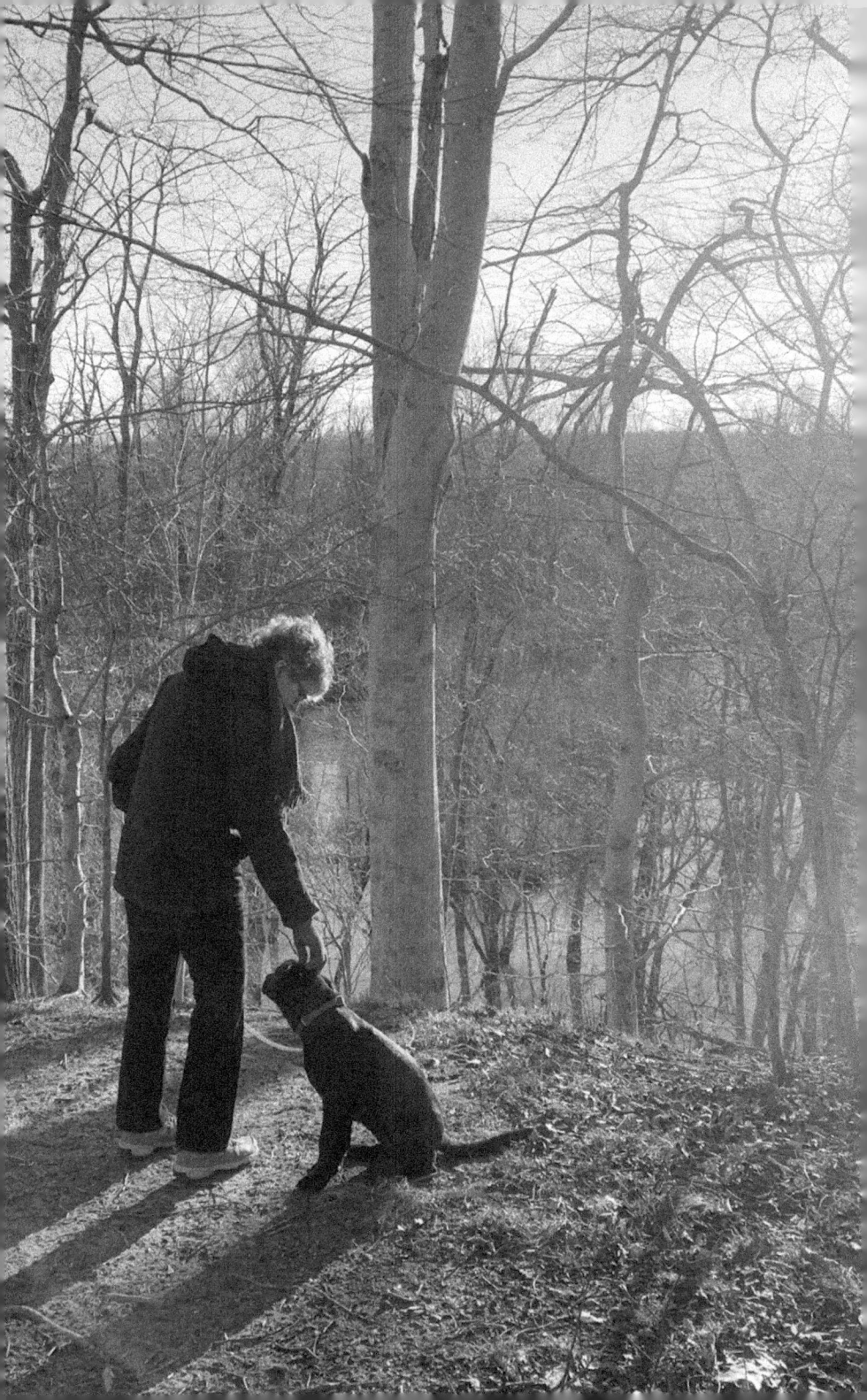

Walk 26

Meet Millie at Davidsonville Park

After nine months of doglessness, we finally gave in and adopted a little Labrador retriever named Millie in February 2021. I say little because she was fairly small at the age of six months and we figured she probably wouldn't get bigger than medium-sized. She's mostly Lab-ish but also a little bit something else that we hadn't figured out yet. Part beaver, by her proclivity for chewing stuff. But she's a sweetheart.

Millie weighs about 40 pounds, has expressive floppy ears, and color that changes with the sunlight like a starling; sometimes black, sometimes brown. Her breast is emblazoned with a white blotch in the shape of a cross. Her bright hazel eyes often have a quizzical look about them as though she's amazed at all the exciting new concepts confronting her—like discovering the buzzy joys of chewing on old coffee filters snatched from the compost heap, digging up cat poop in the tulip bed, and the savory piquancy of the insole of a wading shoe steeped in Chesapeake brine.

We found her through an organization called Operation Paws for Homes, a nonprofit that rescues dogs and cats from overcrowded high-kill shelters in the southern states. Millie, we believe, came from Mississippi. Anyway, the last time we stuck her in her crate I thought I detected a bit of a Blanche DuBois-like whimper. We picked her up from her foster parents in Northern Virginia on my birthday in February 2021 and she's already made herself quite at home.

The cats, on the other hand, have taken up occupancy in the basement. They got along fine with our Irish setter, Bonnie, before she passed away last spring, so we're hoping they'll get used to Millie as well. We shall see.

I'd been taking her to the doggie park at Quiet Waters, where she seemed to get along well with dogs of all sizes, and people, too, though she tends to gravitate toward women like her foster folks. When there are enough pups to play with in the small-dog area, Millie is in her element, positively frolicking.

We've gone on some short walks, but I've been careful not to push her too far too fast. So on one afternoon in early March, my emotional-support spouse, Louise, and I took her to Davidsonville Park, where we figured we'd take an easy stroll. Millie's good in the car, quiet and thoughtful.

On the way, I wondered about how Davidsonville got its name. When we got home, I consulted one of my favorite books, *The Placenames of Maryland, Their Origin and Meaning*, by Hamill Kenny, published by the Maryland Historical Society in 1984. It's a delightful resource. I looked up Davidsonville, and here's what I found:

"Near Birdsville, Anne Arundel County."

That's pretty terse, but the details are a fascinating glimpse into county history. According to Kenny, Thomas Davidson was postmaster in Davidsonville in

1824. The post office was most likely in the general store, which is still there today, serving as the Market/Deli on the corner of Central Avenue and Davidsonville Road. That intersection, it turns out, is all there is of beautiful downtown Davidsonville.

Thomas' father, James, emigrated from England in 1775 and served in the famed Maryland Line under General Smallwood during the Revolutionary War. That's where we got the sobriquet Old Line State. In the War of 1812, James was one of the Old Defenders who turned back the British army at North Point as they marched to attack Baltimore while the Royal Navy bombarded Fort McHenry. James died in Davidsonville in 1841.

And who knew that Davidsonville was a registered historic district? The district consists of just 15 properties gathered around that intersection, including three churches, the Market/Deli, and the 11 closest houses. It was listed on the National Register of Historic Places in 1992, mainly because Davidsonville is among the best-preserved examples of a rural crossroads community remaining in the county. It has managed to maintain its integrity since about World War II despite increasingly intensive development pressure in the rest of the county.

While the historic district is tiny, the actual environs of Davidsonville appear to be vast. Davidsonville Park, for instance, is a full four miles west of the crossroads. It's mainly meant as an active recreation park, with three lighted ballfields, a playground, a restroom that's open seasonally, and about 1.5 miles of paved, ADA-accessible pathway.

But we were there for the unpaved trails that traverse the ridge high above the bank of the Patuxent River. Millie is pretty good on the leash. She pulls a little too much for Louise's taste, but she's sensitive and responsive. And curious. She checked out various aromas along the dirt path, investigating where other critters have left their marks.

Along the way, we were surprised and delighted to hear the "who-cooks-for-you" call of an owl somewhere not far off in the woods, even though it was broad daylight, and then a far-off reply. I recorded the sound and posted it on the Maryland Birders' Facebook page, where several "birdies" quickly identified it as a barred owl with the chirrup of a chickadee in the foreground.

The peepers were prolific in the trees and bushes surrounding a small pond. They're almost deafening that time of year at the bald cypress swamp near the entrance of Quiet Waters. A sure sign of spring. We haven't seen osprey yet, but I've heard they've been starting to appear here and there.

From one prominent overlook, the surface of the Patuxent gleamed in the light of the low afternoon sun, the water brimming the banks with its spring flood. The tulip poplars sported little buds in the highest branches, but the oaks still showed no sign of sprouting leaves.

The path led us from the far end of the playing fields to the stairs leading down the steep hillside to the riverbank below. There's a cartop boat launch down there. The launch, however, is quite a walk from the parking lot, so you definitely need a cart or rollers. And you have to lower and raise your boat up and down a long, long track. It's worth checking out before you commit to a cruise from there. And of course, wait until the water warms up.

We walked Millie back to the car, and along the way, she met up with several larger dogs, sniffed, and got sniffed without being intimidated. We're lucky to have found such a wonderful being to be part of our family. I still hope to take a dog out for a date from the SPCA now and then, just because that's so much fun and the SPCA does such great work, but Millie's my main squeeze from now on. Uh, next to Louise, of course. (Louise edits all of my work.)

Incidentally, I've been asked to recommend walks for folks with some physical restrictions, and I'd recommend Davidsonville Park for that 1.5 miles of paved trail. It winds along the woods and around some pretty little ponds. It's fully ADA accessible.

So are the paved pathways in many of the Anne Arundel County Parks, not to mention the miles of trails. They're a great way to get out into nature, whether you're on a cane, a walker, a wheelchair, or just have gimpy knees. When you get to be 60 years old, you can purchase a Lifetime Senior Citizen Pass for just $40 that will get you into the regional parks that charge admission, but there are miles of paved trails you can explore for free. There's a handy Park Finder app at www.aacounty.org/departments/recreation-parks/parks/.

Davidsonville Park
3042 Patuxent River Road
Davidsonville, MD 21035

Directions: From Annapolis, take US-50 West to exit 16, MD-424/Davidsonville Road. Turn left onto MD-424 South/Davidsonville Road. Proceed south on Davidsonville Road. Turn right onto Double Gate Road. Follow Double Gate Road until the road ends. Turn right onto Patuxent River Road. The park entrance is about a third of a mile up on the left

410-222-7317

aacounty.org/locations-and-directions/davidsonville-park

Open dawn to dusk daily

Plenty of parking on site

Free admission

Toilets available seasonally

Neighborly dogs on leashed are welcome; doggie bag dispensers are available

Easy going, with 1.5 miles of paved trail, fully ADA accessible

Walk 27

Back Creek Nature Park: a Hidden Gem in Annapolis

We used to live in a little cottage on Bembe Beach, right across the road from the Back Creek Nature Park in Annapolis, and I've walked in that park with all five of the dogs that I've had the privilege of sharing a home with over the past 40 years. So when I got invited to give a presentation there for the current class of Leadership Anne Arundel, I thought it only natural to bring Millie along and introduce her, too, to this unique little park so enjoyed by her quadrupedal predecessors.

The 12-acre waterfront park used to be the site of the city's sewage-treatment plant. Some of the buildings, all brick walled and roofed with stately slate, appear to have been built around 1935, like the pretty brick building at the end of Second Street in Eastport, which you'd never suspect was—and still is—a sewage-pumping station. These structures at Back Creek Nature Park are now the headquarters, offices, and classrooms for the Annapolis Maritime Museum's environmental education program.

The Museum signed a 20-year lease in 2016 with the city of Annapolis to expand the education program, which by then had outgrown the old McNasby Oyster Company building in Eastport. The city had created the park in 1990 with funds from Maryland's Program Open Space and named it for former mayor Ellen O. Moyer.

Leadership Anne Arundel was using the site one warm, sunny day in early April 2021 to engage its current class of professionals in the environmental issues impacting the county and the Chesapeake Bay. I was one of several speakers; others represented the Maryland Department of Natural Resources, the Chesapeake Bay Foundation's oyster recovery program, local restoration project contractors, and experts in native plant species. Leadership Anne Arundel is a nonprofit organization that has been conducting a well-respected leadership training and networking institute in Anne Arundel County since 1993. My long-time friend Kris Valerio Shock serves as the organization's president and CEO.

Millie and I met our first group of a dozen or so candidates in the little amphitheater in a glade on the bank of a pond. The seating is made up of a semicircle of stacked granite slabs, remnants from long-ago civil engineering projects around Annapolis. The backdrop is the saltwater pond that separates one edge of Port Annapolis Marina from a wooded bluff topped by one of the city's water towers, its spherical tank gleaming like a colossal robin's egg in the sunshine.

The group politely listened to Heather Wheatley, education coordinator for Homestead Gardens in Davidsonville, as she provided a fascinating discussion of native plant species and how to deal with invasives, while behind and above her, osprey wheeled and whistled, mallards practiced their head-bobbing mating dance, and a pair of

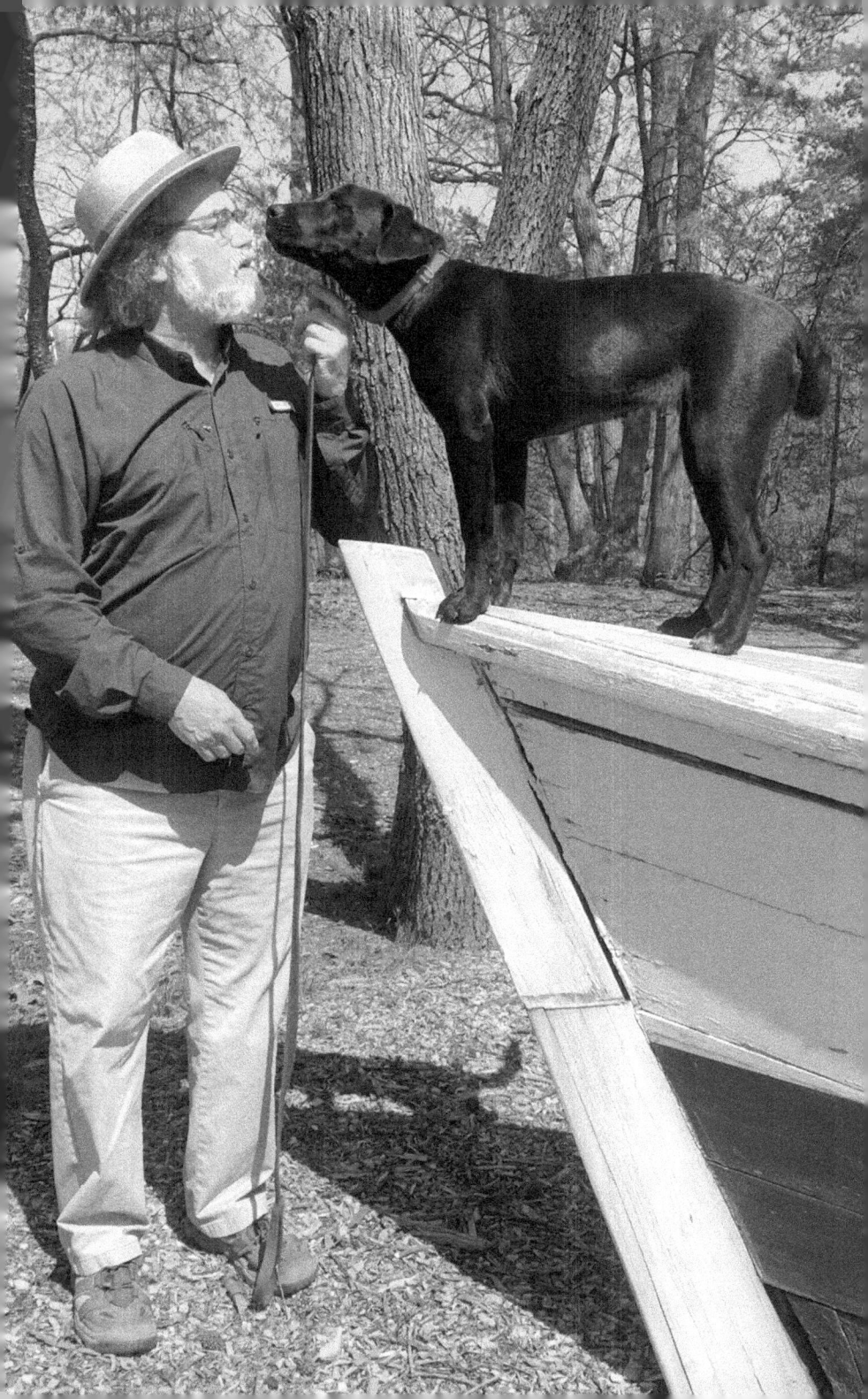

Canada geese splashed down for a landing. Titmice and chickadees fluttered around the branches of the trees overhead, each branch just beginning to show green buds of leaves. It takes a good speaker to keep an audience's attention with such distractions, and Heather is that good.

Then it was my turn. I rambled on about the many opportunities we have here in Annapolis and Anne Arundel County to go sauntering in the woods. Knowing that I would have a hard time competing with the natural phenomena behind me, I invited the group to follow me on a hike up the hill.

In single file, masked and keeping our proper distance, we climbed the tiers of wooden stairs up the slope and into the oak and holly woods. There we discovered another theatrical setting featuring a backdrop of an old wooden deadrise workboat that seemed mysteriously set down on this hilltop like Noah's Ark on the crest of Mt. Ararat after the flood. This boat is one I know well. She's called *Miss Lonesome*, and she was the centerpiece of the exhibit on the oyster industry at the Maritime Museum for more than a decade. Back when I was director of that museum, I had expert boatwrights slice her hull into thirds and mount the sections on custom-built frames, and then had to dismantle doorways in order to wheel the parts of the boat inside the exhibit hall one by one.

A decade later, the museum curator and staff installed a new exhibit, and to make way for that, they dismantled that same door to remove the boat and placed her here in what I consider a reverential setting. I had the group settle down at the concrete picnic tables and talked about *Miss Lonesome.*

I was always taken by that name, ever since I first saw the boat docked at Annapolis City Marina more than 20 years ago. Most watermen name their boats after the women in their lives. The guy who last owned this boat was apparently between girlfriends. She was built in Shady Side in 1921 by a boatwright named Perry Rogers, and like other craftsmen in his profession, he most likely built her by "eyeball," and not from any drawn plans.

She was restored by volunteers in the Eastport Wooden Boat Project in the 1990s, then donated to the maritime museum, where she became an interactive exhibit on how and why such boats are built the way they are. The basic design, a shallow-bottomed hull that's sharp at the bow to cut through the Chesapeake's chop, but that flattens out toward the stern to provide a stable working platform: This is the "deadrise" workboat that's still in use today. Deadrise refers to the V shape of the bow.

The other remarkable characteristic of traditional Chesapeake workboats, both deadrises and skipjacks, is that their bottoms are "cross-planked," meaning that the planks run crosswise from the keel to the edge of the hull, or the chine, rather than running from bow to stern. This method allowed for a boat to be built relatively quickly, lightly, and cheaply, and more easily repaired over time. You can see that clearly on this cut-away boat.

I wrote a song about her that was the title track on one of the Eastport Oyster Boys albums, and luckily, someone had stashed a baritone ukulele on the boat so I could strum it while I sang for the gang.

> *She's called Miss Lonesome,*
> *she's as lonesome as can be,*
>
> *Great blue heron perched upon her bow,*
> *and ducklings nibblin' along her lee*
>
> *If I could find the money and the time,*
> *I'd haul her home and I would make her mine*
>
> *But I'm afraid that that will never be,*
> *and she'll forever be Miss Lonesome*

You can hear the recording on Spotify.

I sang some more songs and told some more stories about the maritime heritage of Annapolis and the Chesapeake Bay, some of which were actually true, and sent them on to their next session. As the group rose to move on, Millie circulated among them, receiving adulation and adoration with aplomb.

Once we had the woods to ourselves, Millie and I walked the paths neatly lined with crushed clamshells (oyster shells are needed to replenish the reefs) and circled around the hilltop, down to the boat ramp and floating dock that's managed by the City Harbormaster's Office.

There's a small boathouse where Capital SUP rents stand-up paddleboards in the warmer months.

We followed the path along Edgewood Road, back to the Museum's education center and then walked along the edge of the salt pond, where the mallards seemed to take a fascination to Millie. The flock swam along the water's edge as we walked along the path, as though Millie had some treats to feed them. Millie, of course, looked to them for the same.

We agreed that this park is a little gem and a charming setting, and I'm happy that our sixth dog enjoyed it as much as the others.

An update: as of 2024, Miss Lonesome was left to rot away and has been dismantled and discarded. All that's left is a sign that says, "Deadrise Park."

Ellen O. Moyer Nature Park at Back Creek
Managed by the Annapolis Maritime Museum & Park
7300 Edgewood Road
Annapolis, MD 21403
www.visitannapolis.org/listing/ellen-o-moyer-nature-park/4032/
Open dawn to dusk daily
Free admission
Plenty of parking on site
Toilets are available in the education building when staff is on duty.
Polite dogs permitted on leash; bring your own doggie bags
Easy going

Walk 28

Taking a Turn Around Terrapin Nature Park

You usually drive through Queen Anne's County to get somewhere else, but you'd be amazed what's right there just on the other side of the Chesapeake Bay Bridge. Take the first exit off Route 50 on Kent Island, head north on Route 8 and turn left into the industrial park and you'll find yourself at the Terrapin Nature Area. It's less than a half-hour drive from Annapolis, but it's a whole other world once you get there.

When Millie and I arrived one muggy afternoon in early May 2021, the large parking lot was almost full, and yet we only met up with a handful of other people and dogs. The other visitors must have been absorbed somewhere in the park's 276 acres or off somewhere on one of the two hiking/biking trails that crisscross the island.

Both of them link to Terrapin Park: the Cross Island Trail that runs six miles east to west along an abandoned rail corridor and the South Island Trail that parallels Maryland Route 8 between Matapeake and Kent Point Road.

There's a trail inside the park that circles a large salt pond. That trail is actually a smooth, flat country lane graveled with crushed shell, perfect for a leisurely bike ride or the afternoon saunter that Millie and I were looking forward to enjoying. There are benches placed at

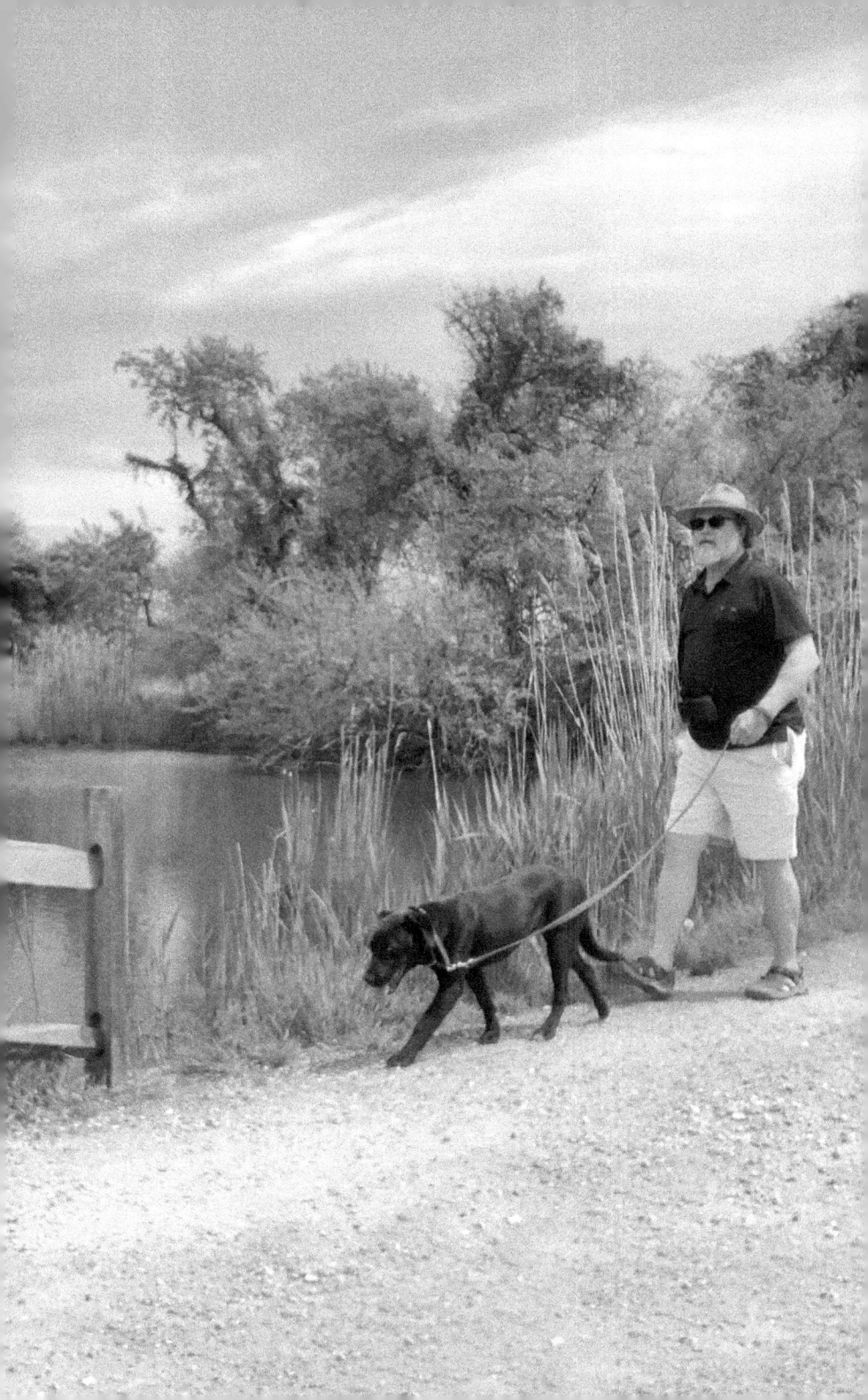

thoughtful intervals, making it an ideal choice for walkers looking for an easy stroll in an exhilarating atmosphere.

The lane starts out in an open meadow, then crosses over the tidal pond on a causeway. We stopped to look for the redwing blackbirds we heard singing in the rushes. Before long, we found a pavilion overlooking the beach.

Walking through the brush and stepping onto the beach felt like emerging through Alice's looking glass, coming out into a mirror image of Sandy Point State Park, which is just four and a half miles away on the far side of the open Chesapeake. The Bay Bridge itself spans the southern horizon. The sunsets over the western shore must be stunning from this vantage point. I doffed my shoes and we barefooted all six of our feet down nearly a mile of beach, me wading ankle-deep in the chilly water and Millie trotting deliberately at the far end of the outstretched leash, stubbornly careful to stay in the dry, loose sand.

Millie's about eight months old now. She has yet to live up to her Labrador retriever genes and let her webbed feet delve into what ought to be her natural habitat. She has only this past week caught on to the concept of tennis balls and their meaning to her existence. Millie is an astonishingly intelligent creature, and it's inspiring to watch her progress from puppyhood. It's almost worth sacrificing a shoe or two. Almost.

This was one of those warm, humid days, a bit overcast with a hint of storm in the clouds. In fact, I was disappointed that it didn't rain to cool things off a bit. It made me think we're in for one of those exceptionally hot summers.

All along that near-mile of beach, we only passed a couple of young moms with their toddlers playing in the sand and just a couple of other people getting a head start on their summer reading. At one point, we crossed over a wooden footbridge that spanned the outlet of the pond as the outgoing tide rushed back into the Bay.

Millie and I were attached by a six-foot strap the whole time, honest; but I still can't see what harm would have befallen the universe if we hadn't been so interconnected. We live in a crazy world. I can get a permit to pack a concealed lethal weapon and carry it down a crowded city street, but I can't get a permit to walk my puppy dog on a beach without a leash.

Queen Anne's County does have such a beach about three miles south at Matapeake (see page 241), and there are others in the area (see "Doggie Parks for the Dog Days of Summer" on page 257).

Dogs are a highly evolved and highly intelligent species. They can be trained to do amazing things: detect explosives and narcotics, sense when someone is about to have an epileptic seizure, help people with poor eyesight navigate urban cacophony, herd sheep by the whistle of a human shepherd from a faraway hillside—even fetch tennis balls.

There should be a system of certifying the level of a dog's training so that it can accompany its human companion on a beach with no leash when there's nobody around to bother. Of course, that means the human must undergo training as well. I always pick up after my dog, and sometimes pick up after other people's dogs so my dog doesn't get the blame.

We had the option of continuing on the trail the rest of the way around the pond, but we decided to backtrack and head home before the storm got a chance to break. By the time we got back to the car, we had logged about 2.7 miles, as opposed to the 3.2 miles we would have walked had we gone all the way around. We beat the rain home.

If you haven't ventured across the Chesapeake Bay Bridge lately, you'll want to be sure you get an E-Z Pass transponder, since the cash toll booths are long gone. I got mine at a Giant grocery store for $25, all of which goes for pre-paid tolls, so the transponder itself is free. Every time you cross from west to east, your account is automatically debited by just $2.50 for your two-axle vehicle. Rides back across the bridge are free. If you don't have the E-Z Pass, a video monitor will record your license plate and you'll get a bill in the mail for $6.

As long as you traverse the bridge mid-week and not during rush hour, you probably won't have much trouble with traffic, but you can always check conditions on the on-line camera at https://mdta.maryland.gov/traffic-cameras-by-facility?WPL=#camera-999.

Terrapin Nature Area
191 Log Canoe Circle
Stevensville, MD 21666

https://www.qac.org/Facilities/Facility/Details/Terrapin-Nature-Area-97

Open from dawn to dusk

Free admission

Plenty of parking on site

Portable toilets are available year-round

Obedient dogs on leashes are welcome; bring your own doggie bags

Easy going

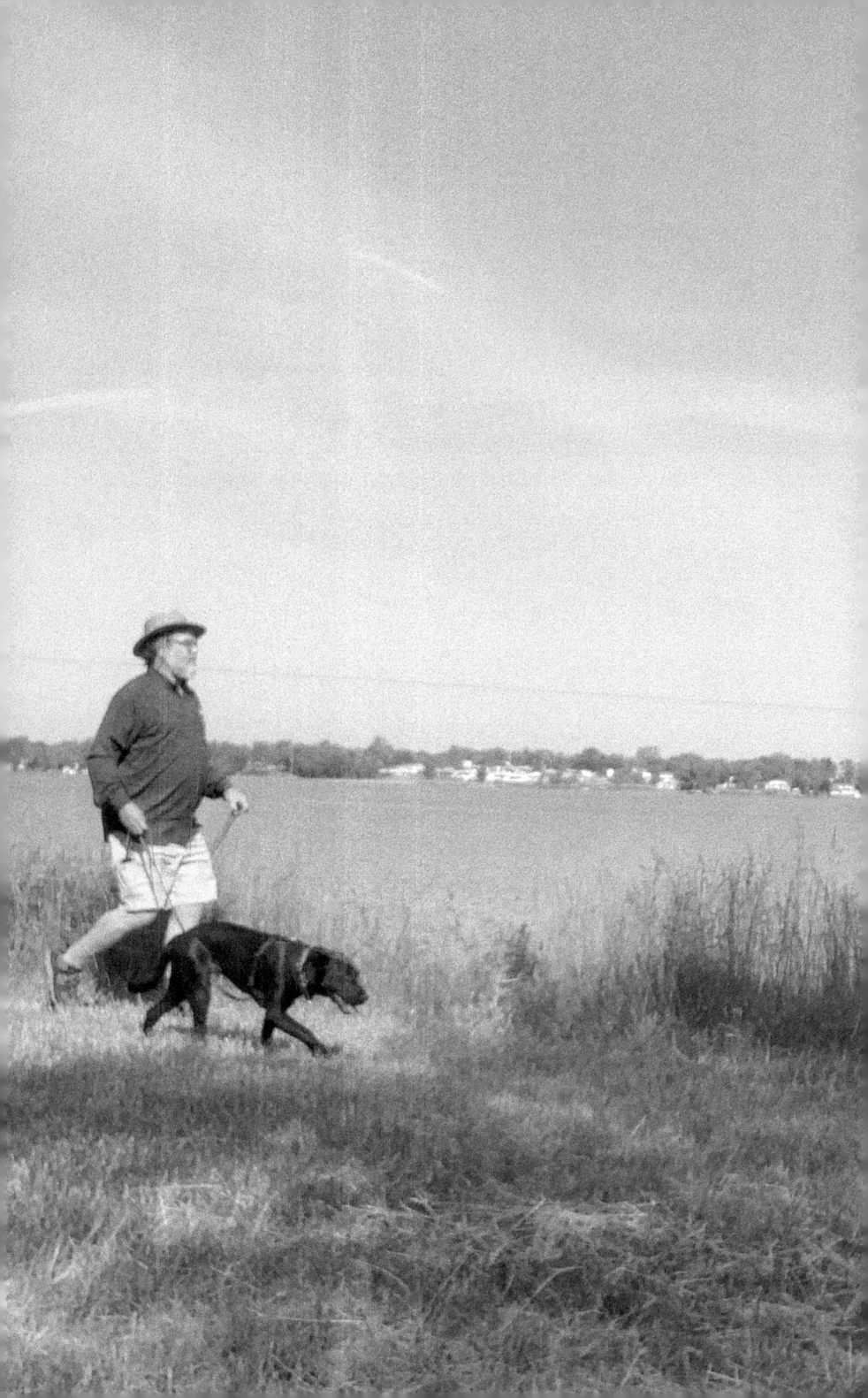

Walk 29

Searching for Palm Trees at Weinberg Park

When I investigated Fort Smallwood Park in Pasadena in 2020, I learned that there was another park nearby, but it took nearly a year before I got around to checking it out. Millie and I found Harry & Jeanette Weinberg Park to be quite rustic but worth a visit.

This park is yet another example of far-sighted civic leaders preserving green space from development for the benefit of the rest of us. Anne Arundel County acquired the 232-acre site in 2003 under the auspices of then County Executive Janet Owens. It's just a quarter-mile south of Fort Smallwood Park on both sides of Fairview Beach Road between White Pond and Wall Cove at the mouth of Rock Creek. There's a gate across the parking lot on Honolulu Lane that may or may not be open on weekends. We were there during the week and parked along the roadside.

Though the park has theoretically been open for nearly two decades, there are no amenities: no portable toilets, no trash containers, no benches, no picnic tables, no nothing. I'm not saying that's a terrible thing; just adjust your expectations and come prepared to be self-sufficient.

You'll be rewarded with a pleasant walk down a shady country lane that runs about a third of a mile from the main road to the edge of the water. There, the forest of locust and maple trees opens up onto a meadow on a bluff overlooking the Patapsco River.

From that point, you can see the skyline of Baltimore beyond Key Bridge* to the left and the White Rocks on the right. The White Rocks are a real curiosity in the Chesapeake Bay, where the only rocks you'll generally find are ones dumped along shorelines as riprap.

The bluff is crowned by towering southern red oaks that must have been saplings when the British fleet sailed by here nearly 200 years ago. I used my new iNaturalist app to learn the names of several of the wildflowers decorating the meadow. One was a tall, spindly plant adorned with what appeared to be tiny purple irises, which the app identified as lyreleaf sage. Another tall plant was called a tufted vetch, this one with more tiny flowers rising up the stem like a deep purple bottle brush.

Millie led me along a path down to the shoreline, where there was a strip of sandy beach separating the river from a tidal pool called Yates Pond. Rising tides are causing erosion along here, toppling lots of trees. There are several places where you have to hop over large fallen logs. Millie was better at that than me.

We watched a little green heron skim across the surface of the pond, and spotted eastern bluebirds, red-winged blackbirds, and brown-headed cowbirds along the way. Once you reach the beach, you can walk about a quarter-mile in the sand before the downed trees block the way. At the far end, someone sometime in the past stacked old car tires to form a bulwark to buck up the bank.

We tried to follow a path that we hoped would take us the rest of the way around the pond, but it petered out into a deer track on the far bluff. We backtracked along the beach rather than bushwhack through the dense brush back to the road.

There was trash, and I had neglected to bring a bag along to take some home with me. Curiously, there were bits of broken bottles here and there, both newly shattered shards and older ones being ground smooth by the churning sand. Someday they'll all be sea glass in somebody's prized collection.

On the way back, we met up with a young mother and her happy little two-year-old son clad in shorts festooned with dancing crabs. This was their first time at the park, though they live nearby. She noted that the beach at Fort Smallwood Park was closed because of the pandemic, so she thought she'd check this one out. "There's got to be an easier beach to get to," she grumbled. No doubt it's tougher to haul a toddler in a wagon full of beach toys all that way than it is to follow a small dog on a leash.

According to a 2003 article in *The Baltimore Sun*, most of the park's 232 acres belonged to Harry Weinberg and his partners since the mid-1960s. They bought the property when the area was still mainly rural. Weinberg, who made much of his money buying real estate in declining areas of Baltimore, died in 1990.

The Harry and Jeanette Weinberg Foundation owned one 35-acre parcel; three-quarters of a second 81-acre parcel; and half of the third and largest parcel, which comprised 116 acres. The Foundation donated its interest in the property—valued at about $2.75 million—to make acquisition of the three parcels possible.

The State of Maryland donated $1.5 million from Program Open Space to buy out the other owners. The park was named for the Weinbergs in recognition of their foundation's donation.

By the time Millie and I got back to the car, we had logged only about a mile and a half, but we had discovered a new place, learned some new plants, spotted some colorful birds, and seen a view of Baltimore that not many folks get to see. This park is not listed on the AllTrails app, so I'm not sure if there are other trails to explore. There didn't appear to be any, particularly on the south side of Fairview Beach Road. Perhaps there will be in the future. This might be a blank canvas for some would-be trail blazer.

A sign at the gate says there's a kayak launch at the end of the road, and that may be the case, but that's an awfully long way to drag your boat and gear. The boat ramp at Fort Smallwood Park would be a better bet.

If you're not up to the challenge of log-hopping, Fort Smallwood has miles of paved walkways, most of which are handicap accessible, and you get nearly the same view across the Patapsco, though you sacrifice the solitude you'll find at Weinberg Park.

*The Francis Scott Key Bridge was destroyed on March 26, 2024, when a cargo ship leaving the Port of Baltimore collided with one of its pylons.

Harry & Jeannette Weinberg Park
1543 Fairview Beach Road at Honolulu Lane
Pasadena, MD 21122

410-222-0088

aacounty.org/locations-and-directions/harry-and-jeanette-weinberg-park

Directions: From Fort Smallwood Road heading for Fort Smallwood Park, turn left on Fairview Beach Road about 1/2 mile before Fort Smallwood Park. Go about 1/2 mile and turn right on Honolulu Lane

Open dawn to dusk daily

Limited parking on Honolulu Lane

Free admission

No toilets

Gentle dogs on leash are welcome; bring your own doggie bags

Moderate, some obstacles to climb over

P.S. And why, tell me why, is a dirt road in Pasadena named for a city in Hawaii? A number of alert readers responded to my bewilderment. It turns out that Harry Weinberg owned so much property in Hawaii that he was known as "Honolulu Harry." An office of the Harry and Jeanette Weinberg Foundation is headquartered there to this very day. Who knew?

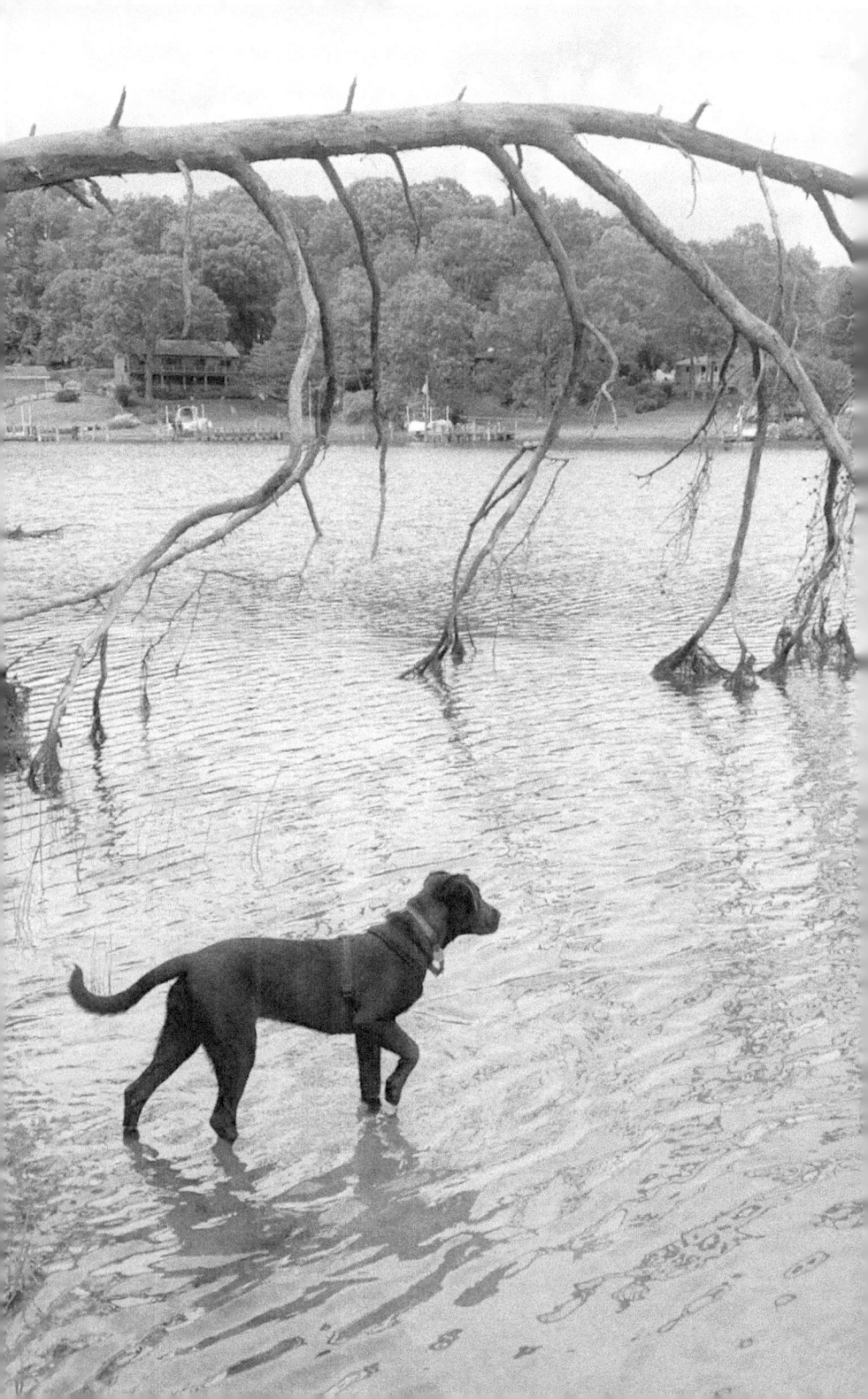

Walk 30

Nursing a Broken Heart at Valentine Creek Trail

June is National Accordion Appreciation month, so of course I took a walk down to Valentine Creek in Crownsville. The connection is that the Annapolis music world had recently lost one of the best accordion players I know, and this trail is in the neighborhood where he lived. I wanted to spend some time alone walking through the woods and thinking about my friend, Randy Neilson. Randy died suddenly at the end of May 2021, after spending the day on the Nanticoke River surveying oyster sanctuaries for the Oyster Recover Partnership.

Of course I wasn't really alone. My sweet little dog, Millie, seemed to be respectful of my contemplative mood. We found the trail on the AllTrails app and followed the GPS to the trailhead in the Arden on the Severn neighborhood. The path leads up a hill into an oak-and-holly forest. It's a little bit steep at first, but Millie hauled me up by the leash attached to her new harness. She can really pull for a fairly young pup still under 50 pounds.

The cicada symphony trilled to a crescendo when we got to the top of the hill. There were mountain laurels everywhere, their clusters of tiny white buds just about to fade. The path seemed to level out and follow an ancient sunken road through the woods. Unlike those made by rolling huge hogsheads crammed with tobacco leaves down to the nearest wharf, it turns out that these narrow ruts were most likely from the time in the late 1800s and early 1900s when this was the site of a sand mine.

Sand is the main ingredient in making glass. This sand was shipped by barge down the Severn River to the Annapolis Glass Works on the Horn Point peninsula, across the harbor from Annapolis City Dock. The factory once occupied the block along Severn Avenue between First and Third streets. Workers melted the sand in brick furnaces. A dozen workers blew the molten glass into molds, creating bottles. The factory also produced china and pottery.

The manager of the glassworks was a Maine native named Charles Murphy. At the time the factory was active, between 1885 and 1902, the surrounding neighborhood had grown to the point where it needed its own post office. Murphy donated one of the townhouses he had built for his workers to the postal service and got the privilege of giving the place a name. Of course, he dubbed it after his hometown, Eastport.

My friend Randy loved the Severn River and the Bay. He volunteered countless hours with the Oyster Recovery Project to survey river bottoms to find suitable places to plant oyster spat. As Millie and I followed the sunken path, admiring the mountain laurel blossoms, I remembered how Randy and I talked for hours while we drove around the state and rambled through the woods finding locations to shoot a video. It was for the song I wrote that we hope will become the new official state song for Maryland.

Randy took my lyrics and ukulele chords and created an elaborate arrangement. To say that Randy was just an accordion player is like saying Bach was just an organist. Randy played the organ, too, at his church every Sunday for 50 years. But he also played no fewer than 19 instruments to accompany the video, which he also produced.

He composed the "Thomas Point Suite" that was performed by the Londontowne Symphony Orchestra (now called the Naptown Philharmonic Orchestra) at Key Auditorium in 2019. He played various instruments in dozens of different groups, including the Eastport Oyster Boys and the Naptown Brass Band, which performed an appropriate New Orleans-style tribute at his funeral.

After about a mile, the path dipped down and touched the Severn River. When you step out of the woods, you can look to the right and see the marsh end of Valentine Creek. Millie waded out into the water and watched with fascination as a great blue heron caught a little fish and gobbled it down its drainpipe neck.

According to the map on the AllTrails app, the path loops around to the left, but we backtracked the way we came in. If you follow the loop around, it's about a 2.5-mile walk. There are plenty of intriguing side trails to make you want to come back and explore some more. The path is fairly flat, but there are enough trip-able roots to keep you on your toes. Despite the recent rain, there were only a couple of soggy spots. This appears to be a popular run for mountain bikers, who have created several improvised jump ramps, but haven't left that many ruts in the mud.

Tucked between the Arden on the Severn community and Herald Harbor, Valentine Creek Trail forest classifies in my book as one of Anne Arundel County's marvelous pocket wildernesses.

Millie and I got back to the car, having logged only about two miles, but that took more than two hours. It was a lovely walk, accented by the mountain laurel blossoms and the cicada accompaniment, the joy of being in the woods with little Millie, and the wonderful memories of my friend Randy Nielson.

One last Randy story. Our daughter's wedding took place this past fall at Quiet Waters Park. I had asked Randy if he knew anyone who could play the cello at the ceremony. He said he didn't and noted with regret that of all the many instruments he had mastered, cello was just about the only one he couldn't play well at all.

On the day of the wedding, Randy showed up, dressed in a tux and carrying a cello, which of course he played beautifully.

Now I want to know how Valentine Creek got its name. If you know, email me at arundelhappytrails@gmail.com.

Valentine Creek Trail
1102 Valentine Creek Drive
Crownsville, MD 21032

410-222-7317

aacounty.org/locations-and-directions/valentine-creek-park

Directions: Take General's Highway, MD Rt. 178 to Sunrise Beach Road, passing the Maryland Veterans Cemetery on your left and Arden Park on your right; then turn right onto Miner Road. Miner Road becomes Plum Creek Drive. Turn right onto Valley Drive. You'll see the trailhead on the right at the bend. Drive slowly.

There is no dedicated parking lot; park politely along the street in this suburban neighborhood

Open dawn to dusk daily

Free admission

No toilets

Sociable dogs on leash are welcome; bring your own doggie bags

Moderate, some topography

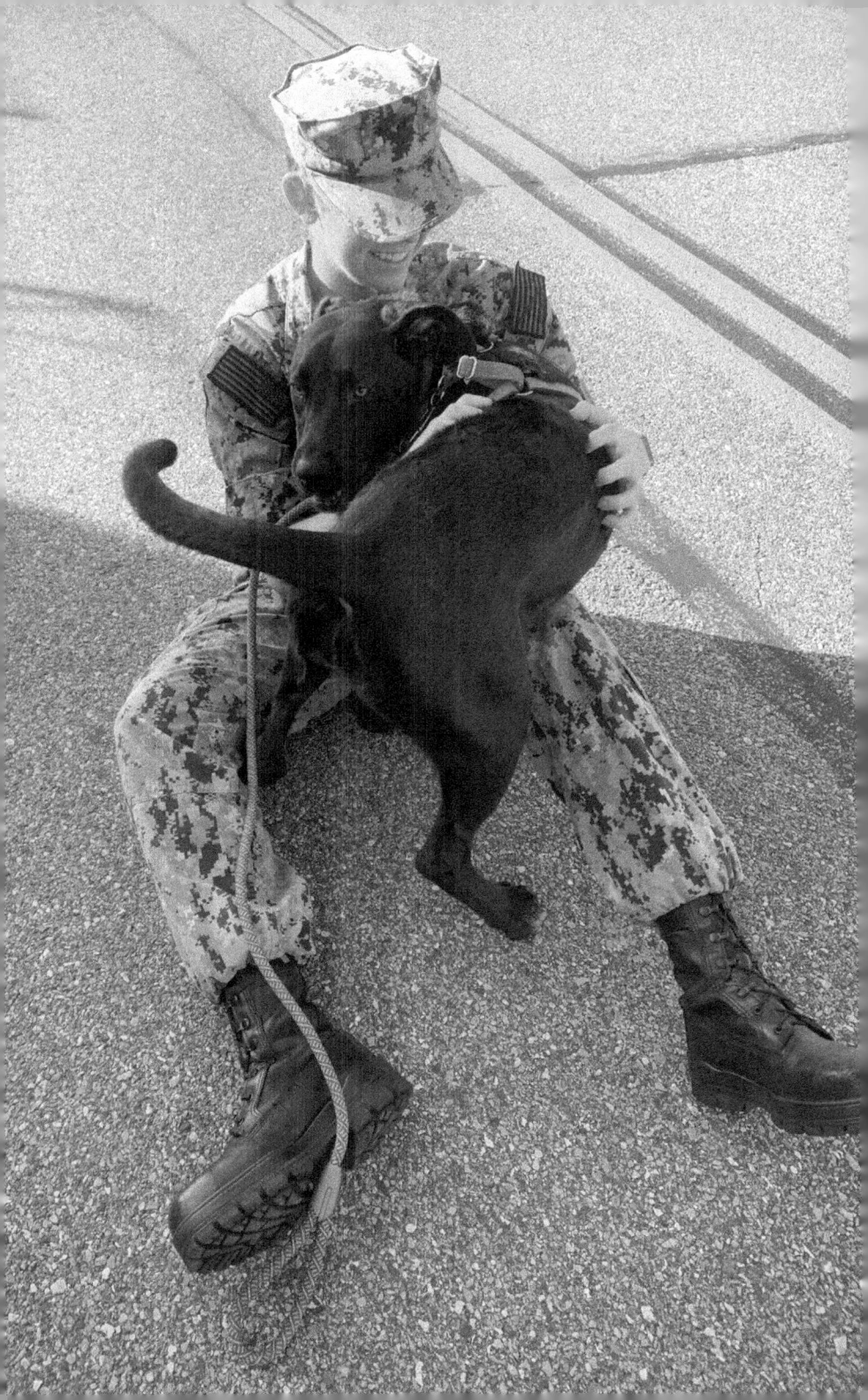

Walk 31

Patrolling the Yard at the United States Naval Academy

Millie and I took a stroll on the grounds of the Naval Academy one early morning in July 2021 after the Yard had been re-opened since the pandemic had finally eased its grip on the world. The U.S. Navy gave Annapolis a huge gift when it launched its school for officers here in 1845, and I wanted to see it again. Of course, as a civilian unconnected with the Navy or the Department of Defense, I couldn't drive onto "The Yard," but there's a relatively new pedestrian gate at the end of Prince George Street. On that mid-week morning, we found plenty of parking on the street nearby.

I wanted to get a close-up view of the newly coppered chapel dome, but the entire area in front of Bancroft Hall is considered ceremonial and off-limits to joggers, bikers, and pets. So we cut straight across behind Bancroft to the Santee Basin and walked along the Severn River.

We passed the historical marker that showed where General Benjamin Butler landed with his Union troops in April 1861, just one week after the surrender of Fort Sumter that launched the Civil War.

The site is remarkable in a number of aspects.

For one thing, the original 1845 Naval School was set on the grounds of an obsolete Army installation called Fort Severn. Those grounds occupied just 10 acres. Today, the Academy grounds cover 338 acres. The expansion was all landfill. The dirt for the fill was dug out of a hole at the bottom of the river off Sycamore Point, near where the Eastport Yacht Club now stands. The original campus ended near the Scott Natatorium and the Wesley Brown Field House, quite a ways back from the modern Annapolis Harbor seawall.

The old circular structure of Fort Severn stood on the point here, where the Severn River met the harbor, and a long pier stretched out into the river. At the start of the war, the USS *Constitution*—Old Ironsides herself—was moored in the mud, serving as a training ship for the midshipmen.

It's not revealed on the historical marker, but according to Jane McWilliams in her definitive history book, *Annapolis, City on the Severn,* when Union Major General Benjamin Franklin Butler arrived in Annapolis with his Massachusetts regiment aboard the steamship *Maryland*, he found the *Constitution* hard aground and a sitting duck for any secessionist sharpshooters that might be lurking in the woods across the river.

The steamship managed to tow the frigate into the channel, but then the *Maryland* ran hard aground and the troops were stuck out there for several days on dwindling rations. I tried to imagine the chaotic scene.

General Butler went on to occupy the town and keep the legislature from voting to secede from the Union only by arresting 31 Democrats, most of whom were held prisoner at Fort McHenry in Baltimore. Ironically, a pro-southern newspaper editor was also arrested and held at Fort McHenry on Sept. 13–14. His name was Frank Key Howard, the grandson of Francis Scott Key, the guy who watched the British bombard that same fort that same night in 1814. (Yes, I know this has little to do with our visit to the Naval Academy, but it's such a stunning historical nugget, I couldn't resist sharing it with you.)

At the same spot where the steamship *Maryland* eventually offloaded its 700 Massachusetts militiamen, I discovered a 109-foot-long Yard Patrol boat, one of the many training vessels in the Academy's fleet, moored at the seawall. A squad of midshipmen—men and women—dressed in camouflage fatigues was lined up ready to board for a cruise. As Millie and I passed by, one of the young women asked if she could say hello to my dog, and of course, the answer is always a hearty "You bet!"

To my surprise and delight, she plopped down on the pavement, her grin beaming from underneath the broad brim of her cap as she grabbed Millie in a bear hug. Millie wriggled with glee. The midshipman introduced herself as Eve Warden with the class of 2023. She was eager to show me a tiny photo on her Apple wristwatch of her two rescue mutts back home in Phoenix, Arizona.

Continuing on our stroll along the riverfront, we passed two women walking a dog. Millie wanted to engage, but the one woman pulled her dog away and said, "He's not as well-behaved as Millie." I guess my dog is becoming famous.

We turned the corner at College Creek. I considered extending our walk across the wooden footbridge that spans the creek to visit the cemetery at Hospital Point and perhaps pay our respects at the late Senator John McCain's grave, but by this point, the temperature was climbing, the concrete walkway was heating up, and Millie was starting to show signs of discomfort.

So we walked up along Worden Field past the bandstand and followed the outer wall to Gate 3, again carefully avoiding the ceremonial area in front of the chapel. There to our relief, we found a coffee shop with some comfy Adirondack chairs on the sidewalk where Millie and I shared a bottle of cold water in the shade. Once we had cooled down, we let ourselves out through the turnstile at Gate 3 and walked down King George Street back to the car.

Now that the Academy is open again, I will be a frequent visitor. I can't wait to get back to the astonishing museum in Preble Hall. But I won't be taking Millie with me. There's too much pavement in the areas where you're permitted to walk with your dog.

United States Naval Academy
52 King George Street
Annapolis, MD 21401

usna.edu

Entrance: Pedestrian Gate 3 at the end of Prince George Street

The Yard is open sunrise to 5 p.m. daily

Armel-Leftwich Visitor Center is open 9 a.m. to 5 p.m.

Free admission, but all visitors need to show an up-to-date driver's license or passport and go through a metal detector

Toilets are available in the Armel-Leftwich Visitor Center

No parking on Academy grounds without authorization

Park on Annapolis City streets or the Hillman garage off Main Street

Patriotic dogs on leash are okay in some areas, but with some restrictions in the ceremonial areas; bring your own doggie bags

Easy going

Walk 32

Kinder Farm Park: A Literal *Kinder-garten*

It had been on my list for more than a year, but it wasn't until we were invited to lead a walk-and-talk program for the Watershed Stewards Academy in late July 2021 that Millie and I finally paid a visit to Kinder Farm Park in Millersville. We were both pleasantly surprised by what we discovered there.

Since it was founded in 2009, the Watershed Stewards Academy has trained more than 280 Master Watershed Stewards in communities throughout Anne Arundel County. These stewards work with neighbors, businesses, schools, and each other to install hundreds of projects every year to reduce pollution in local waterways. These projects range from planting tens of thousands of native trees to restoring streams degraded by stormwater runoff.

At the Academy's request, I led a group of parents and toddlers on a short walk on one of Kinder Farm Park's many trails one muggy evening. As we strolled, we found examples of invasive plant species as well as native species of trees and forest plants. Then we gathered under a grove of ancient maple trees and shared some songs and stories.

Millie, of course, absorbed the attention of the toddlers while she patiently waited in the shade of a picnic table until her service human (that's me, I'm still in training) was done strumming on the ukulele and singing about the Bay.

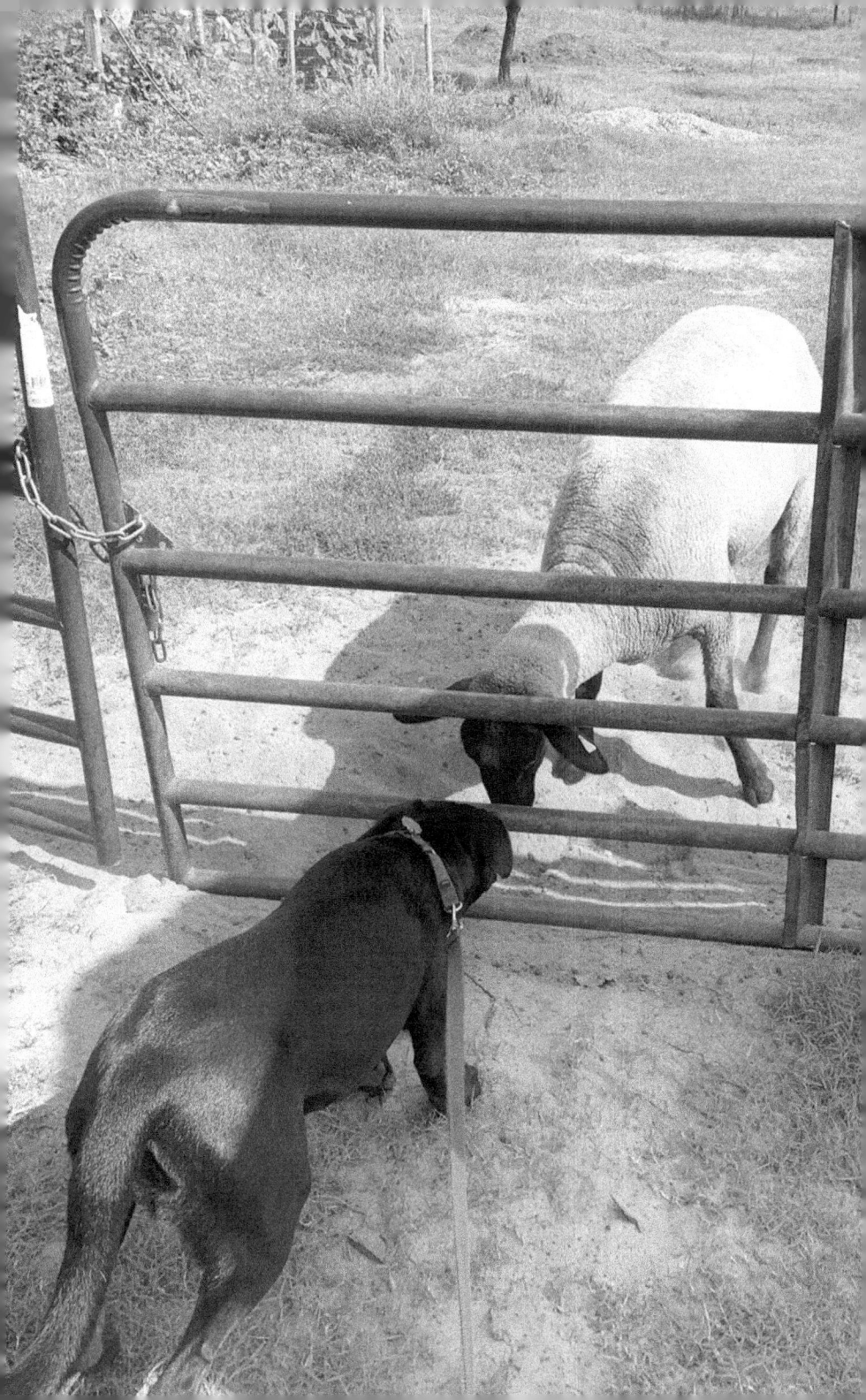

Being there whetted our appetite to see more of the park, so the next morning, Millie and I went back to explore. We got a trail map at the gate and parked by the elaborate playground. Watching the squiggle of kids playing in the park, the curious coincidence occurred to me that "Kinder" means "children" in German. This truly was a "kindergarten."

According to information gathered by the Friends of Kinder Farm Park, Kinder was the family name of brothers Gustave and Henry, who emigrated from Germany and started buying property in 1898. Eventually, they amassed a 600-acre farm where they cut timber and sold milk produced by 15 dairy cows. They also sold ice from the ponds. Imagine nowadays how cutting and selling blocks of pond ice would work as a commercial venture. But mainly, they grew fruits and vegetables that they trucked up to markets around Baltimore until the late 1940s.

Much of northern Anne Arundel County, in fact, was devoted to this kind of "truck farming," that is, until refrigerated train cars and trucks started shipping produce from farms farther south, far earlier in the growing season. The local farmers couldn't compete then. It took 70 years for that trend to turn around and for locally grown produce to become popular again. Meanwhile, after World War II, urban sprawl from Baltimore and Washington, D.C. pressured farm owners to sell off their acreage to developers.

The Kinders managed to keep their farm profitable by shifting from produce to raising hogs, turkeys, and beef cattle. By 1960, the farm was owned jointly by four of Henry's eight sons. They began selling parcels of property to housing developers and the Anne Arundel County Board of Education to build nearby schools. In 1979 the sons sold the remaining 288 acres to Anne Arundel County, yet another example of stellar citizens preserving green space for us all to enjoy.

Many of the farm buildings, including the family home, have been preserved and restored to interpret the county's agricultural heritage. Kids can see real-live cows, pigs, sheep, goats, chickens, and turkeys raised by the local 4-H Club and park volunteers. There's a museum in the visitor center featuring farming tools dating back to the tobacco era.

As you might imagine, Millie was in a state of odiferous bliss as we walked through the barnyard. So many new sights and smells. She was fascinated by a cow lying against a wooden fence, went nose-to-nose with a goat twice her size on the other side of a metal gate, and got stared down by a large black hen in her chicken-wire pen. There were families with kids everywhere, getting a good gander at all the critters, and while this is not a petting zoo, some of the kids did give Millie a tentative pat, which she graciously accepted.

We rambled back behind the barnyard through the woods and fields. On our way, we met one of the park rangers watering a raised-bed butterfly garden and passed a penned-in community garden where a gardener lucky enough to get one of the few plots was busy weeding.

There's a 2.5-mile paved path around the perimeter of the park and a number of unpaved side trails and fence-lined country roads to wander along. The feel is quite bucolic. In the shade of the cottonwoods, a cool breeze came sweeping down the lane as we sat alone and watched a pair of hawks makin' lazy circles in the sky. (Cue the orchestra) *We know we belong to the land—and the land we belong to is grand! And when I say—Yeeow!—* Okay, okay, I got carried away. It's that kind of place.

We made our way back to the car, logging a little more than a mile and a half before it got too hot and muggy to be comfortable.

If you'd like to learn more about the county's agricultural heritage, go to the library and check out a book by the wonderful local historian Will Mumford, who passed away just a few years ago. It's called *Strawberries, Peas & Beans: Truck Farming in Anne Arundel County,* published in 2000 by the Ann Arundell Historical Society.

Speaking of books, here are a few you might enjoy:

In *Finding the Mother Tree*, published by Alfred A. Knopf in 2021, author Suzanne Simard tells the story of her life from a kid growing up in a family of foresters to becoming a professor of forest ecology in British Columbia, and her discovery that trees in a forest—even trees of different species—communicate with one another and even nourish one another through a "wood-wide web" of soil fungi connecting their roots.

Peter Wohlleben's book, *The Hidden Life of Trees: What They Feel, How They Communicate*, published by Greystone Books in 2015, could be considered the companion to Simard's story; in fact, he refers to much of her literally ground-breaking work. However, Wohlleben, who manages forests in the Eiffel Mountains of Germany, takes an approach that is more introspective and perhaps even enchanting.

Eager: the Surprising, Secret Life of Beavers and Why They Matter, published by Chelsea Green Publishing in 2018, follows author Ben Goldfarb's quest to track down the role of this industrious rodent in modern-day America. Curiously, the leading-edge method of restoring streambeds damaged by stormwater runoff is to replicate beaver dams.

If you'd like to share what you're reading or a trail you love to walk, drop me a line at arundelhappytrails@gmail.com. Happy trails!

To learn more about the Anne Arundel County Watershed Stewards Academy and how you can become a Master Watershed Steward, log onto http://aawsa.org/.

Kinder Farm Park
1001 Kinder Farm Park Road
Millersville, MD 21108

410-222-6115

aacounty.org/departments/recreation-parks/parks/kinder-farm/

Open 7 a.m. to dusk daily

Admission $6/car for parking (see web site for discounts)

Plenty of parking on site

Toilets are open year-round

Courtly dogs on leash are welcome; doggie bag dispensers available

Easy going

Walk 33

St. Luke's Restoration of Nature

There are short walks nearby that go a long way toward restoring the soul, and the one at St. Luke's Episcopal Church in Eastport has the double bonus of also restoring nature. The little church's five-acre site was once a tangle of invasive vines with a buried storm pipe that spewed runoff directly into Back Creek. Now there's a new quarter-mile-long stream that drains 28 acres of the surrounding neighborhood and cleanses the water before it reaches a marsh at the edge of the creek. Paths wander through 125,000 square feet of native plantings from Bay Ridge Avenue all the way down to the marsh.

One Sunday in October 2021, Millie the rescue retriever and I attended a blessing of the animals at the church's outdoor amphitheater. The Rev. Diana Carroll led the service. She sprinkled each pet with holy water flicked from a sprig of willow and laid a loving hand on each furry brow. Millie liked that. Of course, she likes any attention she can get, but this seemed special to her. I hadn't been to the church grounds in some time, and I was so taken by the lush flourishing of all the native wildflowers that I had to go find Louise to join me for a walk through the site.

My emotional-support spouse was just as charmed as I was. "This is the kind of place I would have loved to explore when I was a little girl," she said. "We'd build forts and find secret spots to hide." She had her wildflower book in hand and I had the iNaturalist app open on my phone. We started with the little yellow flowers on their towering stalks in the beds surrounding the labyrinth up near the roadway. They looked like black-eyed Susans, only nine feet tall, but the app identified them as narrowleaf sunflowers, a new one for both of us. These beauties, like most of the native plants at this site, are meant to attract pollinators: bees, moths, butterflies, and hummingbirds.

We headed down into the shade of the woods, a mix of red maples, sassafras, and sweetgums along with some saplings of catalpa, pawpaw, yellow poplar, and a few bird-cherry trees. There we discovered low-growing blossoms: American asters with their delicate violet petals and yellow centers, and an elaborate speckled yellow flower that looked like it could take on any orchid in a beauty contest and win. Imagine our disappointment when it turned out to have the mundane name of spotted horse mint.

While the coneflowers had shriveled and blackened, we were amazed that so many of the other flowers were still in such lovely bloom in the first week of October. And there were brilliantly colored berries, like the appropriately named purple beautyberry.

We made it down to the edge of the creek in a little cove between the Watergate apartments and the Severn House condo complex. The stream ends in a 320-foot-wide living shoreline planted with native cattails and marsh grasses. Living shorelines are meant to replicate the natural buffer

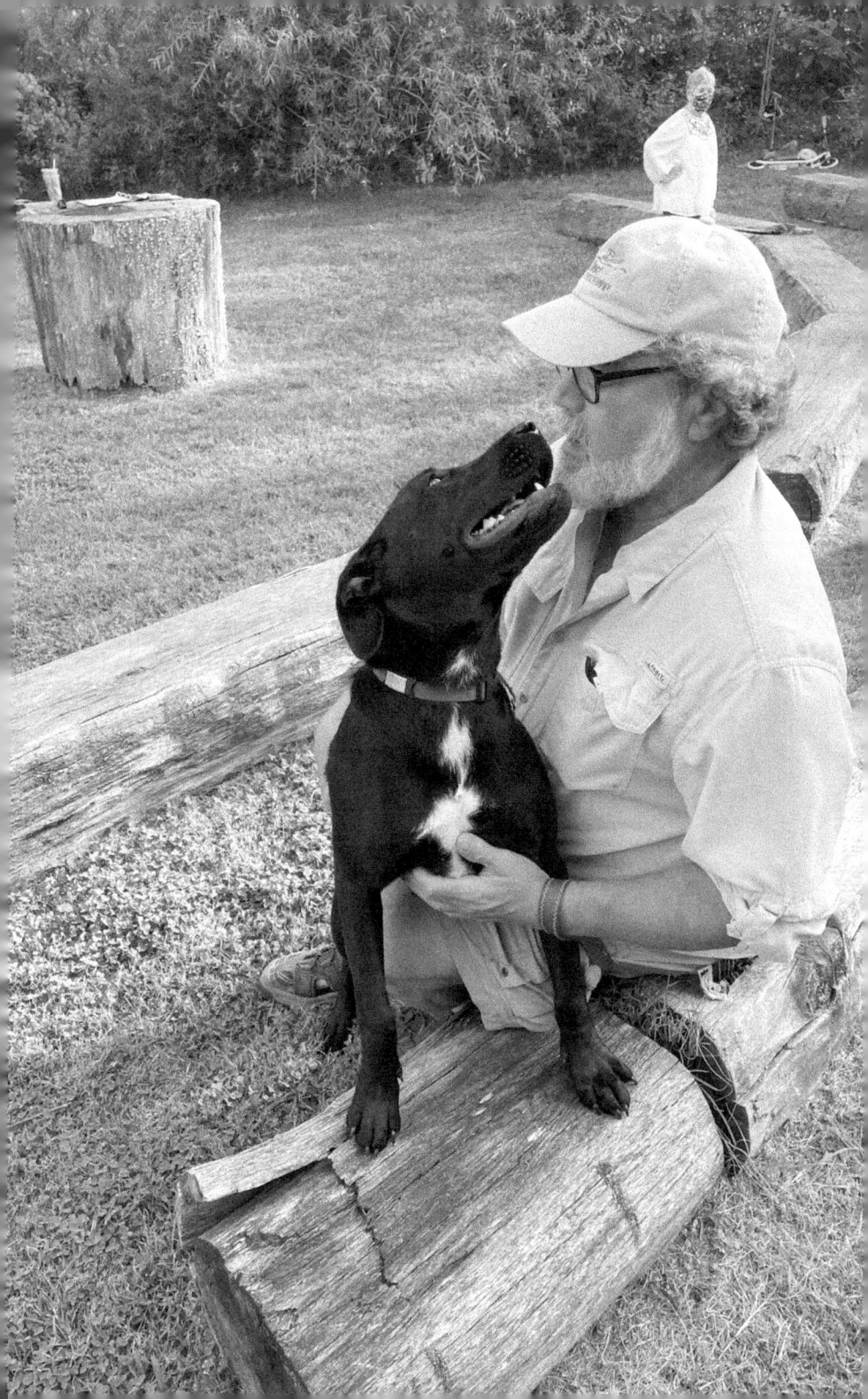

of a marsh, which both filters the stormwater coming off the land before it reaches the creek and protects the shoreline from erosion caused by boat wakes, windblown waves and storm surge. The protective rock barriers have gaps between them to allow critters like terrapins and horseshoe crabs to get in and out of the water.

Millie took in the scene while perched on a large sandstone boulder. I recalled coming to this very spot in 2018, just after the construction of the project had been completed, but before all of the vegetation had been planted. There was a heavy storm that afternoon, and I had donned my foul-weather gear, from my white rubber boots to my Black Diamond sou'wester hat, and trudged down to take a good look at the water flowing along the creek.

Sure enough, the restoration project was already working. The water coming off the street was nearly black with sediment and road pollution, but the step pools, large bioswales, cobble riffles, and log weirs slowed the runoff, allowed the debris to settle into the gravel beds, gave it time to cool, and the water flowing into the creek was clear as moonshine in a Mason jar.

I looked up and gazed through the downpour at the other side of the creek, where I was surprised to see a figure standing in a red rain suit. It turned out to be my friend Elvia Thompson, the co-founder of the Annapolis Green environmental organization. She had come to see the project in action, too. We were both impressed.

The $1.5 million restoration project started in 2013 when Pastor Diana and parishioner Betsy Love started building partnerships with the Anne Arundel Watershed Stewards Academy and RiverWise Congregations.

Funds for the initial design and permitting came from RiverWise Congregations, Interfaith Partners for the Chesapeake, the Watershed Stewards Academy, Maryland Department of Natural Resources, and the Chesapeake Bay Trust.

Funding for the construction was provided by DNR and the Atlantic Coastal Bays Trust Fund, while the Episcopal Church's United Thank Offering funded the amphitheater and other environmental literacy features on the grounds. A Chesapeake Bay Trust Watershed Assistance Grant Program award covered additional costs for the design and permitting. The Annapolis-based Underwood & Associates constructed the project.

Curiously, the offices of the Chesapeake Bay Trust and the Alliance for the Chesapeake Bay are located just a few blocks away in Eastport. All in all, a remarkable effort spearheaded by Pastor Diana and project manager Betsy Love and supported by countless hours of volunteer manpower has resulted in this astonishing gem of a green space for all of us to enjoy.

Millie and I caught up with Louise, who had started heading back toward the church. There we found the hillside covered with a bed of tiny purple flowers shaped like bluebells. Millie seemed fascinated with these for some reason. Ironically, they turned out to be called "obedient plants" apparently because if you bend them, they'll stay that way.

Hmm. Millie's not always that obedient and doesn't always stay when I tell her to stay. What would happen if I harvest a few handfuls, dry them out and sprinkle them into Millie's kibble?

St. Luke's Episcopal Church
1101 Bay Ridge Avenue
Eastport, Annapolis, MD 21403
410-268-5419
facebook.com/restorationofnature
Open dawn to dusk daily
Free admission
Plenty of parking on site
Amiable dogs on leashes are welcome; bring your own doggie bags
No toilets
Easy going

Walk 34

Magothy Greenway Natural Area: a Wonderful Wilderness

I have a friend who winterized his boat using the classic method involving a compass, an anchor, a chocolate bar, and a bottle of rum. He set sail and followed the compass south until the chocolate bar started to melt, then he set the anchor, and opened the bottle. As of January 2022, he and his wife were in Key West, where, they informed me gleefully, it was 82 degrees Fahrenheit.

I am not a winter person, but having no boat longer than my 17-foot canoe, I am stuck here in the snow. Still, I do enjoy a brisk winter walk, though not as much as Millie, our one-year-old rescue retriever. The recent surprise snowstorm left Louise and me huddled in front of the fireplace while watching Millie frolic in the front yard as she searched in vain for all the tennis balls that had disappeared into the drifts.

When the temperature inched above freezing one sunny day, Millie and I took a walk in the Magothy Greenway Natural area with my friend Tom Guay. Tom is the guy who makes things happen in the Severn River Association, one of America's oldest environmental organizations, going on more than 100 years so far.

Tom has activated the organization's comprehensive water-quality monitoring initiative, created an on-the-water environmental education program and fostered an aggressive campaign to plant millions of spat on oyster reefs all up and down the river. Tom's goal is to plant three billion oysters in the river, even, he says, if it takes the next hundred years to do it.

Tom brought along one of his protégés, Jack Beckham, who had recently earned his Bachelor of Science degree in environmental studies at Boston College. At the time, Jack was working with Severn River Association as a paid intern through the Chesapeake Conservation Corps program sponsored by the Chesapeake Bay Trust.

The Magothy Greenway Natural Area has a name that would make you think it's bigger than it really is. Coming in at just around 300 acres, this is one of Anne Arundel County's wonderful pocket wildernesses, a forest surrounded by suburban sprawl, but big enough to absorb you. It comprises two distinct habitats with several miles of trails that lead you through an area dominated by oaks and hollies and then into a dense thicket of tall white pines. The area covers the headwaters of Blackhole Creek on its way to feed the Magothy River.

The trailhead is located on the grounds of Looper's Field, a county recreation park on North Shore Road, abutting the Shore Acres Elementary School grounds in Pasadena. It's not listed on the AllTrails app yet. I was introduced to the site more than a year ago by Paul Spadaro, president of the Magothy River Association, whose volunteers blazed all the trails. The county parks and recreation department

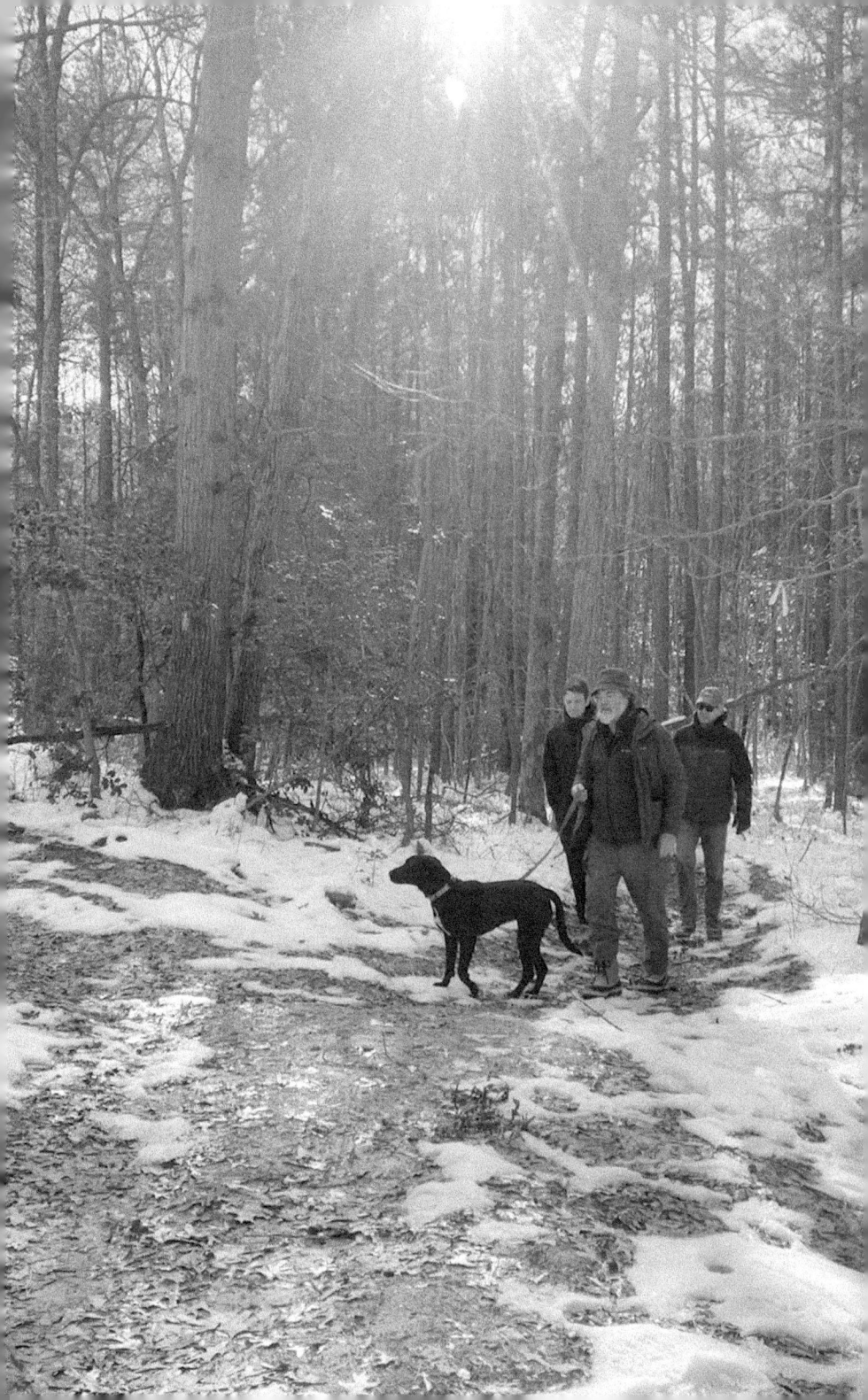

has designated these trails as suitable for equestrians as well as pedestrians. Not to mention us canine-strians. Dogs, of course, must be leashed just as horses, I suppose, must be reined.

The gate is usually chained, but you can log onto the county web site to get the combination for the lock. The trailhead is at the edge of the woods at the far end of the parking lot, marked by a hitching post. Just inside the woods, there's a small black marker near a holly sapling. This is a memorial to my friend Capt. Walter "Jake" Jacobs, who passed away in 2015.

Capt. Jake was a Chesapeake pilot for 44 years, guiding freighters and tankers up and down the Bay. He was a staunch supporter of several local environmental groups as well as the Annapolis Maritime Museum. Any time we got together, we'd sing a rousing duet of "Sailing Down the Chesapeake Bay." I sang that song solo in his memory as Tom, Jack, and I walked past the marker. Millie did not join in.

I have to mention here that in addition to his stellar work saving the Severn River, Tom Guay is also an extraordinarily talented musician and song writer. He plays guitar with the Eastport Oyster Boys and Blue Suede Bop. As we strolled along the level, leaf-matted path, we chatted mainly about music: the new Beatles documentary, a recently published collection of all of Paul McCartney's lyrics, and about the sad passing of our mutual musician friend, Don Cosden of Galesville.

I'd performed with Don and That West River Band at the Chesapeake Music Festival at the Smithsonian Environmental Research Center in 2019, and I was as impressed by his skill on the guitar as I was with his warmth and wit.

Millie led the way as we followed the red-blazed trail through the oak and holly portion of the woods. The path was clear for the most part, with a few puddles here and there glazed over with ice. Snow still covered the forest floor. The temperature was just around 33 degrees, but we were protected from the wind that we could hear rushing through the treetops above us.

I was actually fairly warm as we walked, layered in a flannel shirt, a thick fleece, and a hooded parka. I recently added a pair of fleece-lined trousers to my winter wardrobe, and I've pretty much been living in them this whole past month. I also have a new pair of snow boots with felt liners, and wearing all of that along with Gore-Tex ski gloves and my favorite tweed hat and wool scarf from Scotland, I didn't mind the cold. Millie had no protection at all, but didn't seem a bit bothered as she nosed along the trails.

Soon we made the transition into the pine forest, where we discovered the site of what in the spring would be a vernal pool, but was now just an empty glade. A few swamp magnolias still had some of their shiny green leaves attached. Jack explained that vernal pools are unique microhabitats that fill up with rain or snow melt in the spring and then dry out the rest of the year. They're ideal for fostering critters like frogs, salamanders, and turtles that need to begin their life cycles submerged. The last time I'd been by this one, it was shin-deep in tannic water and teeming with peepers.

We had walked about three miles by the time we'd found our way back to the car. We agreed that this is a pleasant walk, all flat terrain with just a few fallen trees to hitch ourselves over, and remarkable in its variety of habitats. Paul Spadaro informs me that the Magothy River Association volunteers will be expanding the trails into that section of the woods on the far side of North Shore Road in the coming year. He tells me the trails will lead to a bog where pitcher plants can be found. Can't wait to explore some more. When it's warmer.

Where's your favorite winter walk? Let me know at arundelhappytrails@gmail.com.

Magothy Greenway Natural Area
20 North Shore Road
Pasadena, MD 21122
410-222-7317
aacounty.org/locations-and-directions/magothy-greenway-natural-area
Parking: log on to web site for combination to gate lock
Open dawn to dusk daily
Free admission
No toilets
Agreeable leased dogs welcome; bring your own doggie bags
Easy going

Walk 35

Exploring Franklin Point State Park with Senator Sarah

Most of my heroes are people who are older than me—people I want to be like when I grow up. Like Parris Glendening, the former governor who has done so much for the restoration of the Chesapeake Bay. But one of my heroes is considerably younger—Sarah Elfreth, the youngest woman ever to be elected to the Maryland Senate (and as of November 5th, 2024, the youngest women sent by Maryland to Congress).

I was acquainted with Sarah when she worked at the National Aquarium in Baltimore before she was elected to the District 30 seat in 2018, and I was impressed with her energy and vision even then. Since then, she's proven to be a dynamic force for the environment, serving as the Senate chair of the Joint Committee on the Chesapeake and Atlantic Coastal Bay Critical Areas and most recently taking on the mantle of chair of the Chesapeake Bay Commission.

The goal of the commission is to serve as catalyst to coordinate legislation and policy action between Maryland, Pennsylvania and Virginia to restore the Bay. I can't think of a stronger candidate for that role than Sen. Elfreth. Sarah and I got together last weekend for a hike through Franklin Point State Park. She wanted to bring me up to speed on a new piece of legislation she's introducing to boost funding for state parks, The Great Maryland Outdoors Act.

It was on one of those early-hint-of-spring days in February, 2022, when we met at the park in Shady Side. Sarah was as happy to meet Millie, my rescue retriever, as Millie was to meet her. I strapped myself into my new dual harness rig with me on one end of the tether and Millie on the other. I highly recommend this system. It's hands-free dog walking, even more companionable and far more comfortable than a hand-held leash.

As we strolled down the lane toward the water's edge, Sarah noted that over the past couple of years, during the peak of the pandemic, visitation to Maryland state parks increased more than 45 percent. I've seen that myself in my rambles, and not just in state parks, but in county and city parks as well. That's a good thing, she agreed, but it's put a strain on the parks' infrastructure and staff, both of which have been seriously underfunded in the past.

The bill is the result of a year-long study by a commission led by Gov. Glendening, Sen. Elfreth and Delegate Eric Luedtke. The study lists a number of recommendations, including increasing Maryland Park Service staff; supporting projects that mitigate the effects of climate change such as flood barriers and forest buffers; relieving overcrowding by increasing the number of state parks, particularly sites of historic significance and sites that can offer outdoor recreation opportunities to minority communities; improving amenities at existing parks and

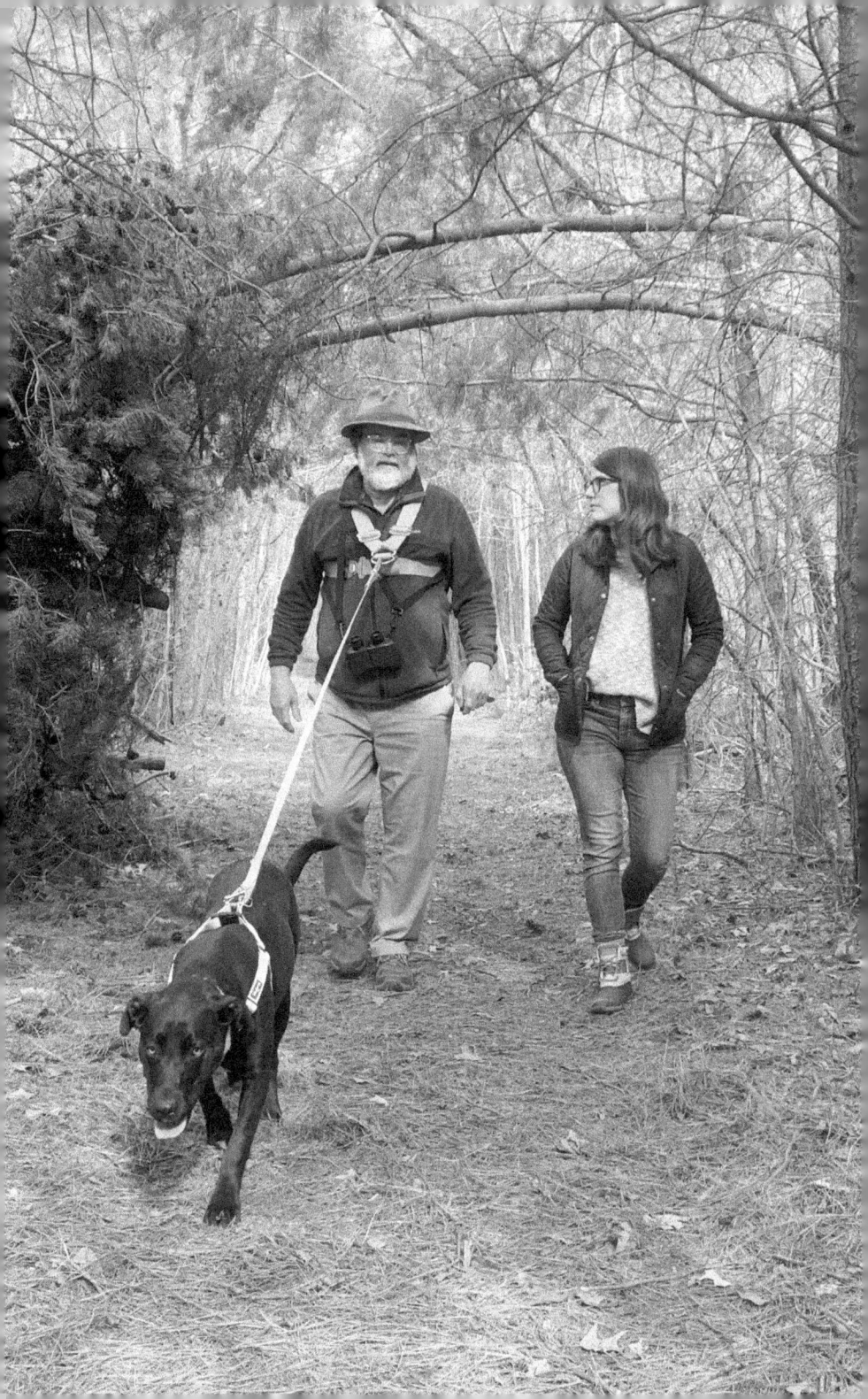

devoting $68 million to catching up on a backlog of needed repairs; and increasing public access to our waterways with paddle-able boat launches and the like.

We stopped in the glade overlooking Deep Creek, which in reality is a tidal pond that's about as deep as a toddler's swimming pool. If ever a site could use some investment, it's Franklin Point. You can launch a canoe or a kayak by tipping it off the edge of the pond, but outside of a portable toilet and a couple of picnic tables, there just ain't much there—except 477 acres of saltmarsh, meadow and forest. The park is maintained and monitored by volunteers.

Sarah and I crossed a raised berm, actually the overgrown landing strip of the family-owned air park that occupied this area up until the early 1990s, like the one at Lee Airport in nearby Edgewater. It's cluttered with the sweet gums there are among the first trees to appear when a meadow transitions to forest.

The property was doomed for development until a group known as the South Arundel Citizens for Responsible Development (SACReD) fought for its rescue. Eventually, the State of Maryland took it over, but lacking the resources to do anything with it, they padlocked the gate and let it lie fallow for 20 years. In 2015, the West & Rhode Riverkeeper organization signed an agreement with the Maryland Park Service to provide the volunteer people power to open the park to the public.

I had the privilege of serving as the Riverkeeper at that time, and I was blessed with a great team of volunteers.

They got busy cleaning up the site, creating trails, and providing monitors to keep an eye on the place. It opened to the public in 2017 and is now open every day, all year long, sunrise to sunset, and free of charge. Still, it needs a lot of work to reach its full potential.

As Sarah and I talked, Millie led us along a grassy path that eventually tunneled through a grove of longleaf pines. The trail peeked out onto the narrow channel that leads from the pond through the marsh and out onto the open Chesapeake Bay. The senator noted how important our parks are, not just for the health of the citizens and the environment of Maryland, but also for the health of the economy.

State parks generate more than $14 billion in consumer spending yearly; 109,000 direct jobs; $4.4 billion in wages and salaries; and $951 million in state and local tax revenue. The senator rattled off these facts from the top of her head. I didn't stop to write all of that down in my reporter's notebook, although I could have, seeing as I had both hands free, but I looked up her testimony in support of the bill when I got home. I concurred that public parks are a good investment all around.

The grassy trail ends in a loop where it touches the marsh, but a side trail marked with a white blaze leads into the oak-and-holly forest. Millie led us into the woods and out onto the open marsh. At one time, the landing strip ended about there in ramps where seaplanes could be launched into the water. Now, it's an expanse of cord grass and bayberry, with a wall of tall invasive phragmite reeds encroaching on the native marsh plants.

Far off to the east, we could see the treetops of Franklin Point proper, a spit of land that extends down from the end of Columbia Beach Road. It's separated from the rest of the park by this marsh and another shallow channel called Flag Pond. The exposed shore of the point on the Bay side has eroded severely over the years. It bears the brunt of wind and waves that can build up with a 100-mile fetch up the Bay. There have been plans in the works to protect this site with a living shoreline, but somehow that project has been stalled. Perhaps the senator's legislation can give it a kick start.

Sarah wondered if there was a way to get from here to there, but there isn't. I've long wrestled with how to connect the two disparate sections of the park. A boardwalk would be nice, but that would be expensive and also block sunlight from any underwater grasses that might be growing below. It wasn't until I got to bed that night that the perfect solution came to me.

I've been reading David McCullough's amazing book, *The Pioneers*, about the people who moved westward in the late 1700s and early 1800s. Early in the saga, he writes about a group of hardy settlers on their way through the wilds of Pennsylvania to the Ohio country. They had crossed Chestnut Ridge in 1788, and on February 14 "they reached Sumerill's Ferry on the Youghiougheny River, thirty miles southeast of Pittsburgh." I dropped the book and picked up my mother's grandfather's book of our family history. That wasn't Sumerill's Ferry, it was Simeral's ferry, owned by one of my ancestors, Alexander Simeral and his brother, John.

It occurred to me that we could connect the main section of the park to Franklin Point with a ferry across Flag Pond. It could be something as simple as an aluminum jon boat and a cable. Wouldn't that be a hoot?

Senator Sarah, see if you can write that into your bill.

Franklin Point State Park is located in southern Anne Arundel County. Access is on the Dent Road entrance off Shady Side Road between Churchton and Shady Side. It's managed by the staff at Sandy Point State Park. Wear waterproof boots and beware of the atrocious plethora of ticks as the weather gets warmer.

Franklin Point State Park
End of Dent Road
Shady Side, MD 20764
410-974-22149 dnr.maryland.gov/publiclands/pages/southern/franklinpoint.aspx
Entrance: Log on for combination to gate lock if launching car-top boats
Parking available in the lot to the left before the gate
Open dawn to dusk, seven days a week
Free admission
Portable toilet in the parking lot
Pleasant dogs on leashes are welcome; bring your own doggie bags
Easy going, with some soggy bits and lots of summer bugs

Walk 36

What's Up at Downs Memorial Park

People who walk with their equines (horses) and ride on them are equestrians. People who walk on their pedes (feet) are pedestrians. I walk with my canine (Millie), so I must be a "canestrian." Given that horses have all sorts of elaborate tack to keep their riders attached to them, I thought it would be good to rig up a new system of connecting me to my dog.

Holding a leash in one hand and a walking stick in the other can be awkward at best, and after a few miles of the dog wanting to walk at one speed and you at another altogether, it can get downright tiresome. Then if you want to use your binoculars to spot a passing bird or simply stop to blow your nose, you can get so tangled up it's like a Laurel and Hardy routine.

Millie has a harness that works quite well. I attach the leash to a ring between her shoulder blades and she can walk along without getting strangled by her collar. That made me think that if a harness works well for her, why wouldn't one work for me, too?

So I dug up an old harness that's been sitting in a bag on a shelf in the garage for 20 years. It's one that offshore sailors use to keep them attached to the boat when a big wave attempts to sweep them overboard. The one and only time I ever used it, I was helping a friend sail his new boat from Southampton, England, across the English

Channel and the Bay of Biscay to Lisbon, Portugal. We encountered several nasty storms along the way, and I was grateful to be strapped into the cockpit so securely. Almost as grateful as I was when we got back to solid ground.

The other day, I wrestled myself into the harness, clicked one end of the six-foot-long tether to the D-ring in the middle of my chest, attached the other to Millie's harness and off we went. Hands-free dog walking turns out to be quite comfortable for both of us.

On a particular January morning in 2022, Millie and I had driven up to Downs Memorial Park in Pasadena, one of Anne Arundel County's premier regional parks. It had been raining earlier in the week, so I figured most of the natural-surface paths in the area would still be a bit squishy, and not wanting to churn up the mud with our footprints, I thought we'd go for a walk where there are hard-surface trails instead. Downs Park is the only major park in the county that we hadn't explored, so that made it a logical choice for this week's ramble.

Downs, as it happens, has more than five miles of paved trail meandering around its 236 acres set between the Chesapeake Bay and Bodkin Creek. It's about a 40-minute drive from our home in Annapolis. The park is named after John "Jack" Downs, a former county councilman who died in 1976, the year before the county purchased the property. The park opened 30 years ago.

The property was the site of an elaborate estate built by a wealthy tobacco importer in 1913. The park's three large picnic pavilions are on the footprints of the estate's guest cottages. The Brightwater pavilion at the north end features the stone chimney from the original cottage. Rangers discovered the remains of a formal garden and restored it to its Victorian splendor, making it a popular venue for weddings.

Millie and I parked by the Brightwater pavilion and strapped ourselves together. We strolled along the park's 2,000 feet of Chesapeake Bay waterfront, enjoying the chilly sunshine and the clear skies. With no leash to hold, I could use both hands to steady my binoculars to view the panorama while Millie searched the posts of a split rail fence for secret messages. The view is astonishing. From there, you can see the Bay Bridge a full eight miles away to the south, or look across to Love Point at the northern tip of Kent Island, another eight miles away to the southeast, and 10 miles across the open Bay to Rock Hall on the Eastern Shore.

A large pylon offshore is one of the two range markers for the Craighill Channel, which light up at night so Chesapeake pilots line up these lights to guide ships into the mouth of the Patapsco River and on to the Port of Baltimore. The next time you're in the passenger seat of your car driving westward across the Bay Bridge, particularly at dusk, look off to your right when you're about halfway across and you'll see the two bright lights of these markers. When the lights converge, you're seeing what the pilot sees when steering straight for the mouth of the river.

We found the gate leading down the wooden steps to the park's doggie beach, where we met a young woman and her energetic American akita, a husky-ish dog who engaged Millie in a friendly wrestling match the minute I let her loose. As the two dogs frolicked up and down the short expanse of sand, we humans chatted. She told me she lives nearby and visits the park frequently. She noted that the salt pond behind the beach is populated with immense numbers of turtles that pop their heads out of the water in the warmer months. Her dog likes to wade in the water, while Millie still hasn't figured out what her webbed toes are supposed to be used for.

Moving on along the trail, we crossed a wooden pedestrian bridge—or should I say, canestrian bridge—over the roadway to the part of the park that borders Locust Cove, a branch of Bodkin Creek. According to a study by the Maritime Archaeological and Historical Society published in 2010, the Bodkin peninsula is long and narrow, vaguely shaped like a knife, "or in a term more common in the 18th century, a bodkin. This resemblance is generally assumed to be the source of the creek's name."

The path led through a pleasant forest of oak and holly, mixed with yellow poplar and loblolly pines. On this mid-week afternoon, we met just a handful of other people; a couple of joggers, a cyclist—or should I say, "cyclestrian"—and a few other canestrians. One older gentleman was accompanied by a brace of corgis. He was on a three-mile hike, while the corgis were walking 10.

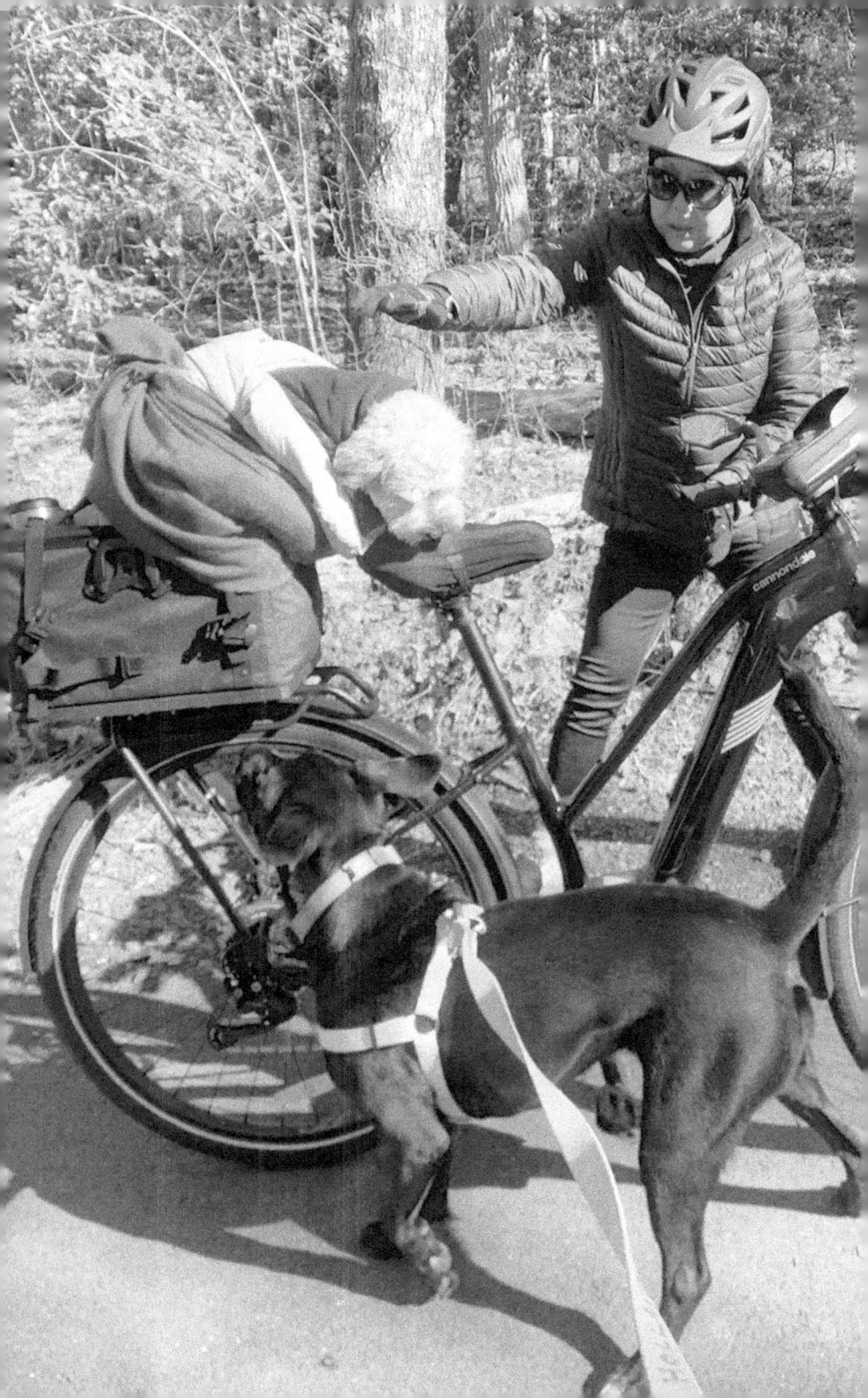

I heard a *ding-ding* behind us and stepped off to the left while a woman on a bicycle passed us in a whirl. To my surprise, she had a fluffy little pooch swaddled in a shawl and stuffed in a box behind her seat. I tried to hail her so we could talk about her pup, but she was off around the bend in a flash. Millie and I stopped to inspect the kayak launch on the creek, and when we returned to the main trail, the woman had looped around and was riding back our way. This time, I waved her down and she stopped to chat.

She introduced herself as Yong Kim. Ms. Kim lives nearby and visits the park almost every day. "My day doesn't start until I take Coco for a ride," she said. Coco, it turns out, is a too-cute cross between a purebred bichon frise and Yorkshire terrier. "She's a 'York-chon,'" Ms. Kim explained. Millie was more interested in Coco than Coco was in Millie. As for me, I was trying to figure out what to call someone who rides a bike with her dog.

Downs Memorial Park
8311 John Downs Loop, Pasadena
www.aacounty.org/departments/recreation-parks/parks/downs/
Admission: $6 per car for parking w/discounts
Plenty of parking on site
Restrooms open year-round
Amiable dogs on leash (or in bicycle baskets) are welcome; doggie bag dispensers available
Easy going

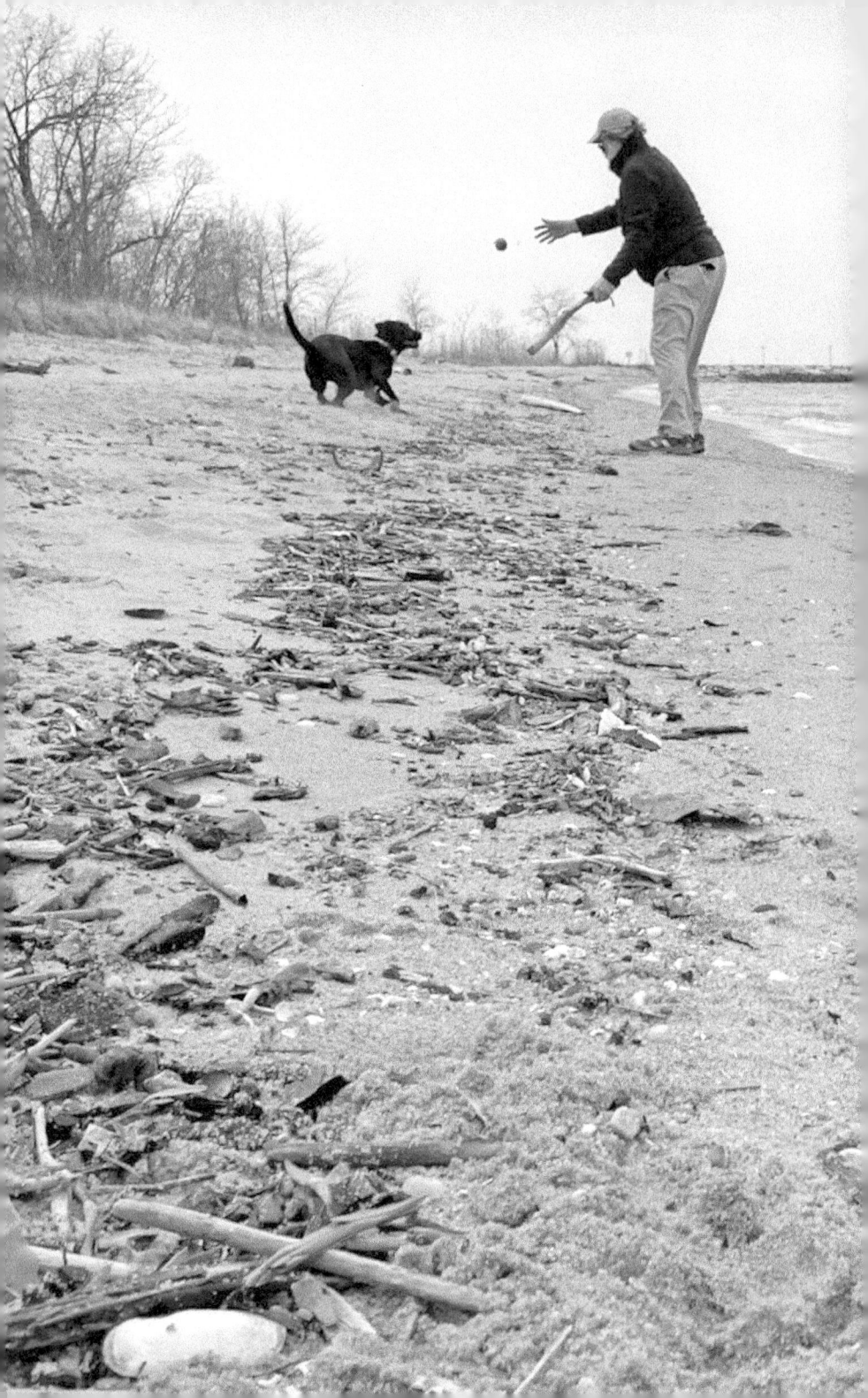

Walk 37

Millie Runs Happily Amok at Matapeake Dog Beach

My friend Eric Smith read the most recent column where I mentioned the walking stick that I had hacked out of a bush. Eric is an artist who has drawn all the witty editorial cartoons in the *Annapolis Capital* newspaper for many years, and when we met for an historic gab session recently, he presented me with a proper stick he had fashioned out of a branch from a witch-hazel tree.

I tried it out this past week on the path down to the Matapeake Dog Beach on Kent Island, and like Eric's drawings, it's quite a work of art. In addition to creating cartoons, Eric also mastered the craft of carving bows from the branches of various trees. This walking stick is eccentric in shape, yet eminently practical – light but stiff, with a suede patch for a handle and a British pound coin mounted as a cap.

So if I'm ever in a pub and short on change for a pint, this stick will come in handy. On top of that, old-time dowsers would use witch-hazel sticks to locate the source of underground water, so I'll never go thirsty no matter what. I discovered later that Indians would brew witch-hazel leaves to make a medicinal tea. We have a brown jug of the astringent liniment extracted from witch-hazel bark in our medicine cabinet. And now, I have a witch-hazel walking stick, thanks to Eric Smith.

Millie accompanied me on my adventure across the Chesapeake Bay Bridge to Kent Island. Millie, of course, is our wonderful rescue retriever. Now that the socks have been burned in the time-honored equinoxical rite that miraculously makes spring appear, Millie has ventured into the water and discovered what the webbing between her toes is for. I've been taking her to the doggie beach at Quiet Waters Park and tossing a tennis ball into the water for her to fetch, just a few feet away at first, then farther and farther and deeper and deeper until she finally caught on.

I had heard that Queen Anne's County had its own dedicated dog beach and decided to give it a try. Curiously, it's located where the ferry from Sandy Point used to dock before the first Bay Bridge was built in 1952. It's just a half-hour drive from our home in Annapolis.

When we arrived at Matapeake Beach on a mid-week mid-day in March 2022, ours was the sole car in the lot. There's a chain-link fence with a gate leading onto the grounds of the people-only part of the park. This is the county's one public swimming beach. In addition to an outdoor amphitheater and a family picnic area, there's also a clubhouse on the bluff overlooking the Bay.

You can rent the clubhouse for family gatherings. The building is actually the old ferry terminal, built in 1936. According to the Queen Anne's County Parks and Recreation web site, the clubhouse operated as a ferry terminal and restaurant for the next 16 years until the opening of the Bay Bridge in 1952. That's about the time that the Natural Resources Police started using the site as a marine academy and shooting range. The county acquired the property in 1999 with the help of DNR's Program Open Space, renovated the clubhouse and opened the beach to the public.

The path to the dog beach runs along the outside of the fence and into the loblolly pines. About halfway down the mile-long trail, the path descends a steep bank and the forest changes from pines to yellow poplars and other hardwoods. It soon opens up onto a breathtaking panorama of the Chesapeake Bay. That view alone is worth the trip.

The full 4.5-mile length of the bridge forms the northern horizon, while the massive stone jetty protecting the NRP boat basin juts out into the Bay along the southern horizon. I used my binoculars to scan the opposite shoreline in between. You can plainly see the Eiffel-shaped towers on Greenbury Point, and all the domes and spires that make the Annapolis skyline so unique: the Naval Academy Chapel, the State House, St. Anne's and St. Mary's steeples.

While the beach is 23 miles away by car, City Dock is less than seven miles away as the osprey flies. And there were osprey whistling overhead now that they've finally returned to the Bay. How wonderful that the view of the "Ancient City" hasn't changed all that much in at least a hundred years. Oh, except you can also see tops of the skyscrapers all the way out at Parole Towne Centre on the far horizon.

Closer in, I could see two of the 12 freighters at anchor in the middle of the Bay, an area known as Annapolis Roads. They're waiting for space to open up at the Port of Baltimore, 35 miles to the north. Ironically, as we headed back across the bridge, I could see the massive hulk of the 1,000-foot-long container ship that's run aground off Gibson Island.

The beach itself is more than two football fields long, and we had it all to ourselves. I found a piece of driftwood and used it as a baseball bat to hit a tennis ball for Millie to fetch, and we spent the next hour running up and down the shoreline, enjoying the 60-degree breeze. While the South River has been quite placid on our recent visits, the wind was kicking up the waves on the open Bay, and Millie was too spooked to wade into them. So we kept our frolicking up on the dry sand.

Millie is quite the athlete when it comes to chasing the balls I bat for her. She'll leap into the air like an outfielder snagging a homer heading for the stands. She'll dive for grounders like a shortstop with a man sprinting for third. When she gets the ball, she'll do a little victory prance before she gets around to bringing it back to me. Then she'll drop it and I'll whack at it again. My batting average is fairly good, too.

We kept this up until she discovered a half-sized tennis ball that was a pretty pink color. She seemed taken by this novelty. She dropped her green ball and sniffed at the little pink ball, went back to the green ball, then decided she would play with the pink ball after all. She brought it back to me and though it was a bit of a challenge to hit with my ersatz bat, she chased and fetched it several times and liked it so much, she brought it home. I'm sure the next dog to come along will enjoy the green ball we left behind. My new walking stick worked well on our walk back up to the parking lot.

Of course, I had to find out about the name Matapeake. When we got back, I consulted my cherished tome, *The Placenames of Maryland, Their Origin and Meaning* by Hamill Kenny. Matapeake, he notes, was the name of the Indians who lived on that section of Kent Island when the colonists started showing up in the early 1600s. The name could be translated from ancient Algonquian as "Junction of Waters." Matapex, which is likely a plural form of Matapeake, is the name of a community and a portion of Shipping Creek on the eastern side of the island.

It was there that the very first English settlement in Maryland was founded in 1631, when William Claiborne established a fort and a trading post to buy furs from the Indians. He was a loyal Virginian and this eventually led to armed conflict with the Marylanders who arrived three years later. But that's a story I'll save to share with my friend Eric Smith when we get together for our next historic gab fest.

JEFFERSON HOLLAND | 245

Matapeake Clubhouse and Beach
201 Clubhouse Drive
Stevensville, MD 21666

Queen Anne's County Parks & Recreation

Open 8 a.m. to dusk daily

Plenty of parking on site

Free admission

Portable toilet in the parking lot

Congenial dogs are allowed off leash; bring your own doggie bags

Easy going

Walk 38

Stroll Horn Point on the Eastport Walking Tour

It turns out I've got a dog that performs tricks, but not just normal dog tricks. No, Millie does this amazing vanishing act. This generally happens around the night of the full moon. She de-materializes from the back yard and presto! She re-appears on the other side of the fence so she can go play with the foxes. How she does it, I don't know. She must be some sort of Houdini-esque hybrid pedigree, what a writer on the fursnpaw.com blog calls a Labracadabrador.

When not being lured away by wily foxes, Millie is quite obedient and eager to please. She was perfectly well behaved when we went for a walk around the Eastport peninsula the other day. Eastport is the maritime district on the Horn Point peninsula across the harbor from Annapolis proper. There are more marine-related businesses there than anywhere between Newport, Rhode Island, and Fort Lauderdale, Florida.

It's a very walk-able neighborhood. In fact, it's got its own walking tour, with 20 interpretive panels scattered about the six-by-four block area between Annapolis Harbor and Back Creek. The tour got its start in 1998 as a project of the Eastport Historical Committee, which evolved into the Annapolis Maritime Museum in 2000. The late Peg Wallace was the dynamo behind both organizations. Peg was an inspirational being,

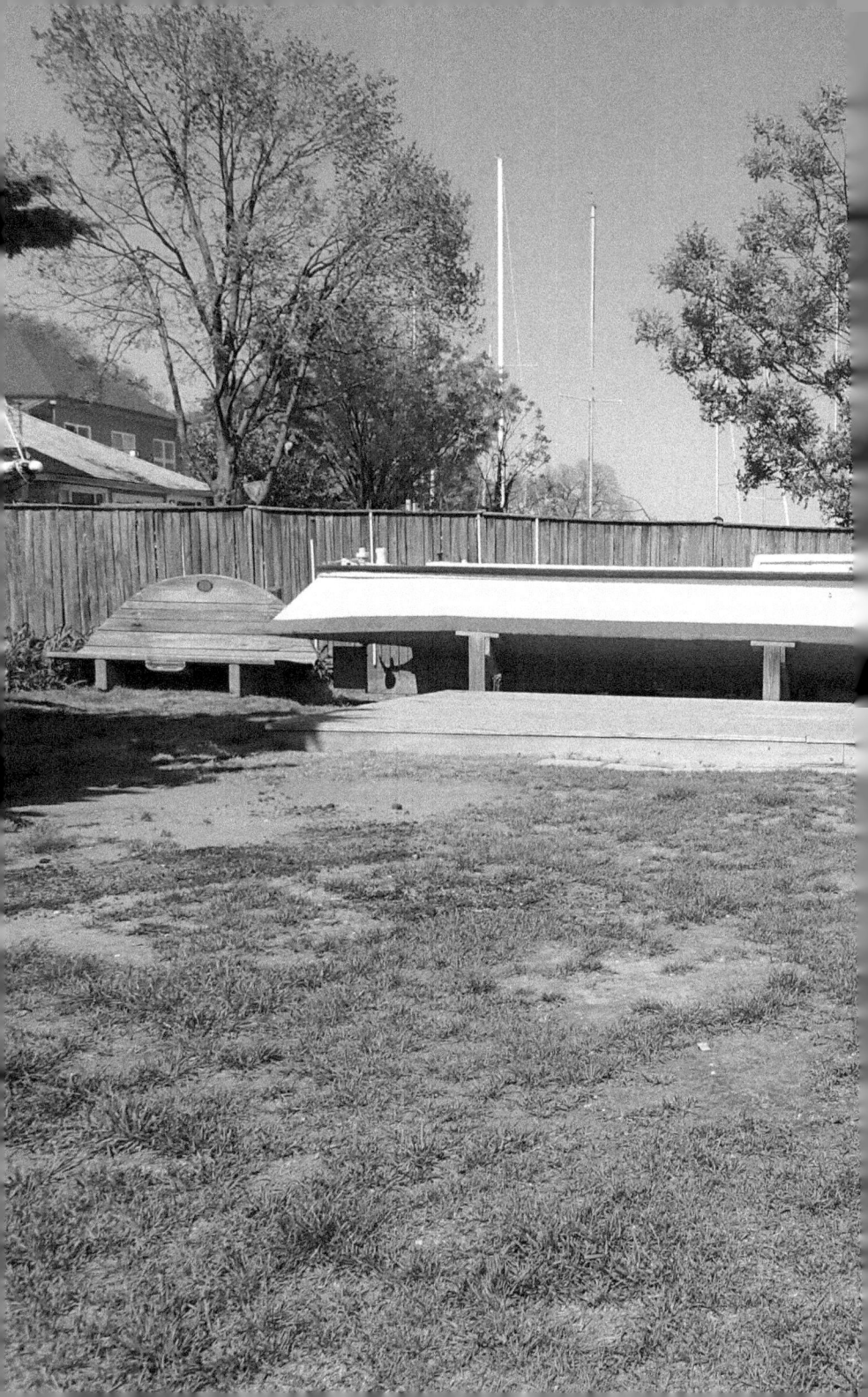

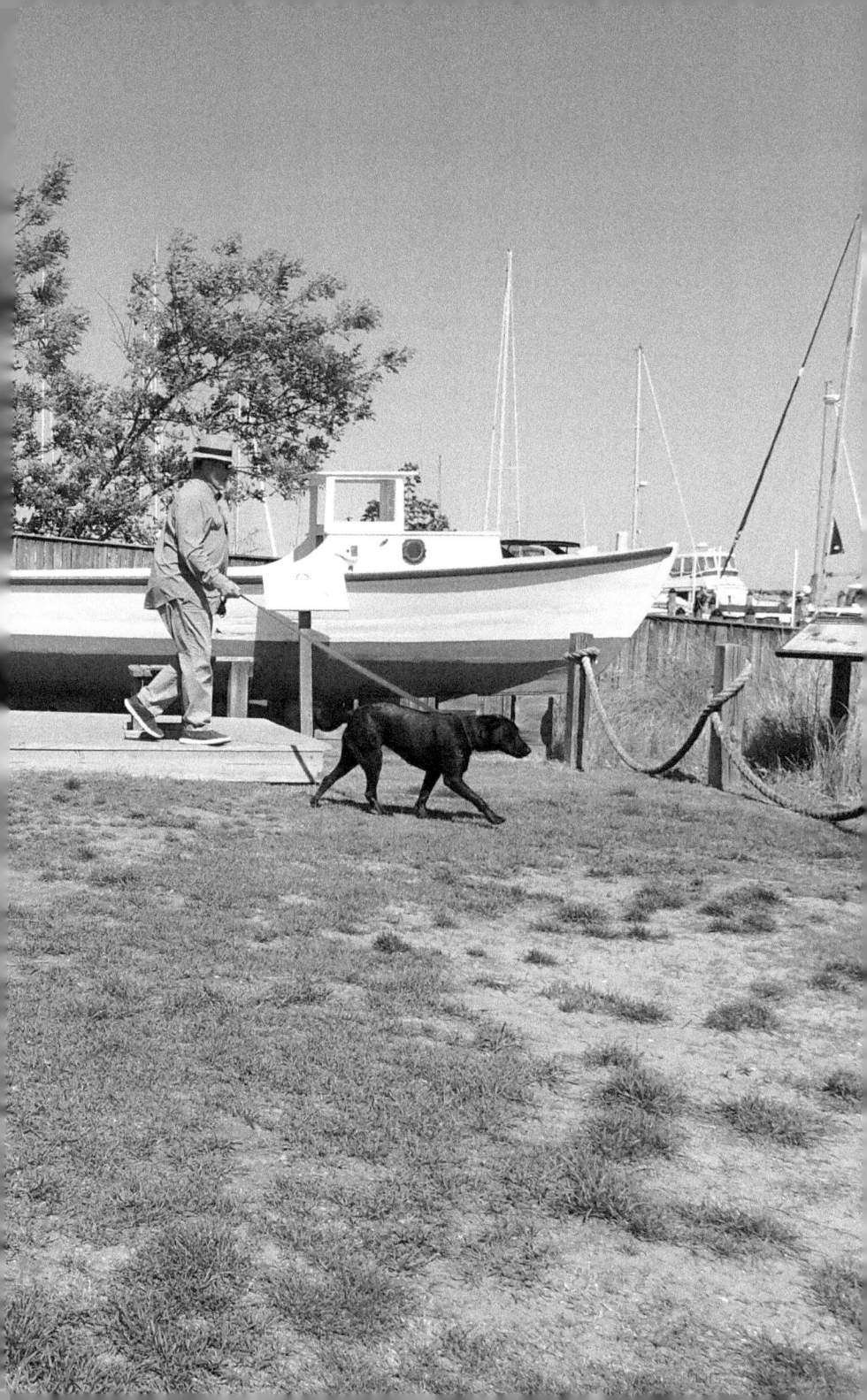

one of my true heroes. I had the privilege of working with her as the first director of the museum. She had a bumper sticker on her old Mercedes sedan that read, *Well behaved women seldom make history.*

The original sign panels were created by Peg, along with Elizabeth Reed and the late Mike Miron. Several were damaged by Hurricane Isabel in 2003, and Elizabeth and I helped Peg update all the panels in 2005. Many of these succumbed to the sun and weather over time, and they were replaced last year, mainly through the efforts of Mark Hildebrand. There's no linear logic to the route, so you can start anywhere. There are orientation panels at the foot of the Spa Creek Bridge and at the museum at the Back Creek end of Second Street.

That's where Millie and I started our tour. The museum occupies the former McNasby Oyster Company building. In 1918, William McNasby Sr. built the first structure on this site, which was damaged by an unnamed hurricane in 1933. It was renovated and expanded to serve as an oyster and crab processing plant until the business closed in the early 1970s following the death of William "Mac" McNasby Jr.

The structure briefly served as a waterman's co-op, but that venture folded when the oyster population plummeted in the early 1980s. It had been abandoned for years before the museum leased it from the city of Annapolis in the year 2000.

The building was nearly destroyed by another hurricane in 2003. Yes, I know that Isabel had technically been downgraded to a tropical storm by the time it hit Eastport, but I was there and I'm calling it a hurricane. We rebuilt the building, making it as storm-resistant as possible, and reopened it in 2008 with a new exhibit on the oyster industry and a new environmental education program, both of which are still running strong.

But that day, we weren't there to visit the museum. Millie and I were there for the adjacent waterfront park at the mouth of Back Creek. I had forgotten to bring my new junior league baseball bat, but I did have a tennis ball, which I hurled into the creek, much to Millie's delight. There are two traditional Chesapeake Bay workboats on display in the park, a small skipjack and a drake-tail workboat named in honor of Peg Wallace. The workboat works as the backdrop to a popular summer concert series.

After Millie had worn off at least some of her energy swimming after tossed balls, she shook off and we headed down Chester Avenue to the end of the Horn Point peninsula. One of the wonderful things about Eastport is that there's a miniature waterfront park at the end of nearly every street, or at least a spot where you can view the water.

The beach at the end of Chesapeake Avenue is particularly lovely. The marker there describes Fort Horn, which stood on the bluff at the end of the point and protected Annapolis from attack by the Royal Navy during the

Revolutionary War and the War of 1812. I lounged in one of the Adirondack chairs while Millie took another swim. The beach looks out over the mouth of the Severn River and the Eiffel-tower-shaped antennas hovering over Greenbury Point on the far side.

Around the corner from here, there are row houses on what's now called Jeremy Way. These served as housing for workers at the glass factory that occupied the corner of Severn Avenue and Second Street around the turn of the 20th century. They were built by the factory's manager, Charles Murphy. One of these town houses was designated as a post office for the village that had been growing on Horn Point since the end of the Civil War. The new post office needed a name, and Murphy provided one. He named it after his hometown in Maine: Eastport.

Millie dried off as we strolled down Severn Avenue. The shoreline of the harbor from Horn Point all the way up past the Spa Creek Bridge is packed chock-a-block with modern marinas. An enterprising cat could make his way by hopping boat-to-boat from First Street to Sixth Street without ever getting his feet wet.

From the late 1800s up to after World War II, these marinas were working boatyards where craftsmen built and maintained wooden workboats, skipjacks, bugeye schooners, and proper yachts. As the oyster industry dwindled, so did the golden age of wooden boats. In the 1950s and '60s, fiberglass boats proved to be more affordable and easier to maintain, and that's when the boatyards devoted to workboats evolved into marinas catering to modern recreational sailboats and powerboats.

There's a plaque at the end of Fourth Street dedicated to the late Arnie Gay, who was instrumental in that transition and who was perhaps the one person responsible for Annapolis' claim to be America's Sailing Capital.

That phrase was actually coined by the venerable naval architect Melbourne Smith, who designed the original Pride of Baltimore. He noted that while Newport may have more sailboats, it's not the capital of Rhode Island. Annapolis might not be the Sailing Capital of America, but it surely is America's Sailing Capital. Though Melbourne died in 2018, he's still got a stool dedicated to his memory at the Boatyard Bar and Grill just a few blocks down Severn Avenue.

Millie and I got to the Spa Creek Bridge, where two significant historical events occurred over the centuries. In 1781, the Marquis de Lafayette and his troops encamped here on their way to help General George Washington defeat the British at Yorktown. Then in 1998, the citizenry of Eastport revolted and seceded from the City of Annapolis to form the Maritime Republic of Eastport. Some say they're still revolting. You can see the yellow MRE flags proudly waving all around the peninsula.

MRE volunteers stage annual fundraising events like the Tug of War across the harbor on the first Saturday in November. Over the years, they've raised more than $500,000 for local nonprofits like the Eastport Elementary

School and the SPCA. Every year, on a Saturday in mid-May, they host the ".05K Bridge Run" that starts on the Eastport side of the Spa Creek Bridge and goes all the way over to the Annapolis side, with a water break in the middle. I once ran that—or hobbled it, anyway—six weeks after knee replacement surgery. I didn't win that year.

Millie and I hardly covered half of the Eastport Walking Tour that afternoon. Next time, we'll concentrate on Second Street and Chester Avenue, where many of Eastport's black families have lived for generations. These panels interpret the community's deep roots in the church, the school, and the Chesapeake Bay.

Eastport Walking Tour
www.allaboutannapolis.com/eastport-walking-tour.html
This is a free, self-guided tour on public streets in the Eastport neighborhood of Annapolis.

Ben Ogle's Bones

In 1999, I read a quote from then Mayor Ellen O. Moyer that she was launching a tongue-in-cheek search for the unmarked grave of Benjamin Ogle, one of Maryland's first governors. He had married Henrietta Margaret Hill, known as "Henry." She had inherited much of what we now call Eastport, and Ben used the Horn Point Peninsula to raise his stock of thoroughbred racing horses.

I was surprised to read further that the mayor was pleased to announce that the Poet Laureate of Eastport was writing an ode to commemorate the search. Hmm…I was that poet and this was the first I'd heard of the commission.

I figured I'd better get to work on this command performance, so I sought inspiration in a churchyard in Baltimore, where I found the gravestone of one of my favorite poets, Edgar Allen Poe. This is the result:

Show me the bones of Benjamin Ogle,
Search in the gardens and under the bridge,
Find me the grave of that real estate mogul
Who owned all of Eastport and half of Bay Ridge.

Nobody knows where they buried the gentleman,
Chaser of steeples, breeder of steeds,
Once he was governor over our merry land,
Now no one knows what his epitaph reads.

Ben's father, Sam, was lain 'neath St. Anne's
Along with Ben's infantile brother;
They were moved to make room
    for the new church's plans,
But to just where, no one's yet discovered.

So there's oodles of Ogles,
    but no one knows where,
No monument commemorates them;
They might be interred on the grounds of Bel Air,
Their Prince George's County estate, then.

Or they might be out there on the Ogleton Farm,
A place long since renamed Bay Ridge,
Or they might be where Lafayette's troops
    stacked their arms,
Right there by the Eastport bridge.

Ben let it be known that none should despair
When fate cut his noble life short;
If eternal contentment were Ben Ogle's plan,
Where else would he lie but Eastport?

So if your dog's digging about in the yard
And he unearths a stick or a stone,
Be careful of what you're about to discard—
It just might be Ben Ogle's bones!

Walk 39

Doggie Parks for the Dog Days of Summer

Summer started wimpishly this past week on a cool, damp day. Still Millie, my rescue retriever, needed to get out and get some exercise. She does not accept inclement weather as an excuse to not go for a walk. We're fortunate to live in a community near Quiet Waters Park, where there are not just one but three dog parks: a fenced-in area for small dogs, another one for big dogs, and a fenced-off section of sandy beach right on the South River.

Almost every day, I hit tennis balls into the river with my baseball bat, and Millie dashes merrily after them. On this day, I looked out the window. "Let's not go in the rain, Millie, you might get wet." Millie gave me that look, curiously the same look my wife gives me when I say something really stupid. So, reluctantly, I scooped my car keys out of the basket, slipped into my rain jacket and snatched Millie's leash. She sat patiently at the top of the stairs, waiting for my command. I called to her and she bounded down, barely touching a step, then dashed through the door and headed for the car. Off we went to the park.

On any sunny day, you can see cars heading for the park with a back window rolled down and a furry head sticking out, ears and tongue all flapping in the breeze in eager anticipation of a visit to the dog park. I've often thought that would make a delightful photo essay. On this rainy day, we drove with all the windows up. I showed my old-guy lifelong pass at the gate—one of the best investments you can make—and we drove to the far end of the park. We leashed up and walked to the South River Overlook, took the stairs down the steep embankment, and headed for the dog beach. There's a new fence and gate guarding the beach, which comprises a short crescent of sand in between stone jetties. You can look out the mouth of the river from there, and on a clear day, see the southern tip of Kent Island across the Bay.

Millie and I had the beach all to ourselves. I hit balls into the river, and Millie swam out and brought them back. We repeated the exercise until I figured that she had had enough. Millie disagreed, but allowed me to click her leash back onto her collar and we headed back up the hill. We passed by the large dog park, where a solitary owner was sitting on a bench watching a lonely pooch wander about. On most days, this is a lively, happening spot, with people standing around chatting while their dogs scamper about.

Dogs need to socialize with one another, just as they need to run and run and run. Thankfully, there are plenty of places here in Anne Arundel County and across the Bay in Queen Anne's County where you can let that happen off the leash. There are just a few rules, in addition to common civility:

Scoop your poop. I usually have a spare plastic bag in my back pocket, but there are plenty of bag dispensers in

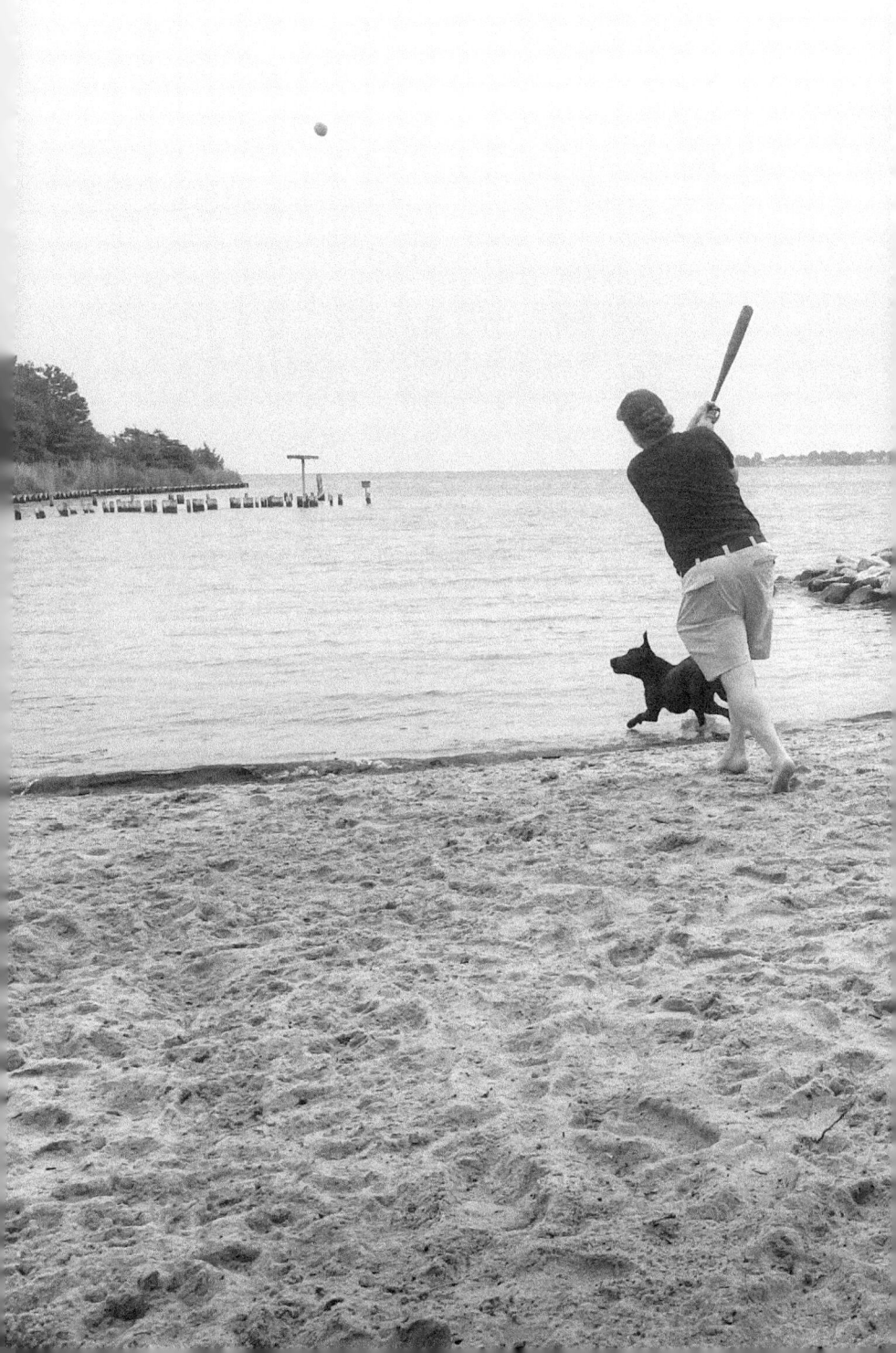

the parks. Once, out of desperation, I fished around in a trash can and found an empty cardboard coffee cup with a plastic lid, and it worked great. Leaving dog poop lying there isn't just rude; it makes the rest of us dog owners look bad. And it's against the law. Not only that, but especially on the beach, nasty bacteria can wash into the water that can make people sick.

When you're not in the confines of the dog park, keep your dog on a leash. You might have the sweetest dog in the world, but they're bound to meet up with one that isn't. And there are plenty of deer and other distractions in the parks to lure your pup away. The last time we took a hike on Wye Island, a dog got loose and disappeared, chasing after a herd of white tails. The owners assumed it was gone for good. Fortunately, it was found the next day, and there was a happy reunion. The lesson learned was to use the leash at all times.

Here's the most important one: Do not leave your dog unattended in your vehicle, even for a few minutes. On a hot day, the temperature inside a closed car can become deadly very quickly.

In addition:

🐕

All dogs must be vaccinated

🐕

Puppies under 3 months of age are not permitted

🐕

Enter at own risk; not all dogs get along

Anne Arundel County Dog Parks

Most open dawn to dusk:

A. Bell Branch Park
1150 Barbara Swann Way
Gambrills, MD 21054

B. Broadneck Park
613 College Pkwy.
Annapolis, MD 21409

C. Downs Park
(fenced-in areas and dog beach)
8311 John Downs Loop
Pasadena, MD 21122
Park entry fee

D. Loch Haven Park
3424 Pocahontas Dr.
Edgewater, MD 21037

E. Maryland City Park
565 Brock Bridge Rd.
Laurel, MD 20724

F. Quiet Waters Park
(fenced-in areas and dog beach)
600 Quiet Waters Park Rd.
Annapolis, MD 21403
Park entry fee

G. Towsers Branch Park
1405 Jackson Rd.
Odenton, MD 21113

Queen Anne's County Dog Parks:

H. Matapeake Dog Beach
201 Clubhouse Drive
Stevensville, MD 21666
(See "Millie Runs Happily Amok at Matapeake Beach" on page 241.)

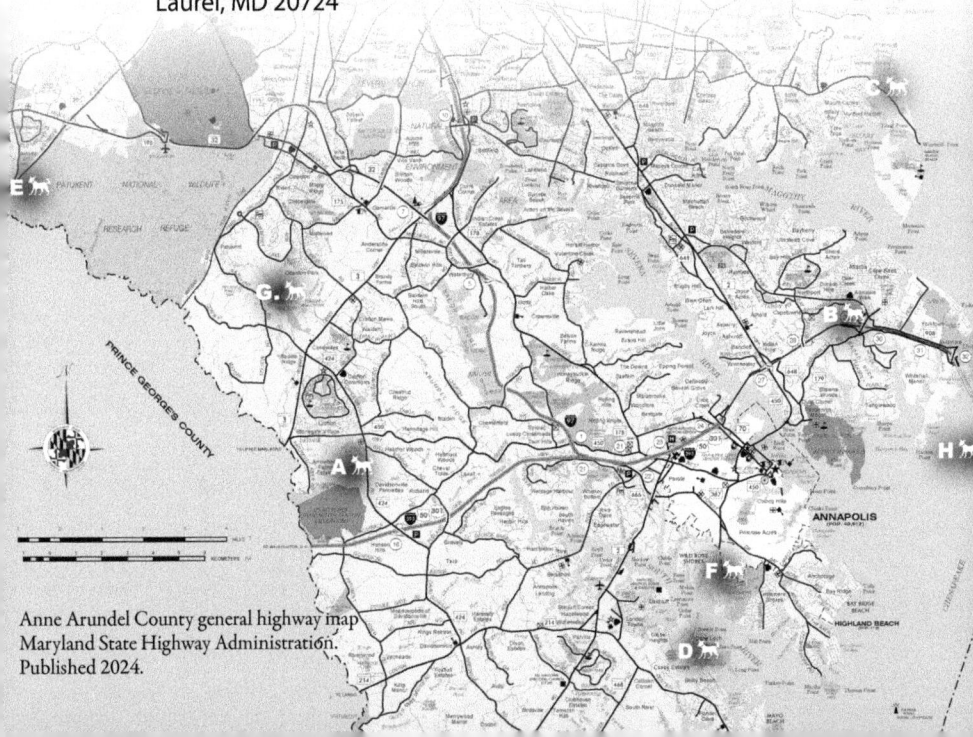

Anne Arundel County general highway map
Maryland State Highway Administration.
Published 2024.

Walk 40

Hooray for Butterflies at Tawes Garden

The third week of June is National Pollinator Awareness Week, and to celebrate the occasion in 2022, my wife Louise, our rescue retriever Millie and I toured the Helen Avalynne Tawes Garden in Annapolis. The garden is a five-acre oasis of pond and forest tucked in behind the Tawes State Office Building, headquarters for the Department of Natural Resources, and though we've lived in town for decades, this was our first visit. It will not be our last.

The garden is perhaps Maryland's most intimate state park. It even has its own ranger, Jay Myers, who's been nurturing the site for more than 40 years. Louise and I met Ranger Jay in front of the main entrance to the office complex on the corner of Taylor Avenue. Along with him, we met Suzanne Weber, the horticulturist for both the Tawes Garden and Sandy Point State Park, as well as Meg Hosmer, a certified Anne Arundel County Master Gardener who lives nearby in the Murray Hill neighborhood.

Jay is a gentle and jovial guide. He led us around the corner of Herbert Sachs Drive to what he referred to as the "weekend" entrance to the garden. Over the years, in doing a good deal of business with various departments within DNR, I always entered the building through the front

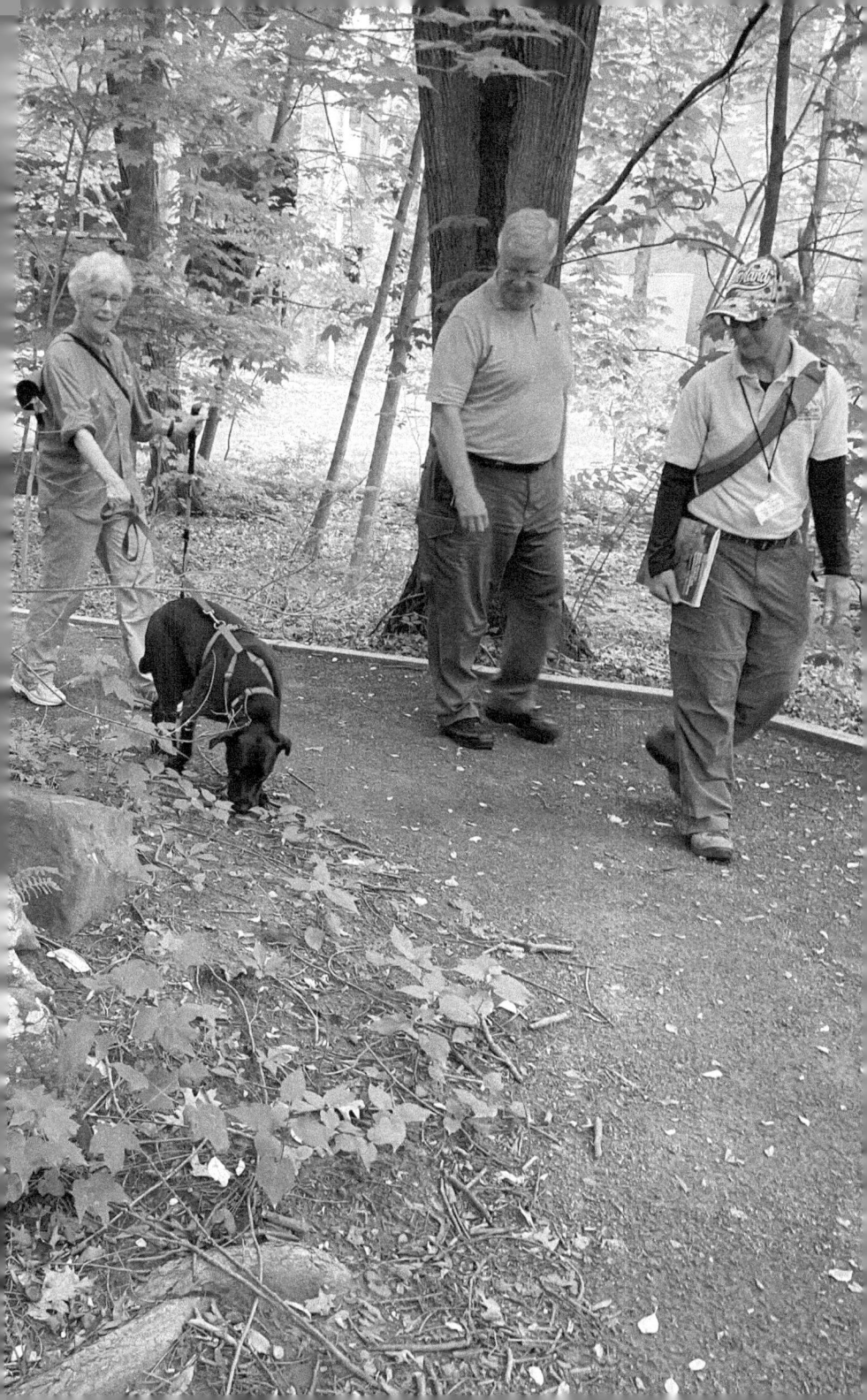

door and checked my ID with the guard at the desk. You can still get to the garden this way, but it's not necessary. The garden is accessible from dawn to dusk simply by walking around to the back of the building.

There, Jay explained that in the early 1970s, a woman named Stevie Lyttle, president of the Federated Garden Clubs of Maryland, enlisted the aid of her friend, the legendary state comptroller Louis Goldstein, to help her find a plot in the city of Annapolis where she could create a garden that would demonstrate all the habitats of the state of Maryland, from the mountains to the piedmont to the coast, a sort of "Maryland in miniature."

Goldstein led her to a vacant lot on the site that would become the DNR office complex. For years, it had been the home of the West Annapolis carnival. Ranger Jay explained that dirt excavated from the foundation of the buildings got piled up on the lot, where it was sculpted into hills and ponds. The soil needed heavy conditioning to make it suitable for planting. The Federated Garden Clubs, DNR and the Department of General Services cooperated on the planting, and it's astonishing how the completely man-made garden has blossomed over the years.

Native trees that were planted as saplings a mere three or four inches in diameter hardly 50 years ago have grown to tall, mature oaks, maples, loblollies, and even bald cypress. Jay, who has watched all these trees grow all these years, led us along the paths that meandered around the edges of the ponds through several distinct habitats, from a streamside environment to an Eastern Shore peninsula and up into a Western Maryland forest—a full 18-foot rise in elevation—complete with boulders imported from Catoctin Mountain. If it weren't for the hum of the traffic on Rowe Boulevard, you'd swear you were 100 miles west and 1,000 feet up a mountainside. We strolled by a raised planter, offset to accommodate visitors in wheelchairs, planted with flowers and herbs of different textures, tastes, and fragrances to stimulate all the senses.

The garden is named in honor of Mrs. J. Millard Tawes, a former first lady of Maryland from 1959 to 1967. Helen was born in Crisfield on the Eastern Shore in 1898. She met young Millard on a hayride when she was 16, and they eloped when she was only 17. Like Teddy Roosevelt, Gov. Tawes was a keen advocate for public parks. He made Assateague Island a national park and doubled the area of land covered by the state parks system. He and Mrs. Tawes broke ground for the garden in 1975.

All along on our stroll, Suzanne Weber and Meg Hosner shared their knowledge of the flowers, shrubs, and trees we encountered in each of the habitats. We were surprised to see a prickly pear cactus in the dunes of the coastal plain section, with its bright yellow blossoms. Suzanne stepped off the path to inspect a small ash tree that had somehow evaded the ash borer beetle that has devastated most of the others of its kind. We stopped at a pollinator habitat demonstration garden set off by a pergola with stately columns. Flowering shrubs with blossoms ranging in color from coral to lipstick red adorned the raised bank that curved around the edge of the garden.

This section of the garden is designed to attract the butterflies, bees, beetles, wasps, moths, flies, ants, birds, and even bats that collect and spread pollen from plant to plant. Up to 80 percent of all plants depend on these pollinators to fertilize their fruits and seeds.

Some scientists say that pollinators are responsible for one out of every three bites of food we eat.

"Anne Arundel County Master Gardeners like Meg Hosner are key partners in the garden's ongoing viability," Suzanne explained. Meg and other volunteers perform most of the maintenance in the Tawes Garden. The nonprofit Unity Gardens organization provided a grant for the pollinator habitat demonstration plantings. They're designed to give you ideas on how to plant your own garden at home.

In addition to serving as the horticulturalist for the Tawes Garden, Suzanne also works at Sandy Point State Park. At both sites, she's promoting the Maryland Park Service Project Butterfly and Bumblebee program as well as Park Quest Pollinators. These are ongoing slates of programs and activities designed to educate the public about the role pollinators play in maintaining diverse ecosystems and the nation's food supply.

If you'd like to help, you can donate to support butterfly and bumblebee habitat and education in state parks.

Projects supported by these donations include planting and restoring native gardens, field edges, and meadows that benefit a wide variety of species and connect park visitors to the beauty and wonder of nature. You can also participate in ongoing educational programs and visit existing gardens, fields, and meadows at parks that support thriving pollinator populations.

Tawes Garden
580 Taylor Avenue
Annapolis, Maryland 21401

To schedule a guided tour, call 410-260-8189

Open sunrise to dusk

Free admission

Parking is available at the Navy/Marine Corps Stadium in the Gold Parking area, with a $5/day fee

No toilets unless you check in at the main entrance of the office building during office hours

Munificent dogs on leash are welcome; bring your own doggie bags

Easy going

Walk 41

Tour a Restored Stream at Broadneck Trail

It's interesting to witness the evolution of trails over time. One of the first trails we explored way back in the early days of the pandemic was then called the Arnold Loop. It circled around a forested tract owned by the Anne Arundel County School Board. I referred to it as a "pocket wilderness."

As the area became more and more popular with hikers, dog walkers, and mountain bikers, the AllTrails app started calling it the Forked Creek Trail. And indeed, the tract covers the headwaters of Forked Creek from where it begins near Broadneck Elementary School. Beyond the boundaries of the forest, the creek flows northward and joins the Magothy River by the Ulmstead Gardens community.

That first time I was there, I was with my emotional-support spouse, Louise White, and our wonderful Irish setter, Bonnie. I recall that the creek had cut into the bank of the steep hillsides over the years, excavating a 15-foot-deep gully that must have been shooting tons of sediment and nutrients downstream to pollute the river every time it rained.

I revisited the site at the invitation of avid reader Lois Findlay, who wanted to show me the newly completed project that restored a good stretch of that creek. Lois was waiting for me at the trailhead along with her black Labrador retriever, Bella, who looked curiously similar to my dog, Millie. The dogs greeted each other in a happy tangle of leashes, and if it weren't for the color of those leashes—Bella's being blue and Millie's yellow—it would have been difficult to tell them apart.

Both dogs have a white blaze decorating the breast and a dab of white on one foot. Bella's slightly narrower snout hinted that greyhound roots may make up part of her family tree. Millie? Still not sure of her roots, but based upon her propensity for chasing tennis balls, I started calling her a Spalding retriever until I found out that Spalding makes a ball for every sport except tennis. Both dogs were eager to get moving, even though the morning was already beginning to get muggy.

Lois led me past a carefully hand-painted sign that read Broadneck Trail and pointed out the new markers, wooden posts along with 2022 carefully stenciled with the name of the side trail and topped with a spiffy-looking custom logo. Somebody was taking pride in maintaining this path.

Along the way, as we chatted, I learned that Lois has a career as a consultant for tech firms, though she's taking time off this summer to explore some of the more spectacular national parks out west with Bella in her RV. When she's not working her day job, Lois serves as the volunteer treasurer for the Bicycle Advocates for Annapolis & Anne Arundel County.

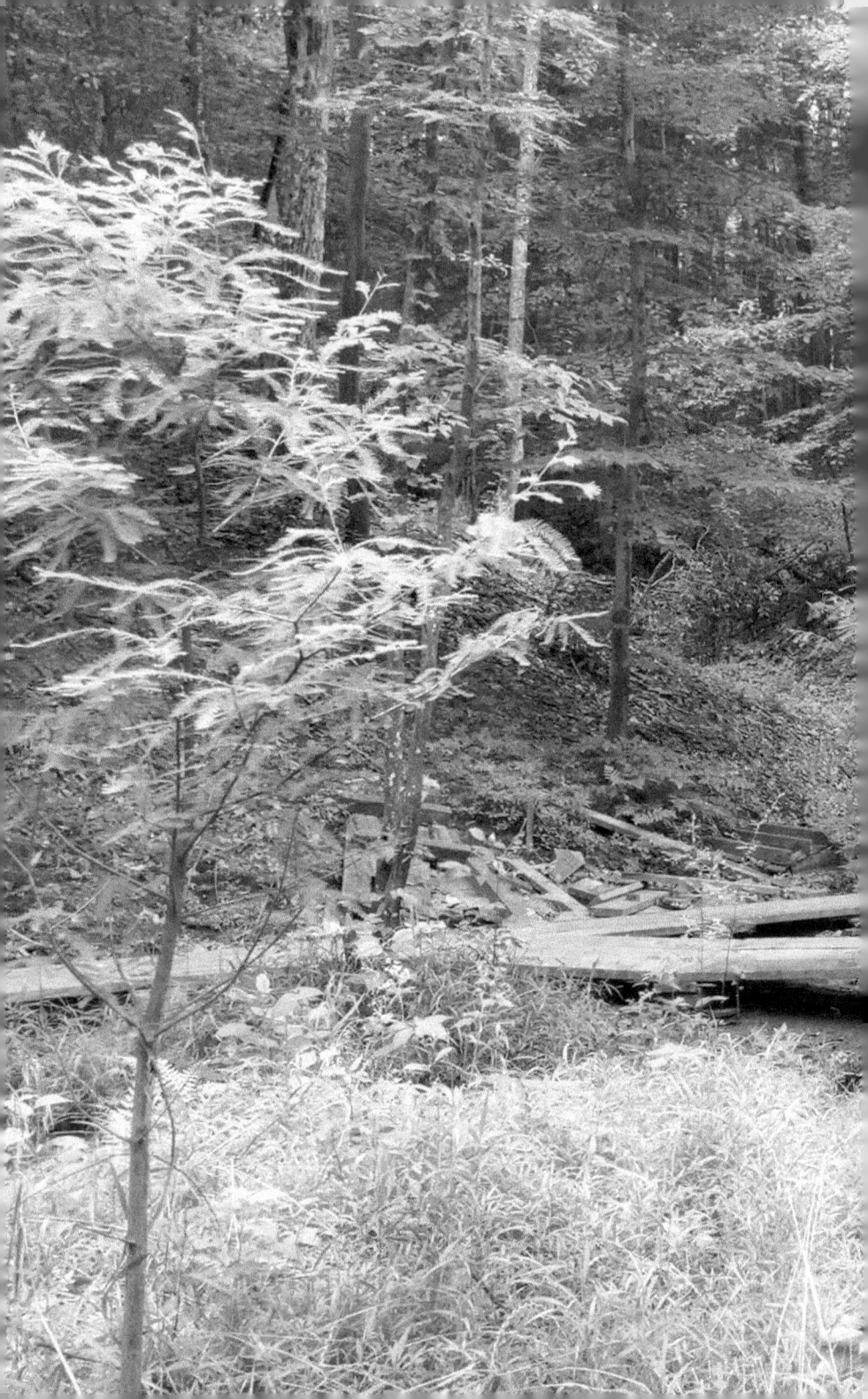

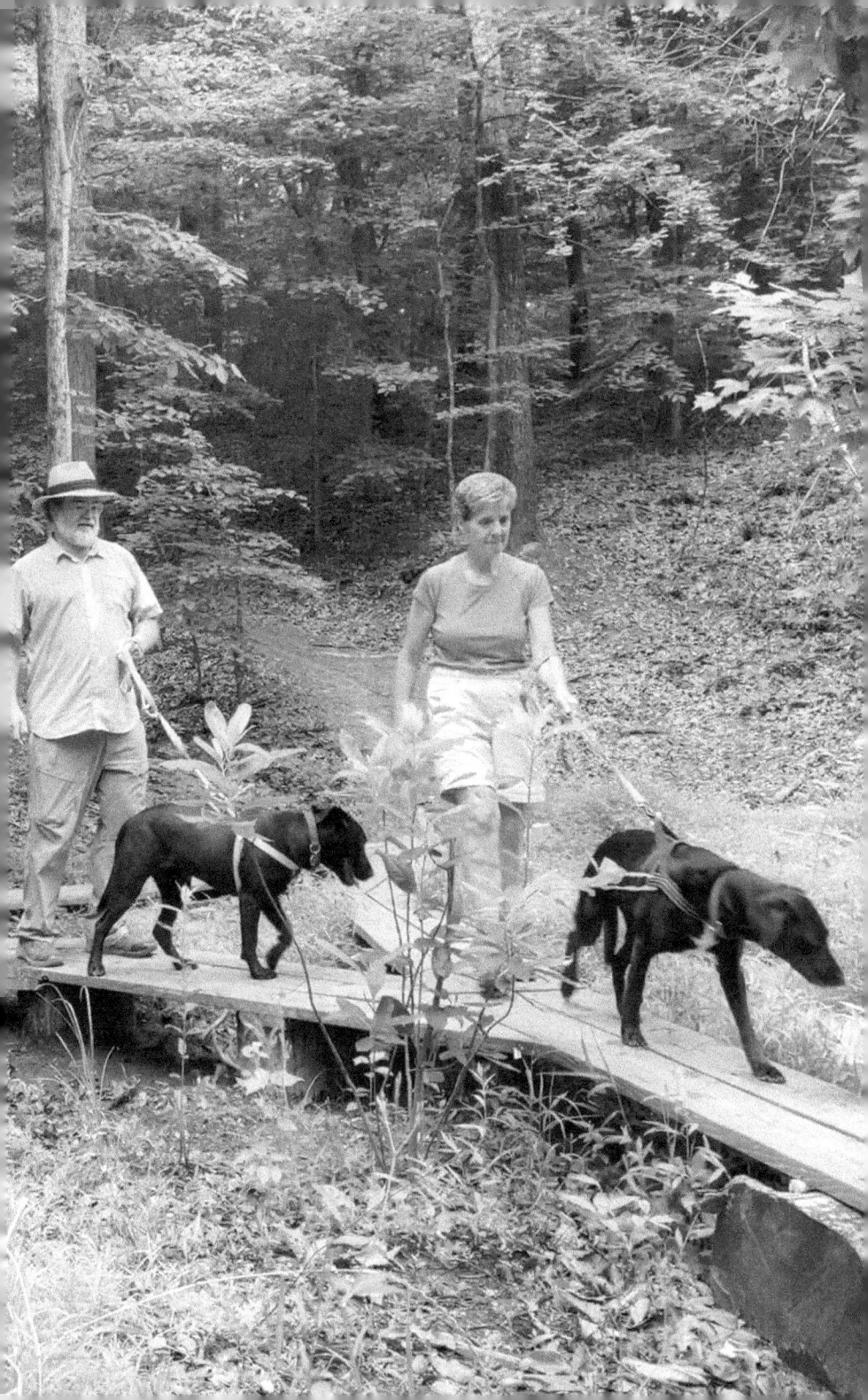

BikeAAA is a non-profit organization dedicated to promoting safe cycling. I was happy to learn that. I ride my bike to work several times a week these days.

We walked, single file, Bella leading the way, along the trail through a forest comprised mainly of enormous yellow poplar trees, their trunks towering into the leaf canopy, round and straight as Roman columns. The path sloped down to the stream bed, and there what used to be a deeply cut gully had been transformed into a series of step pools, each girded by rock and surrounded by newly planted saplings.

An interpretive panel along the trail identified the project as the work of the Anne Arundel County Bureau of Watershed Protection and Restoration, which made a lot of sense to me. This is the group responsible for making sure the county meets its goals in reducing stormwater runoff that pollutes the Chesapeake Bay. It's funded by a fee authorized by the Bay Restoration Act signed by Gov. Robert L. Ehrlich Jr. in 2004. Every household in the county chips in an average of $89.25 each year. We were looking at a prime example of our tax dollars at work.

The project restored about 1,400 linear feet of eroding channel using a method called a Step Pool Storm Conveyance. The pools were mostly dry when Lois and I were there, but you can readily imagine that during a storm, rainwater would fill the upper pool, overflow its lower edge to fill up the next pool and the next, on and on downstream. In each pool, the stormwater gets slowed down to allow it to seep into the soil. The eroded dirt that gets suspended in the stormwater has a chance to settle out. The surrounding native trees and shrubs soak up the excess nutrients that would otherwise feed the algae in the Bay, leading to dead zones and fish kills. The storm surge that used to scour the channel into a deep gully has now been tamed.

After Lois and Bella and Millie and I roamed along the length of the restoration project, we were all pretty much done in by the heat and humidity, so we cut the rest of the hike short and made our way back to the parking lot.

I wanted to find out more about the creek restoration, and I knew just who to ask. Once at home, I contacted Joe Ports, the county's project manager for the Magothy River watershed. Joe and I had worked together for several years in the West and Rhode Riverkeeper organization.

"This was an interesting job that was a great partnership between the County's Bureau of Watershed Protection and the Bureau of Utilities," Joe reported in an email. "The channel used to be so eroded that it had exposed a 16-inch diameter pressurized sanitary sewer main several times over the years."

The partners managed to figure out a way to design the project so that the sewer main didn't have to be re-routed, which saved county taxpayers millions, he said. The project has a 65-acre drainage area, five acres of which are impervious, meaning that the rain can't seep directly into the ground because of the school buildings and paved parking lots. The drainage area is designed to capture and treat the rainfall from a storm that drops as much as 1.27 inches of rain over that area, which amounts to an astonishing total of about 450,000 gallons for such a storm. The step pools will absorb hundreds of pounds of nutrients and keep 458 tons of sediment from polluting the Magothy River every year.

The total project cost, including design and construction, Joe reported, was roughly $2.2 million. The county Bureau of Utilities contributed $850,000 for construction, and a grant from the Department of Natural Resources' Chesapeake and Atlantic Coastal Bays Trust Fund brought in another $827,000. So our tax dollars got leveraged quite dramatically.

And then, thanks to Lois, I got to meet one of the guys who's been maintaining the trail all these years. I spoke over the phone with Brian Shannon, a mechanic at the Bike Doctor shop in Severna Park.

"I've lived in Arnold for 40 years," he told me, "and I've lived in Ulmstead Gardens for 15 years, only about 100 feet from the park."

He's done a lot of trail maintenance on the Broadneck Trail as well as at Bacon Ridge and Waterworks Park. "I'm out there all the time," he said. "I've been riding mountain bikes for some time, but these days, I do more hiking with my dog."

Brian said he is just one of a group of 10 to 15 people who volunteer their time to take care of the trail. "These are people from hikers to runners to mountain bikers, some are environmentalists and naturalists, and we want to make sure the park is protected. It's a small community of people putting what we can into it. Overall," he said, "there's well over six miles of trails."

And so there you have it: a remarkable pocket wilderness tucked in behind a school, where public funds are used to restore the waterways and where private citizens donate their time and talent to give us a wonderful place to walk in the woods with our dogs.

Broadneck Trail Broadneck Elementary School
470 Shore Acres Road
Arnold, MD 21012
The trailhead is located in the southwest corner of the parking lot
Free admission
Plenty of parking on site
Open dawn to dusk
No toilets
Friendly dogs on leash welcome; bring your own doggie bags
Easy going

Walk 42

Smelling the Begonias at Historic London Town and Gardens

The last time we visited Historic London Town and Gardens was in March 2020, just before the pandemic seemingly shut the whole world down. I remember the camellias were in magnificent bloom then, and our Irish setter Bonnie was still with us, and blooming as well.

When we returned in mid-May 2002, the site had only recently come back into full public mode when I visited with my emotional-support spouse, Louise White, and our latest canine companion, Millie, the rescue retriever.

It was on one of those brilliant May days we get after a cold front passes through, cool and clear. We checked in at the visitor center and paid our admission. Millie was welcomed into the lobby and got fawned over by one of the volunteers. She tolerated the attention, but she was eager to get out and go for a walk through the gardens, and so were we.

If you've never been to London Town, you've been depriving yourself of a wonderful experience. It occupies a 23-acre park on a bluff set between South River and Almshouse Creek in Edgewater, just a 20-minute drive from Annapolis. Much of the site is devoted to what amounts to a horticultural zoo, with collections of native and ornamental flowering shrubs and trees.

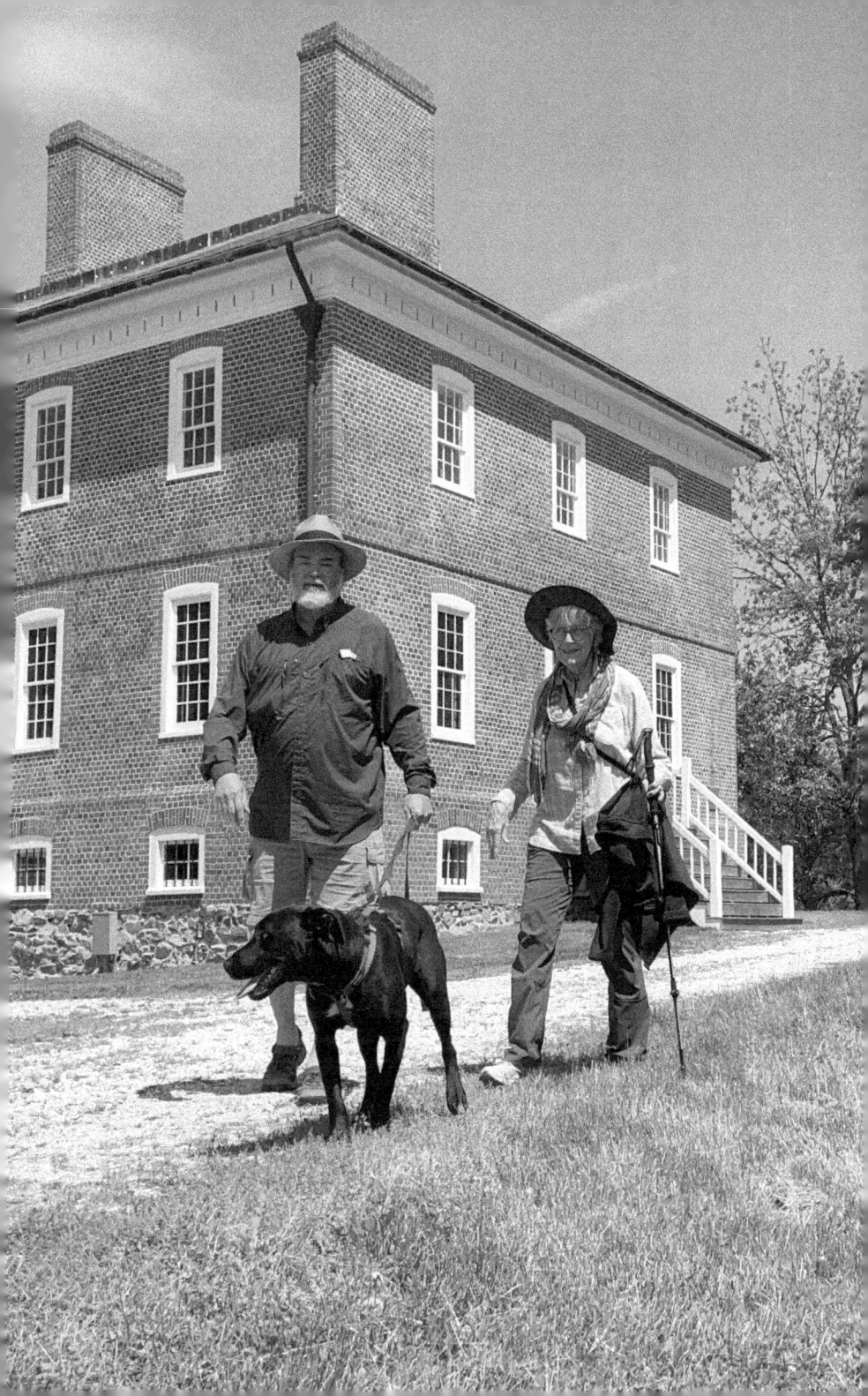

The visitor center houses a world-class museum where one of the many exhibits of local history tells the story of the enslaved people who were essential to the tobacco economy throughout the Chesapeake. At one point in time, all ships sailing the South River were required to "Unlade and put on Shore, all Negroes" here at the tobacco port of London Town.

One of the original buildings of that historic town, the William Brown House, is open for guided tours. The large brick Georgian house was built as a tavern around 1760 by William Brown, a carpenter and slave owner who ran the ferry across the South River. If you were traveling between Williamsburg and Philadelphia in that era, as the likes of George Washington and Thomas Jefferson did many times, you would have passed through London Town and ridden its ferry across the river and on to Annapolis.

By the 1780s, the town's prominence was ebbing as Annapolis grew. Brown lost the house to his creditors. In 1828, the county purchased the building to use as an almshouse to shelter needy citizens. It served that purpose until 1965. London Town and Gardens was established in 1971, and since then the Brown house has been lovingly restored to its 18th century elegance and now serves as the centerpiece of the park.

Other buildings, like a tobacco barn, a tenement house and a carpenter's shop, have been authentically recreated in period style on foundations uncovered by archaeologists from Anne Arundel County's Lost Towns Project.

The park is owned by the county and managed by the nonprofit London Town Foundation.

We took a stroll around the historic buildings, but we were really there to see what was blooming in the gardens. The Woodland Garden section features towering native trees, including some truly magnificent willow oaks, one of our favorites. As you wander along the graveled paths, you can appreciate the collection of flowering trees and shrubs whose blossoms count out the months through the seasons. The camellias were already past bloom, and most of the dogwoods had dropped their white petals, but we were pleased to see that many of the rhododendrons and azaleas were still in full, glorious color.

We also came across beautiful wildflowers like the spider wort, with its miniature purple flowers. We were astonished to find the largest jack-in-the-pulpit I've ever seen, its three-part leaves looking like giant poison ivy, and underneath the leaves, we saw its green blossom in the middle demurely draped over itself like a shy toddler hiding under her blanket.

The path led us to a brick portico overlooking the South River where it meets Almshouse Creek. We descended a set of stairs that led down to a charming glen with a little bridge arching over a brook. A huge willow oak was silhouetted against the silver glow from the surface of the river. As we approached the water's edge, Millie suddenly perked up and lunged to the end of her leash. Her attention was riveted on something there in the marsh at the mouth of the stream. We followed her point and saw a brown furry head pop up through the reeds.

"It's a muskrat!" came from both Louise and me at the first glance. But then as the critter crawled out of the marsh and onto the rock seawall, we saw that it did not have the hairless, possum-like tail of a muskrat, but the bottle-brush tail of a groundhog. I've only seen groundhogs—what we called woodchucks when I was a kid—always in dry fields, never in wet marshes, so I was surprised, especially when he hid behind a rock, poked his head up to give Millie the evil eye and then let out a piercing, one-note whistle as loud as any angry football ref about to let fly a penalty flag. We took the cue that we were not at all welcome and headed up the steps on the far side of the glen.

At the top of the bluff, we found ourselves in the more formal Ornamental Gardens. In previous visits, we've seen daylilies, hydrangeas, roses, and crepe myrtles in summer, and the asters, mums, and salvias that bloom in the fall.

On the way back to the visitor center, we bumped into Rod Colfield, who served as London Town's executive director at the time. As we chatted, he mentioned that the organization had received several new grants to help make the site more ADA accessible. As it is now, the paths are either soft gravel or covered with wood chips, and there are stairs up and down the banks in the gardens. He also told us that the pier at the bottom of the hill will be rebuilt to provide room for visiting tall ships and recreational boats.

As Louise and I wandered the grounds of Historic London Town and Gardens with Millie, our thoughts turned toward our wonderful Irish setter, Bonnie, that gentle creature who loved going for walks with us and never once got whistled at by a woodchuck.

Historic London Town & Gardens
839 Londontown Road
Edgewater, MD 21037
www.historiclondontown.org
Open Wed.–Sun. 10 a.m.–4 p.m.
Admission (see web site)
Plenty of parking on site
Restrooms in the visitor center
Amiable dogs on leashes are welcome

Walk 43

Who's Who at St. Anne's Cemetery

The gravestones at St. Anne's Cemetery in Annapolis bear the names of many of the town's populace dating back centuries. "I see it as an historic document," explained my friend Ginger DeLuca, chair of the committee dedicated to the graveyard's preservation. "It's really here for the living to remember their ancestors. All these people were alive at one time."

Ginger was kind enough to take me on a tour of the cemetery in mid-September 2022 and extended the invitation to my rescue retriever, Millie. We met on one of those sunny, warm late summer days, perfect for a walk. Ginger was eager to show me the work she and her volunteers are doing to eradicate invasive vines from the trees and shrubs, but she's also passionate about the astonishing history of the place and the people buried there.

The cemetery is located along the banks of College Creek, which bears the name Graveyard Creek in the old maps. It sits on a grassy hill between Rowe Boulevard and Northwest Street. It's been there since 1790.

The original St. Anne's Church on Church Circle was built around 1704, and many citizens of Annapolis were interred in the surrounding church yard. By the time of the Revolutionary War, the structure had become too rickety and too small to accommodate the growing congregation.

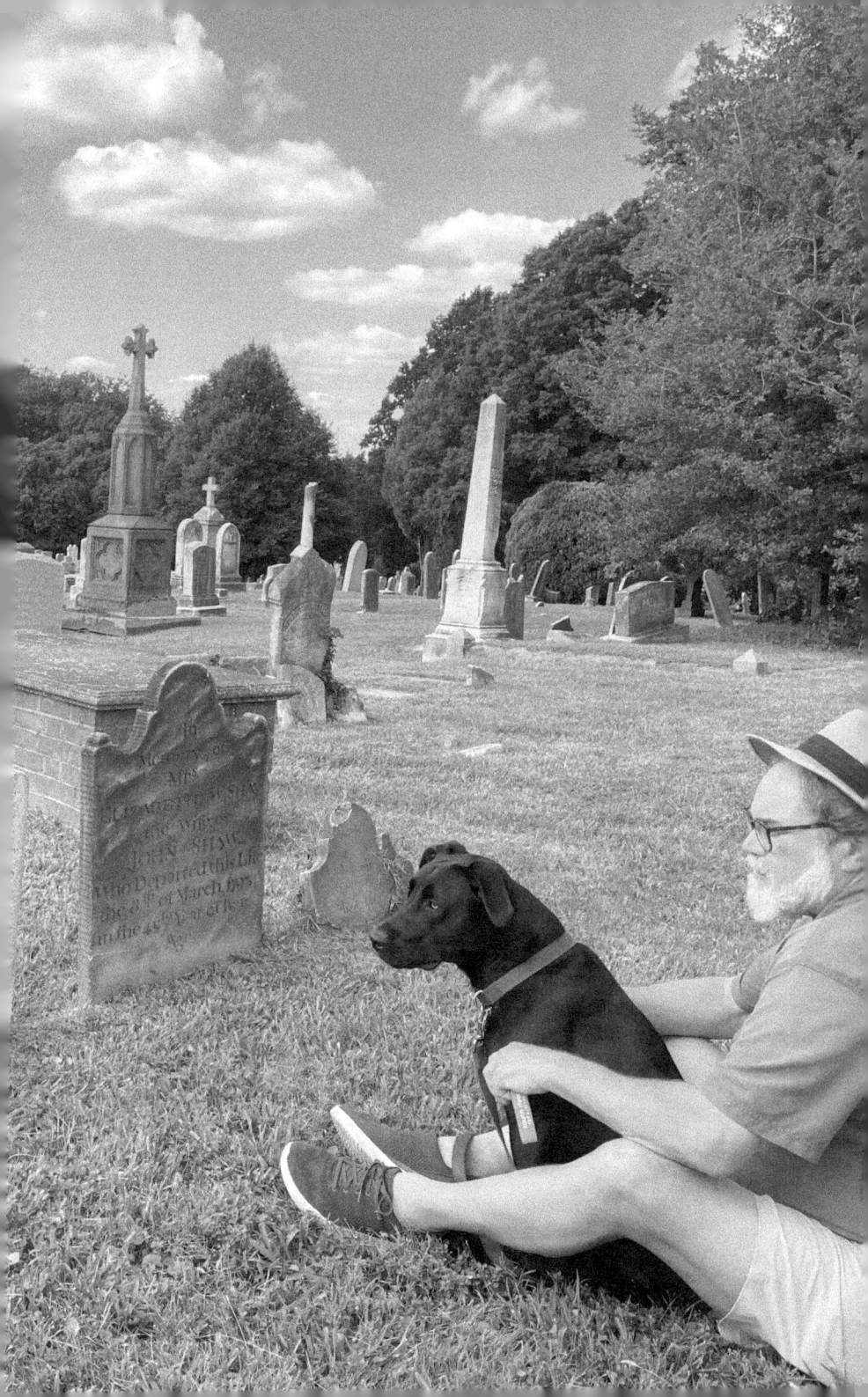

So the first church was razed in 1775. The construction of the second church was delayed by the war, but since the building itself was planned to be larger than the first, a number of graves had to be displaced to make room for the new structure. Some of those graves are still in the graveyard at Church Circle, but others were moved to the new cemetery in 1790.

Curiously, that second church building burned down in 1858 when a new-fangled central heating furnace caught fire on St. Valentine's Day. Just as its construction was delayed by the Revolutionary War, the rebuilding of its replacement, the third church, was delayed by the Civil War. A portion of the bell tower from the second church was incorporated into the new structure, the one standing in Church Circle today.

Ginger showed me a modest mound where it's thought that anonymous bones disinterred during the construction of the second church were reburied. As we strolled among the tombstones, Ginger pointed out some decorated with Stars of David, others bearing the names of prominent Annapolis Black families, like the Bishops and the Prices. The cemetery was always meant for everyone and anyone in the city, she noted, not just members of St. Anne's.

We stopped by a trio of headstones, weathered with age. The middle one was the grave of Henry Price, the well-known free Black community leader who served as the pastor of what is now Asbury United Methodist Church on West Street from 1838 to 1863. He was also the grandfather of Dr. Daniel Hale Williams, who performed the world's first successful open-heart surgery in 1893.

Ginger showed me a mammoth willow oak tree at the center of the cemetery. Its 22-foot diameter might have made it a certified champion tree if not for the fact that its top half was lopped off by some ancient storm. It must have been growing strong when the first graves were dug here. Ginger and her core crew of eight or nine volunteer stewards conduct work parties every Thursday morning to clear ivy and other vines from this and all the other trees on the site.

Periodically, she'll call in as many as 30 other volunteers to tackle bigger jobs. They're working to create a meditation garden sponsored by the Nature Sacred program of the Annapolis-based TKF Foundation. It would be part of a "scatter garden" where the ashes of loved ones could be sprinkled. The Anne Arundel County Watershed Stewards Academy and the Unity Gardens foundation are assisting with that project. Ginger noted that maintenance at the cemetery itself is funded by fees families pay to have their relatives buried there. The cemetery is not financially supported by the church itself.

We passed by a number of stones that had tumbled over. This is not the result of vandalism, Ginger explained, but of time and gravity. The actual grave sites and the stones are the responsibility of the individual families, she said.

She showed me another trio of stones shaped like the headboards of a bed. "People back then viewed death like a long sleep," Ginger explained. "That's why so many gravestones are shaped like that. You'll also see small footstones on some graves for the same reason."

The middle one of these stones was that of John Shaw, the noted Annapolis cabinetmaker who died at the venerable age of 84 in 1838. In addition to crafting exquisite furniture, Shaw was responsible for maintaining the State House from the 1770s up to the early 1800s. Millie and I sat in the grass and wondered what he would think of the State House, now shrouded in scaffolding and what looks like gauze. I'll bet he'd be very curious about the restoration project going on there.

Ginger noted that there are no less than 119 graves of Civil War soldiers in the cemetery. "About half served in the South, half in the North," she said, which reflects the loyalty of the general populace in Annapolis and most of Maryland at that time. At least one family had sons fighting on both sides.

One of the most prominent examples is the obelisk of James Iredell Waddell. I'm not one to condone public monuments to Confederates, but I do think a cemetery is a suitable setting. Waddell commanded the CSS *Shenandoah*, a commerce raider that swept the northern Pacific Ocean of Yankee whaling ships. Waddell went on a spree, capturing, burning, and sinking whalers, yet he never took a single life. His captives were dropped off safely in neutral ports. Eventually, he met up with a British ship whose captain showed him a newspaper revealing that Lee had surrendered at Appomattox in April, 1865. This was August.

Knowing he'd be strung up from the nearest yard arm if he'd been captured by the U.S. Navy, Waddell sailed the *Shenandoah* the rest of the way around the world by way of Cape Horn and turned himself in to the authorities in England.

After the war, he settled in Annapolis with his wife, Anne Iglehart, daughter of a local businessman, and they built the Victorian stone house that still sits on the corner of College Avenue and Prince George Street.

Waddell was the only Civil War captain on either side to circumnavigate the globe. He fired the last shot in the war, even though the war had been over for months; and he devastated the Yankee whaling industry, doing more to save the whales than anyone in history. The entire world economy shifted from whale oil for illumination and lubrication to petroleum, which had just recently been discovered in Oil Creek, Pennsylvania.

Oh, the stories the St. Anne's Cemetery can tell. Ginger DeLuca leads occasional historic tours of the cemetery. Keep an eye out on the web site stannes-annapolis.org/news/cemetery-tour.

St. Anne's Cemetery
Northwest Street
Annapolis, MD 21401

Open dawn to dusk

Free admission

Limited parking available on the street

No toilets

Cordial dogs on leashes are welcome; bring your own doggie bags

As Poet Laureate of Eastport in 2018, I wrote this ditty inspired by Captain Waddell, not meant in any way as a tribute to the Confederacy he fought for, but in recognition of this one Annapolitan's remarkable career.

BALLAD OF THE CSS SHENANDOAH
Let's sing a rousing chorus now for Captain James Waddell,
He sank the Yankee whaling fleet and burned 'em all to hell,
It's a fascinating story and a stunning one to tell,
Of the Anglo-Rebel pirate, Captain James Waddell

Sing ho! For Shenandoah! Confederate colors furled,
Fired the final cannon shot and followed it 'round the world,
Never a soul was lost, and all his captives left alive
On Shenandoah's voyage of 1865

A man without a country, a rebel without a cause,
Kept fightin', never knowing that the war'd been done and lost,
He cleared the North Pacific of the Yankee whaling fleet
Till he met ship with a newspaper clip that told of Lee's defeat

The Old Man had surrendered back in April, Waddell read,
The leaden columns filled his heart with melancholy dread,
For months he'd been a-pirating, when all was done and said,
If the Yankees caught him now, they'd put a noose around his head

For he'd captured six Yankee whaling ships
    on his way to the Cape of Good Hope,
Burned four New Bedford whalers on route to the Sea of Okhostk,
And then in only nine cold days upon the Bering Sea,
He took two dozen more on his epic blubber-blazing spree

With Union ships patrolling all the oceans of the globe,
And nowhere else to turn, and not a place to call his home,
He lowered her flag and stowed her guns and steamed
   around the Horn,
Doomed, she was, to never see the land she'd battled for

He could have run to Mexico, or beached on the nearest shore,
But he voyaged 17,000 miles around the tip of Cape Horn,
At last, on the second of November, he arrived at Liverpool
And surrendered to the British there, the entire Union Navy fooled

Sing ho! For Shenandoah! Confederate colors furled,
Fired the final cannon shot and followed it 'round the world,
Never a soul was lost and all his captives left alive
On Shenandoah's voyage of 1865.

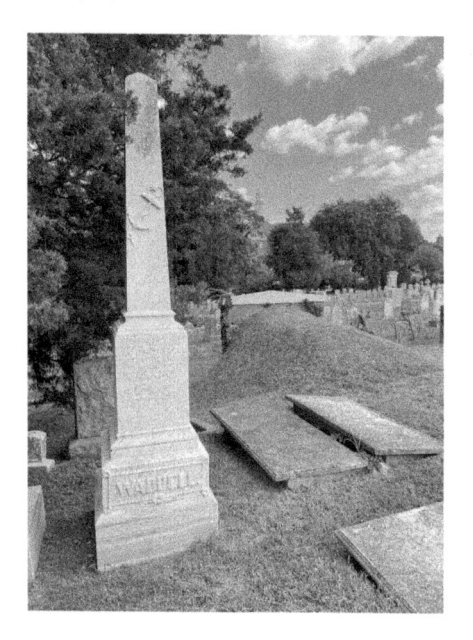

Walk 44

A Free Morning at Annapolis City Dock

I'll bet you're one of those people who has vowed never to go to downtown Annapolis again. It's just too crowded, and there are never enough parking spaces. Well, hah! In July 2022, I spent a couple of hours strolling around the City Dock and there were just a few people around and acres of free parking. Of course, I was there at 8 o'clock in the morning, but that's the secret magic time to go.

It was 10 degrees cooler than later in the day. Each morning, the sun rises up over Kent Island and beams down the mouth of the Severn River, turning Annapolis Harbor into a sea of shimmering silver, silhouetting the sailboats in the mooring field.

Millie and I took our pick of hundreds of empty parking spaces and began our morning stroll. Our first stop was to inspect a tall ship tied up to the pier at the end of Prince George Street. This long dock has recently been acquired by the city, and the Annapolis Harbormaster rents space to non-profit vessels that promote educational, historical, or heritage pursuits. The ship's deck was swarming with kids, and I knew by the rigging that it must be the Schooner *Sultana*.

The original *Sultana* was a merchant vessel built in Boston in 1767. It was the smallest schooner ever commissioned in the British Royal Navy. The *Sultana* here at the dock is a reproduction built in Chestertown in 2001 by the Sultana Education Foundation. She sails as a school ship, taking more than 4,500 students out onto the Chesapeake Bay each year for hands-on programs in environmental science and history.

Millie and I sat on a shady bench at the end of Prince George Street as I finished my coffee while she flirted with a couple of young women on a morning walk. Next to the park there's a small grey wood-framed building that looks out of place in red-brick Annapolis. This is the Burtis House, the sole-surviving waterman's home located on City Dock. Cap'n William H. Burtis worked the water and rented boats from this pier.

From the mid-1800s to the mid-1900s, City Dock was known as Hell Point. The houses were mainly two-story frame dwellings like the Burtis House. This was a neighborhood of working-class families whose livelihoods depended upon one of the industries along the waterfront: the coal and lumber yards, sawmills, oyster-packing houses, warehouses, steamboat wharfs, and boat houses.

In 1941, the Naval Academy expanded, annexing the properties north of Prince George Street and condemning the existing residential and commercial buildings there. One of the streets that disappeared in the annexation was called Holland Street. The athletic field house with its distinctive oversized Quonset-hut-shaped copper roof was completed in 1957.

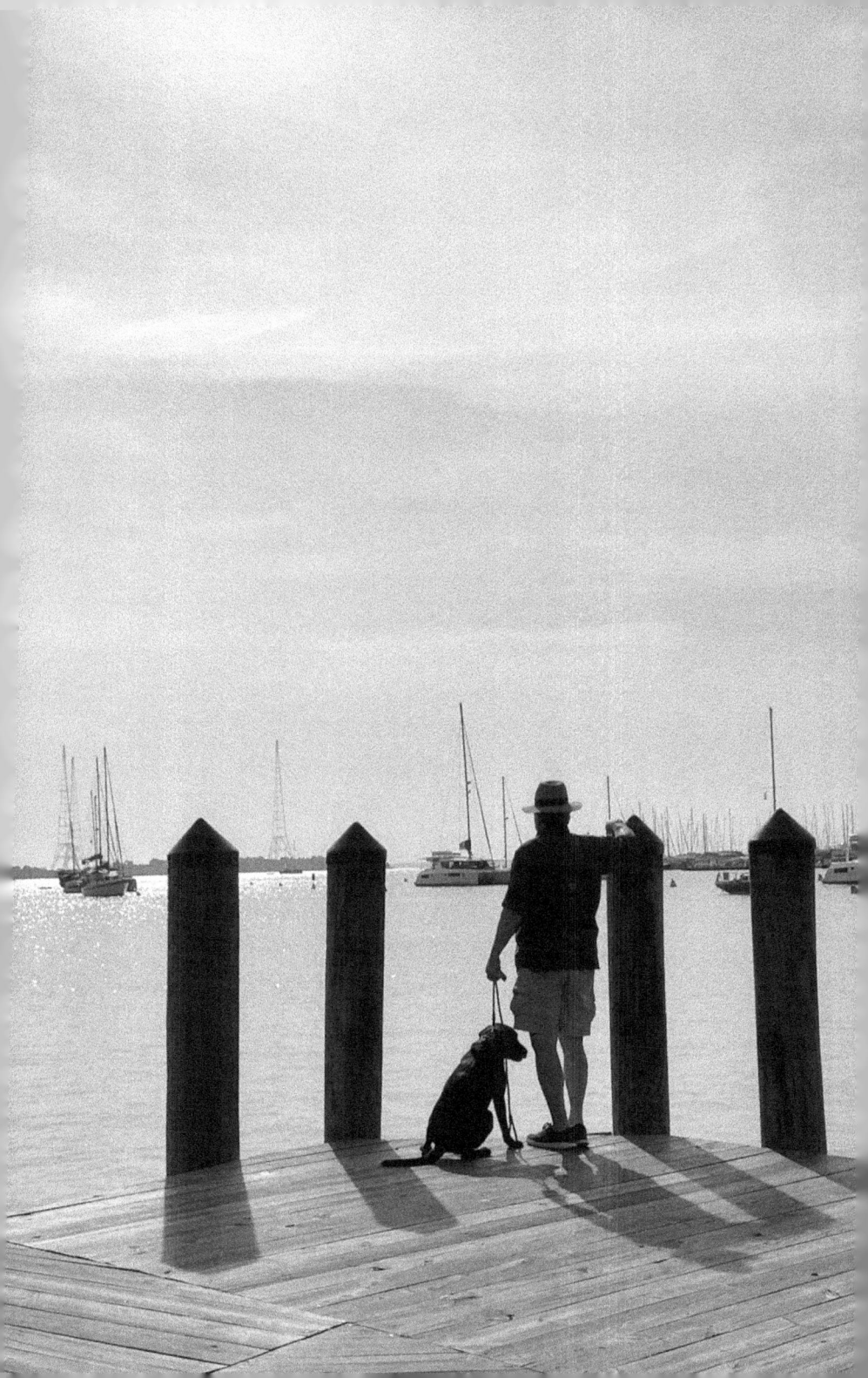

The Burtis House is all that remains of the Hell Point era in the maritime heritage of Annapolis, except for the house at the far end of the block on the corner of Craig Street. The Chesapeake Bay Office of the National Park Service is working with Preservation Maryland and the city to restore the Burtis House and raise it above the high-tide line.

Once restored, the Burtis House might serve as one of the official Gateways welcome centers for the newly envisioned Chesapeake National Recreation Area; as an extension of the Annapolis Maritime Museum; or perhaps as new headquarters for the Annapolis Harbormaster.

Millie and I strolled around the brick-paved Susan Campbell Park at the end of City Dock. To debunk a common misconception, this is not Susan B. Campbell Park as in Susan B. Anthony. It's named after the daughter of former Annapolis alderman and mayor pro tem Robert Campbell, an auctioneer by trade and a legendary character in his own right who lived nearby.

I looked back at the city skyline, which from this vantage, hasn't changed all that much in 250 years, except the State House dome, which at the time was cocooned in shroud-wrapped scaffolding while undergoing a $1.5 million restoration.

The expanse of parking lot between the bricked park and the Market House will also be renovated to the tune of another $50 million. Work is scheduled to begin once the new Noah Hillman Garage is completed. The new City

Dock park will have the same amount of green space as one and a half football fields. There will be three flexible plazas that can have around 60 parking spaces or be cleared of cars for events like the boat shows. While some parking will disappear, there will be a total of about 200 spaces left, including the 50-car lot at 110 Compromise Street.

The main goal of the plan is to raise City Dock above the high-tide line. Global warming has caused sea level rise and day-to-day nuisance flooding that has a negative economic impact. Nuisance flooding is when the tide rises high enough to disrupt daily activity. This is flooding that's not necessarily associated with any storm but caused by the direction of the wind, the phase of the moon, or the time of year and so it's sometimes called "sunny-day flooding" or a "king tide." In 2017, a study showed that Annapolis businesses suffered between $86,000 and $172,000 that year in lost business due to nuisance flooding at City Dock.

In 2017, the National Oceanic and Atmospheric Administration reported that Annapolis experiences the greatest increase in average annual nuisance flooding of any U.S. city. While there were only 3.8 days of nuisance flooding between 1957 and 1963, there were 39.3 days of floods between 2007 and 2013, a whopping 925 percent increase. It's only getting worse. The Union of Concerned Scientists predicted that Annapolis will experience as many as 200 annual flood days by 2030 and 350 annual flood days by 2040. In November 2021 the

City Dock was flooded shin deep and kayakers paddled past the restaurants on Dock Street.

Yet on this day, the tide was at its normal level, the sun was in the sky and all was well at City Dock. Millie and I strolled past a coffee klatch of a half dozen seasoned gentlemen sitting in the shade of the trees and solving the problems of the world. A lone cyclist zipped past, and a jogger or two. A local dad had brought his grown-up son visiting from California to see the harbor. The son confessed he needed a "doggie fix" and asked if he could say hello to Millie. I readily agreed, and Millie happily succumbed to a heartfelt hug and a scrub behind the ears.

Annapolis is a great town for walkers, and I met one of the most devoted just them: my friend Tom Mullen from across the harbor in Eastport. Tom walks five miles a day, six days a week—though in the summer, he gives himself a break and walks only five days a week. Still, you'll see him in his red T-shirt and baseball cap all around town. We posed for a photograph, then Tom strode off on the rest of his walk while Millie and I headed for home. It was almost 10 o'clock, the hour that the parking meters must be fed.

Annapolis City Dock
One Dock Street
Annapolis, MD 21401

Free admission

Plenty of free parking until 10 a.m.

Toilets available in the Harbormaster's building

Companionable dogs on leash are welcome; doggie bag dispensers available

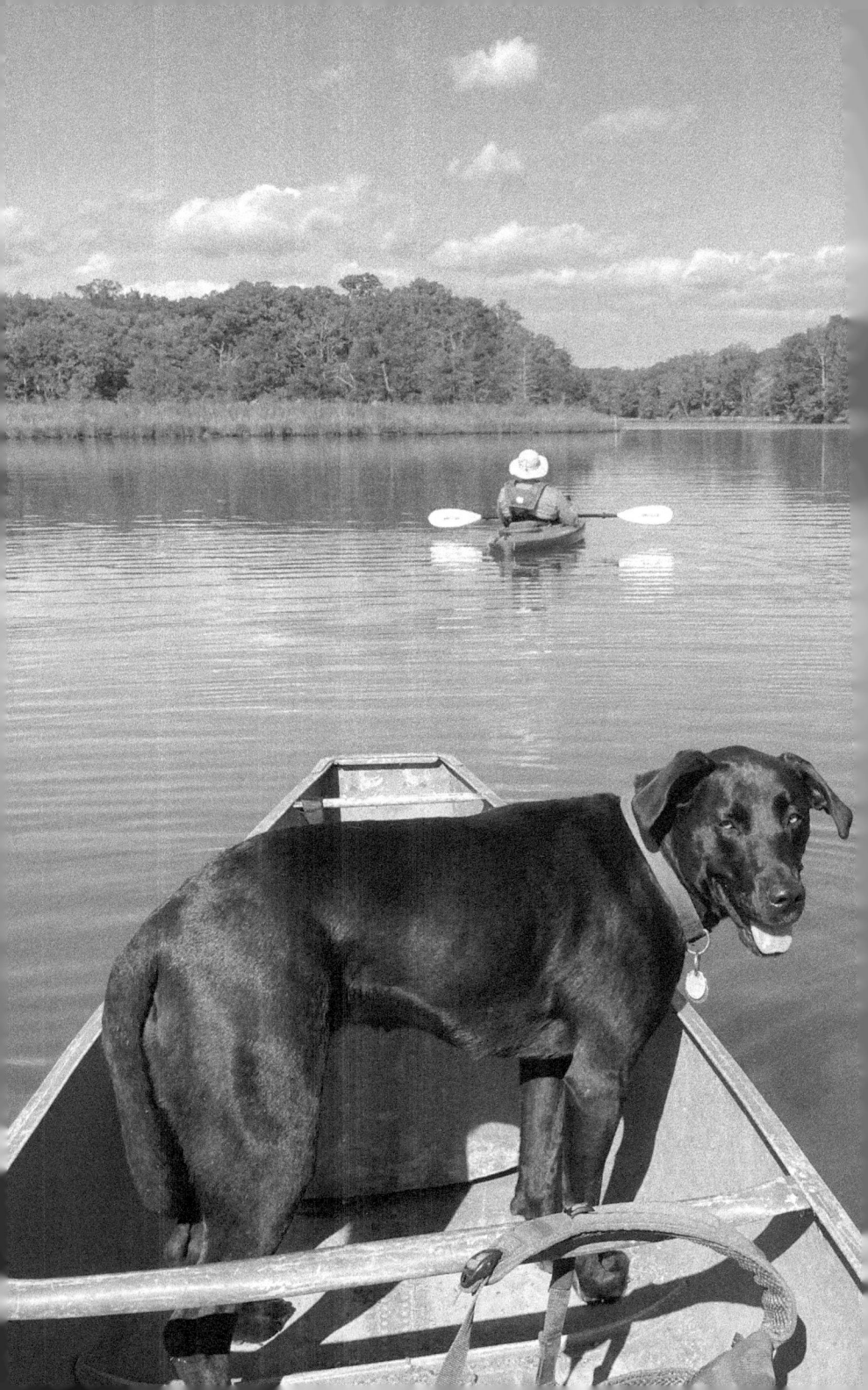

Walk 45

Paddling the Rhode River

It was good to get my old canoe out on the water for the first time in a long time, thanks to help from my new friend Jon Chapman, who picked me up at my house with his dandy trailer one fine day in mid-October 2023. The canoe is a 17-foot square-stern Grumman aluminum that my dad bought when I was six years old. Over the years, it's been paddled down the length of the Allegheny River in Pennsylvania, explored a long stretch of the Russian River through the Napa Valley in California, and bumped into alligators on the Peace River in Florida. Here on the Chesapeake, I added oarlocks to row it on the open waters of the Bay. It weighs 94 pounds, so it took the two of us to load it up.

Chapman, who lives in Annapolis, recently retired from the Maryland Environmental Trust where he served as Stewardship Manager, overseeing more than 1,300 properties protected with conservation easements statewide. He's a cheerful sort of fellow, and we had a good chat on our drive down to Mayo to launch my canoe and his kayak at Carr's Wharf on the Rhode River. My good dog Millie came along with us. She behaves well in a small boat, and she's the perfect weight to act as ballast.

This was one of those stellar early fall days. The trees were just beginning to show a hint of color. The air temperature was right around 70 degrees. I looked up data from the National Oceanic and Atmospheric Administration's "smart buoy" anchored off the mouth of the Severn River, where the water temperature was about 64 degrees. This is important to know, because if the water's much colder than that, it can be dangerous if you were to tip over. The main hazard comes from hypothermia. The longer you're in the water, the harder it is to rescue yourself. But there's also the danger of the gasp reflex when you first plunge into cold water. It's difficult to breathe when you've filled your lungs with a pint of brackish creek water.

Fortunately, we chose a calm day with a light breeze out of the south, and of course we both wore life jackets. Carr's Wharf is an Anne Arundel County park located on the southern edge of the Mayo Peninsula. The county recently rebuilt the 309-foot-long fishing pier, where we found one lone fellow chicken-necking for crabs. The boat ramp is mostly sand, which is great for launching paddle-able boats.

Millie settled in the stern of the canoe, and I shoved off. I'm quite familiar with this area, having served as the Riverkeeper for the Rhode River and the West River for six years. I've patrolled every inch of shoreline while monitoring water quality and serving as the eyes, ears, and voice of the rivers. It was a fun job and I enjoyed all the time I spent out on the water. The office of the little nonprofit organization was at Discovery Village in Shady Side for several years, then we moved to the campus of the Smithsonian Environmental Research Center in

Edgewater. Several years ago, my old organization merged with Arundel Rivers Federation, whose headquarters are now in Mayo.

The Smithsonian owns a good deal of the shoreline as part of its 2,600-acre property. As we pulled away from the launch site, the contrast was striking: the shoreline of the Mayo Peninsula side of the river was lined with million-dollar mansions, while the rest of the shoreline owned mostly by the Smithsonian and YMCA Camp Letts hasn't changed a whole lot since Capt. John Smith sailed by more than 400 years ago.

We paddled and rowed across the mouth of Bear Creek and checked on the living shoreline at Camp Letts. This was a restoration project managed by the Riverkeeper organization while I was there. Wave action had eroded the shore, creating a sheer bluff. Contractors installed low-rock breakwaters and backfilled them with sand and gravel. We got school groups and local families to come and plant marsh grasses and native trees to hold the sand in place. I told Chapman about what happened the very day after the contractors removed their heavy equipment. It was early spring, and I watched a female horseshoe crab crawl up the new beach to lay her eggs. Build it and they will come, I think I heard somebody say one time.

We paddled up past the Camp Letts marina and poked into the mouth of Selman Creek. I pointed out an eagle's nest high up in a tree on the far bank, and sure enough, we saw one and then two bald eagles soaring above the tree line. One year, I counted no less than four eagle nests on the Rhode and West rivers.

I've never figured out how the rivers in Anne Arundel County got their names. Capt. John Smith named most of the rivers on the Chesapeake after the people he met living there, people like the Choptanks, the Susquehannocks, and the Nanticokes. But he seems to have skipped by our rivers, mainly because at that time, the Susquehannocks to the north of here were at war with the Piscataways to the west of here, and this area was a sort of no man's land, so there was nobody living here for Capt. Smith to meet and name the rivers after.

I can see why the first Welsh settlers copied the name of the Severn River on the Western Shore as well as the Wye and Tred Avon Rivers on the Eastern Shore, but I'm mystified by how the South River and West Rivers got their names. I do have a theory about the Rhode River, though. It doesn't seem to be associated with a family name like Carr's Wharf and Selman Creek, but it could be a divergent spelling of the word "road," which is another word for a ship anchorage.

In colonial times, when tobacco was the mainstay of the economy, ships would sail across the Atlantic from England to load up casks or hogsheads tamped full with "sot weed." The ships would stop at the wharf of each plantation, and when their holds were filled, they would gather together in one spot to sail across the ocean as a fleet to be able defend themselves from the predations of pirates and French and Spanish privateers. What better place to anchor out than the Rhode River? It's protected from bad weather no matter what direction it comes from. And it's one of the prettiest anchorages on the whole Chesapeake Bay.

With the wind so calm, Chapman and I could chat easily on this and other diverse topics as we paddled along. It turns out that we have a lot of acquaintances and former colleagues in common, both of us having served in the environmental community. On our way back to Carr's Wharf, I pointed down the main channel toward the West River and told Chapman about the time I saw that whole square half-mile of water swarming with a huge pod of dolphins. That was before Millie's time, but I wonder how she would have responded. I'll bet she'd have jumped in to play with them. What good dog wouldn't?

Rhode River
Carr's Wharf
1001 Carrs Wharf Road
Mayo, MD 21037
Open dawn to dusk daily
Free admission
Free parking for 10 cars
Portable toilet on site
Cheerful dogs on leashes are welcome; bring your own doggie bags

Walk 46

Elktonia Beach: Walking a New Park with a New Walking Buddy

I'm going to have to change Millie's name. Now that our granddaughter, Lyla, has been learning to talk, she calls Millie, our rescue retriever, "Mimi!" (Always with an exclamation point). Mimi—that is, Millie—is always very excited to see Lyla and our daughter, Anna, when they come to Annapolis to visit us. And last week, Lyla took a walk along with Millie and me at Elktonia Beach.

Yes, at nearly 18 months old, Lyla is walking and talking; at least she's beginning to figure it all out. And we had a ball together, the three of us.

Elktonia Beach is the newest park in the city of Annapolis, occupying a five-acre bit of waterfront on the Chesapeake Bay at the mouth of the Severn River.

It's the last remnant of the 180-acre property that Black entrepreneur Fred Carr bought in 1902. His daughters, Elizabeth Carr Smith and Florence Carr Sparrow, owned and operated two side-by-side resorts for their Black patrons between the 1930s and the 1970s. They provided rare access to the water at a time when most other beaches were segregated.

When we first moved here in the 1980s, before the Chesapeake Harbour complex was built, I walked among the rusted skeletons of the pavilions at Carr's and Sparrow's Beaches where people from all around the region gathered

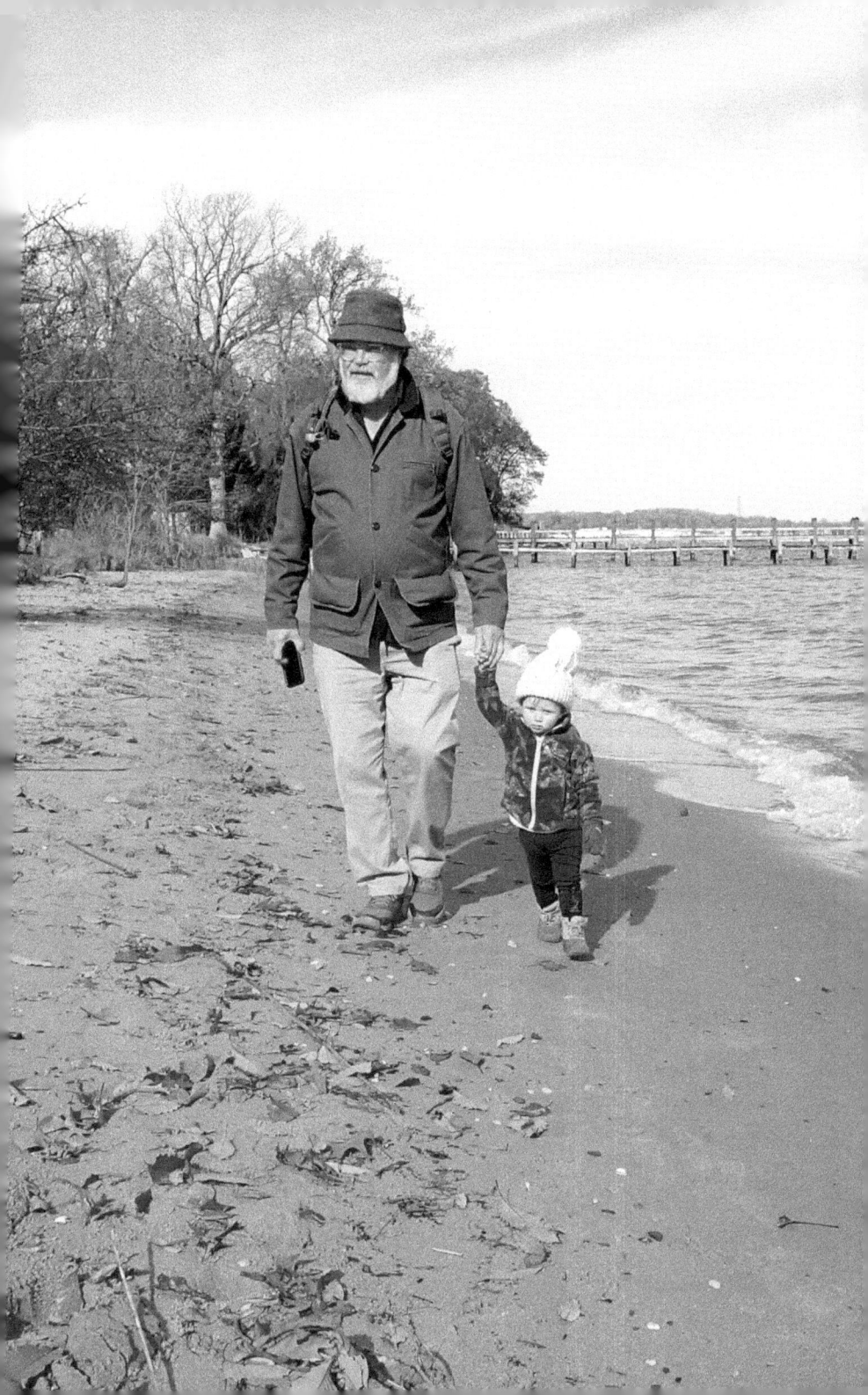

to hear and dance to the music of such renowned stars as Ella Fitzgerald, James Brown, and Otis Redding.

I'm convinced—with absolutely no facts to back me up—that Otis Redding wrote "Sittin' on the Dock of the Bay" here on this Bay, and only changed the setting to San Francisco when his agent feared that a song about the Chesapeake would never get airplay. I have yet to have anyone prove me wrong about this notion.

My friend Vince Leggett, founder of the Blacks of the Chesapeake Foundation, spearheaded a drive to save the last five acres of The Beaches. Last year, the Foundation signed an agreement between the city of Annapolis, Chesapeake Conservancy, the state of Maryland, and The Conservation Fund to purchase the property with federal, state, and city Program Open Space funds.

Former Governor Larry Hogan and the Maryland Department of Natural Resources also helped, along with federal funds, thanks to U.S. Senator Ben Cardin as well as a state grant, thanks to the support of State Sen. Sarah Elfreth. There are plans afoot to protect the beach from erosion with a living shoreline and to conserve the adjacent property to expand the park and create an area for interpretation for Blacks of the Chesapeake.

The beach is just a short drive from our home. I strapped Lyla into her car seat, and Millie hopped into the back. We parked in the lot of the Annapolis Maritime Museum and Park, formerly the Ellen O. Moyer Nature Park on Edgewood Road. With Lyla's mittened hand wrapped firmly around my little finger, we crossed the road and walked the tree-lined lane to the beach. There's no sign for the park on the road yet, but you'll find the lane across from the entrance to Port Annapolis Marina.

There are four large interpretive panels at the end of the lane explaining the site's historic significance, but it's when you emerge from the woods and see the open vista of the Chesapeake Bay that you really appreciate what the place is all about. You should have seen the look of delight on Lyla's face, eyes bright blue and cheeks cherry red from the 50-degree chill. She strode right down to the water's edge—or did the toddler's rendition of a stride, anyway—where the waves lapped gently up onto her rubber boots.

We walked up and down the short stretch of beach where there were smooth white stones to sift out of the sand, a slab of driftwood to teeter on like a balance beam, an old tennis ball that had washed up into the reeds to toss to Millie: no end of fascinating distractions for a one-and-a-half-year-old to discover. Then we sat together on a lone wooden bench to admire the view of the Eiffel-shaped towers on Greenbury Point across the mouth of the Severn River, the low white arch of the Bay Bridge gleaming in the sun and the ships at anchor way out in the middle of the Chesapeake.

Lyla couldn't have known that her mother, Anna, grew up on this same beach just a few hundred yards from this site, on the other side of the Bay Woods retirement community. We used to rent a little cottage on Bembe

Beach where Anna was born and where we lived until she was middle-school age. But it made me happy to see Lyla appreciating being at the beach with the same joy as Anna.

Lyla and I got along fine that chilly afternoon, even after she lost her balance right as a rogue wave splashed over the toes of her boots and she landed bottom-down in the wet sand. We even re-discovered the mitten she had shucked along the way.

By the time Lyla and Millie and I got back to the car, we had walked about three quarters of a mile all told, but then I realized that as tall as she is for her age, her little legs are only about one third the length of mine, which means that she walked an equivalent of 2.25 miles!

I'm grateful for my time with Lyla, and grateful that she and her parents live near enough for us to get together so often. It's been astonishing to watch this little human evolve and grow so fast. She seems to achieve some new level of ability, dexterity, and mental agility every time I see her. I'm not sure if she'll ever call Millie anything other than Mimi!, but I will tell you how my heart flip-flopped the first time she pointed at a picture of me and murmured, "Pops!"

Another thing I'm grateful for is the opportunity to have written the column on which this book is based. It's so nice when people stop me in the aisle of the grocery store to tell me how much they enjoy reading it and going on the walks I've written about. Here's a mystery that some alert reader might solve for me: What's the origin of the name Elktonia? Was it somehow related to the Elk's Club?

If you know, please send me a note at ArundelHappyTrails@gmail.com.

Elktonia Beach
7131 Bembe Beach Road
Annapolis, Maryland 21403

annapolis.gov/1972/Elktonia-Carrs-Beach

Limited parking across the road at the Annapolis Maritime Museum and Park (formerly Ellen O. Moyer Back Creek Nature Park)

Free admission

Open dawn to dusk

No toilets

Toddlers and convivial dogs on leashes are welcome; bring your own doggie bags (and diapers)

Walk 47

Chasing the Chill at Chesapeake Bay Foundation

It hadn't snowed in so long I couldn't find my old snow shovel. And me with a 100-foot-long driveway. The last time it snowed, I think it was three years ago, we got dumped on and I had to dig us out. After I'd cleared four or five yards of driveway, I started hearing the bass voice—deep as a coal mine—of Tennessee Ernie Ford rumbling in my ears, singing, "Shovel 16 tons, and what do you get? Another sore shoulder and a crink in your neck. St. Peter, don't you call me, 'cause I can't go—I still gotta dig through all of this snow…"

Fortunately, the drive runs down a south-facing slope, so if there's only a few of inches of snow, like that first snow in mid-January 2024, most of it disappears all by itself as long as the sun shines. So, thankful to be relieved of that particular chore, I allowed nature to take its course while I took my good dog Millie for a walk. In the snow. That morning started out at 18 degrees Fahrenheit. I waited until it warmed all the way up to 26 degrees.

I've got a good pair of snow boots, waterproof with thick felt liners, and I bundle up in layers, so I'm generally quite comfortable out in that sort of weather, even though I'm not a big fan of the cold. Millie, on the other hand, doesn't just tolerate the snow; she lathers in it.

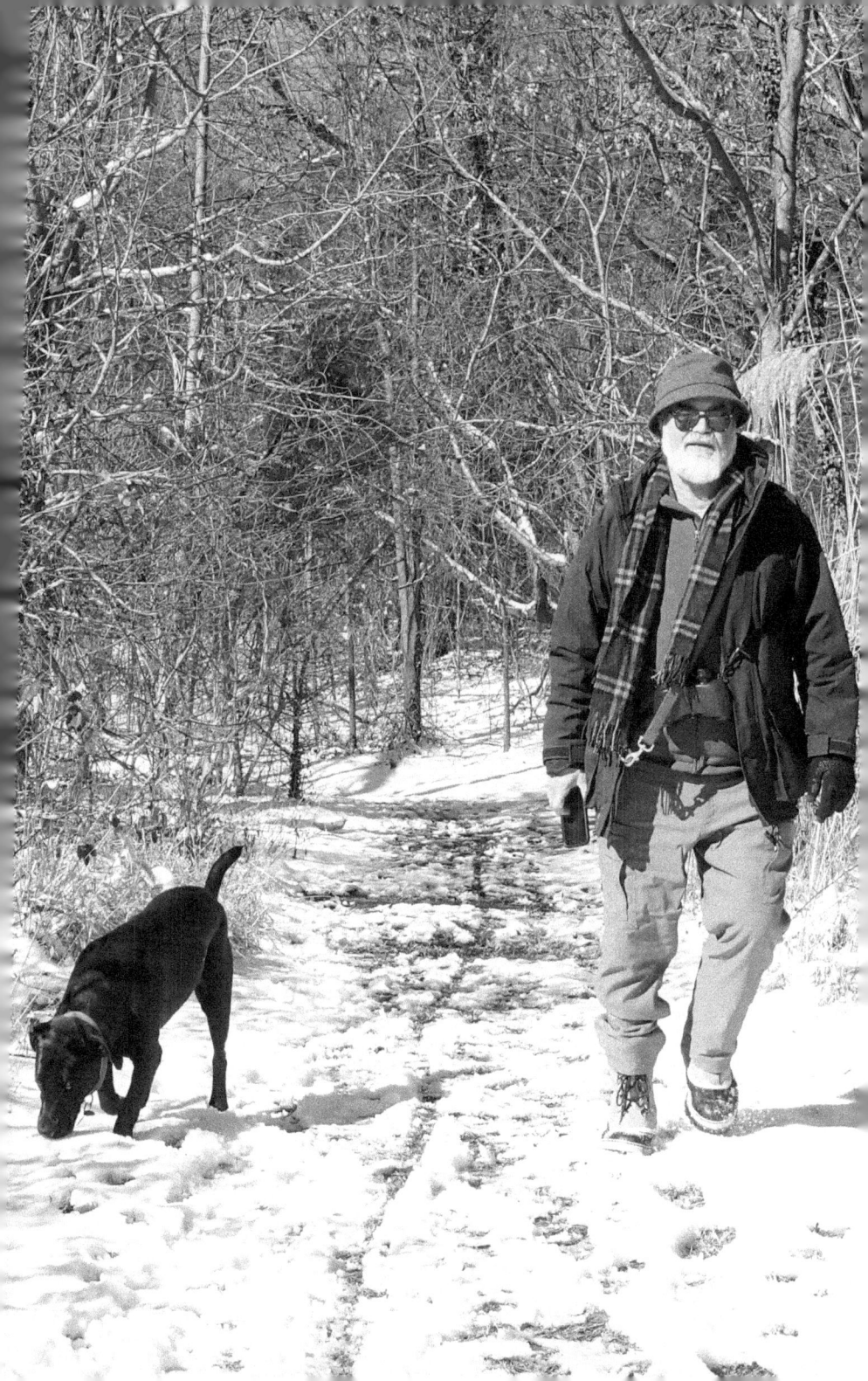

I was hoping to catch sight of one of the flocks of tundra swans that hang around these parts. Sometimes they're gathered near the beach on the South River in our community, which sits next door to Quiet Waters Park. Other times they raft up on one side of Thomas Point or the other. We drove to Thomas Point Park, which is open to the public free of charge until the end of March, but we saw only a handful of swans and some canvasback ducks. The last time we were there, just a week before, we saw a raft of at least 50 swans off the end of the point and just as many in another bunch on the river side near the park entrance.

Since we'd recently been to that park, I decided to try something different. It turns out that the public is welcome to walk around the property at the Chesapeake Bay Foundation's headquarters in Bay Ridge during office hours. We parked in the upper lot in front of the Phillip Merrill Environmental Center. When it opened more than 20 years ago, it was the first building to receive the U.S. Green Building Council's Platinum rating for Leadership in Energy and Environmental Design. It's named for the diplomat and philanthropist who also happened to have owned and published the *Annapolis Capital* newspaper before his untimely death in 2006.

Founded in Annapolis in 1967, the Chesapeake Bay Foundation now has offices in Maryland, Virginia, Pennsylvania, and the District of Columbia and 15 field centers where they provide environmental education for thousands of students. It's one of the leading nonprofit organizations restoring the Bay and its rivers and streams.

On the day we visited, the sky was clear and blue, and the sun gleamed a shimmering silver across the surface of the Bay. The wind was calm, so the cold was not oppressive. Millie and I crunched through the snow and walked the sandy beach from the pier to the inlet of Black Walnut Creek, an intriguing channel that winds back from the Bay through a marsh and opens up onto a broad saltwater pond.

On the far side of the creek, you can see the houses of the Highland Beach community. Historically, this started out in the 1890s as a rare summer resort for Black families from Washington, D.C. Highland Beach was founded by Frederick Douglass' youngest son Charles, and the cottage Charles built for his father now houses the Frederick Douglass Museum and Cultural Center.

Legend has it that Charles built the house with a deck on the second floor so his father could stand there and look across the Bay to see the Eastern Shore where he grew up. He was born in a little cabin on the banks of Tuckahoe Creek in 1817 or 1818. I've kayaked by that spot. I'd like to come back here and kayak Black Walnut Creek when the water gets warmer.

Millie led me along a trail through the woods that paralleled the near shore of the pond. I was disappointed that the only birds we saw were the little songbirds flicking about in the bushes. What I took for a great blue heron turned out to be a branch protruding from a submerged log.

The trail led us into a thicket of Virginia pines, their paired needles forming a "V" for Virginia. We came across several inviting benches along the way with splendid views of the pond. There in the woods, the air was still and it was actually quite pleasant despite the cold. By the time the path circled us back to the parking lot, we had logged about a mile and a half, just the right length for a quick winter outing.

Millie and I drove back home, where I warmed up over a bowl of soup with ham and black-eyed peas, but she insisted on being let out onto the screen porch where she plopped down on her day bed for a chilly nap.

The Phillip Merrill Environmental Center
6 Herndon Ave.
Annapolis, MD 21403

Open 8:30 a.m.–5 p.m., Mon.–Fri., except holidays

Park in the upper parking lot

In the summer, you need to get a pass to use the beach

No toilets

Compatible dogs on leashes are welcome; bring your own doggie bags

Walk 48

Discovering History at Jonas and Anne Catharine Green Park

Annapolis has celebrated many important women over the course of its venerable history, but one particular stand-out is Anne Catharine Green. Her husband Jonas died in 1767, leaving the widow with her husband's debts to repay and six children to feed. Others with the same plight, but not the same backbone, might have given up and begged for alms from the parish priest, but not Anne.

Jonas' print shop sat behind their rented home on Charles Street, and Anne pulled up the sleeves of her gown and took up her late husband's work publishing the Maryland *Gazette*, forerunner of the very newspaper where these essays were first published. Under her diligence and drive, the business thrived, and soon she could afford to buy her house and even commission a portrait of herself by none other than Charles Wilson Peale. Before she died in 1775, the Maryland *Gazette* became instrumental in shaping the political landscape that led to Maryland's fight for independence from British rule.

Jonas was quite the guy in his own right. Like his mentor, Benjamin Franklin, Jonas was a brilliant man of many talents. Historian Elihu Riley wrote that Jonas Green was not just a "dignified publisher," but also one of the leading wits in the Tuesday Club, Annapolis' mid-18th-century version of the Algonquin Round Table. Green's disparate titles were recorded in the club's annals as "P.P.P.P.P." or "poet, printer, punster, purveyor, and punchmaker."

Each weekly meeting at the stately home of one or another member began with a series of toasts, followed by a hearty meal and entertainment in the form of music, poetry, bad jokes, and riddles; and apparently, Jonas Green was adept at all of those pursuits. Truly a man after my own heart, or more appropriately, I am a man after his own heart.

I read up on Jonas and Anne after visiting their namesake Anne Arundel County park on the north side of the Naval Academy Bridge on one of those chilly, overcast, early-March days in 2024. My wonderful rescue retriever, Millie, came along, of course. The park is known locally as Jonas Green Park, but the actual name is Jonas and Anne Catharine Green Park. It doesn't cover a lot of ground, only six acres, but the site has dramatic views across the Severn River of the U.S. Naval Academy, with the city's age-old domes and spires sprouting above the skyline.

The park lies within the shadow of the Naval Academy Bridge, built in 1994. This bridge replaced a beautiful bascule drawbridge that was opened for new-fangled automobile traffic in 1924. There's a remnant of that older bridge that juts out into the river a full 288 feet, providing fishermen with a high pier to dangle their lines from. (Note to the grammar police: Merriam-Webster recently declared that it's "permissible" for people speaking

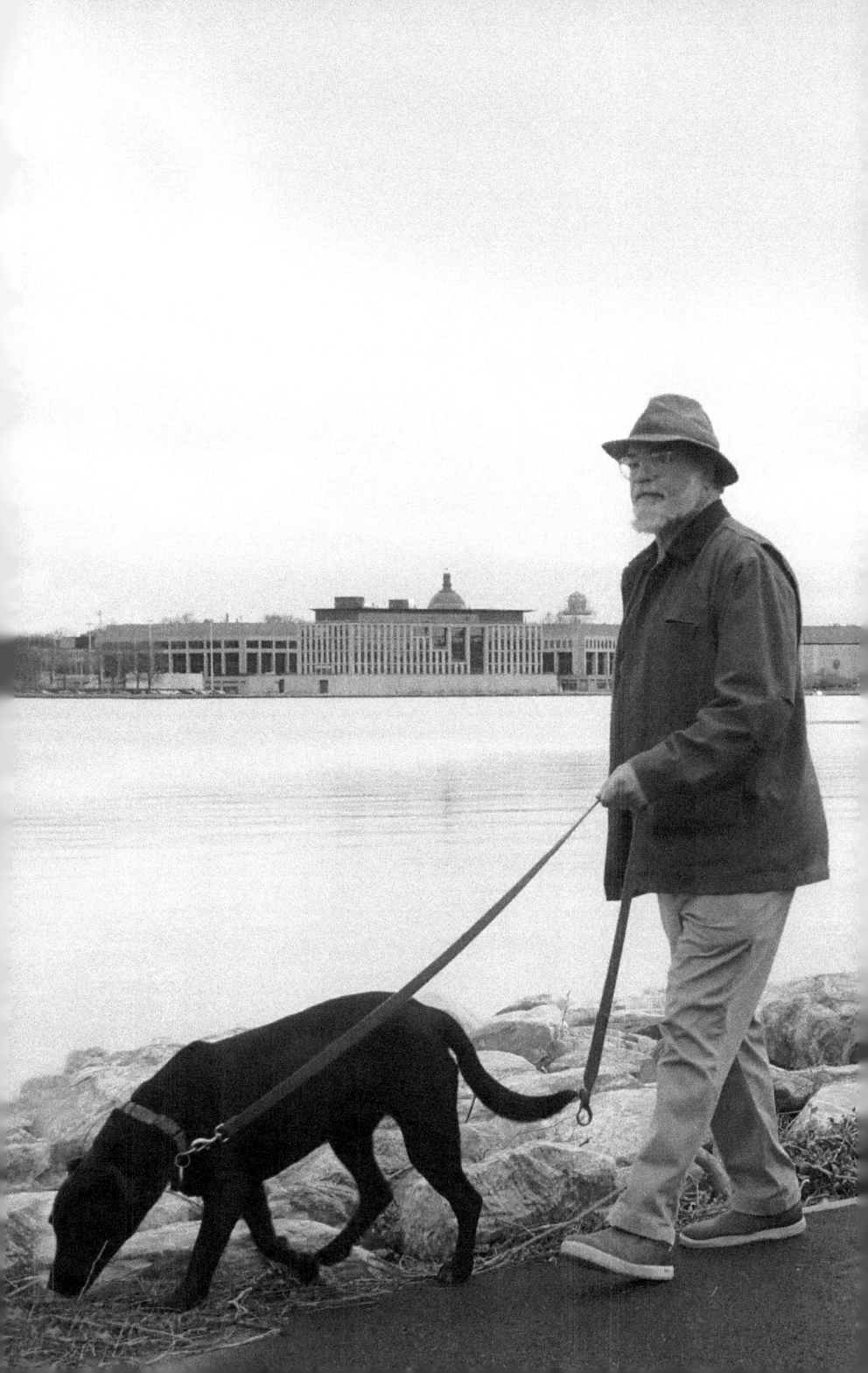

English to end sentences with prepositions. What's next, permission to dangle participles?)

I've been up and down this river thousands of times over the years in everything from the governor's yacht to a staysail schooner, but I'd never seen the Severn from this vantage point. From there, you can see the other bridge spanning the river more than a mile upstream. That's the U.S. Route 50/301 Bridge, which opened in 1953. You can also see a huge white mansion with a broad staircase leading down to the river's edge. That's Manresa, which began as a spiritual retreat for Jesuit priests in the late 1920s. It became an assisted-living facility in 1995.

Millie led me on the short loop around the park grounds, cheerfully greeting a number of other well-behaved dogs, large and small. Most of the walkways are paved, and the whole park is handicap accessible. As we strolled, we noticed a squad of T-shirted midshipmen and women jogging across the bridge above us and a crew of other middies racing up the Severn in a pair of rowing shells. The path winds underneath the deck of the old bridge and links to a short stretch of beach, where a young couple were lounging on lawn chairs with their big, beautiful rottweiler. You can launch a canoe, stand-up paddleboard, or a kayak from here, but whatever you do, don't go in for a swim. The current can be treacherous.

There are several interpretive panels explaining the site's living shoreline and stormwater runoff pond habitats. A muddle of mallards paddled in a puddle, much to Millie's amusement, but apart from a stray herring gull, we didn't see much other wildlife. Lately, I've heard of osprey sightings in the area, but haven't seen or heard any myself yet. The osprey returning from Central and South America are a sure sign of spring, along with the bright yellow daffodils sprouting up through the grass here and there.

Millie seemed to linger on the beach, wistfully eyeing the river with its still-clear winter water. Soon the water temperature will be warm enough for her to start swimming regularly. I'm sure she'd love to do it now, and I'm sure she'd be fine—I once had a retriever who would break through the ice for a chance for a swim—but I'll keep her dry for another few weeks until spring arrives for real.

The visitor center at the park doubles as the headquarters and trailhead for Anne Arundel County's extensive network of recreational trails that include the B&A Trail, BWI Trail, Broadneck Peninsula Trail, and the WB&A Trail. Just think, you can hop on a bike here and ride all over the northern section of the county. That would be fun, if I could figure out a way to bring Millie along.

Reading about Anne Catharine Green, I couldn't help imagining a bronze statue of her with her printing press adorning the Westgate Circle. I can't think of a better way to honor an amazing woman, creative and determined and intelligent, the first female publisher in America at a time when few women worked outside of the home, editor of the first newspaper in Maryland and one of the first in the Colonies. It would be a monument to all of the strong women in Annapolis' long history.

Jonas and Anne Catharine Green Park
2001 Baltimore Annapolis Blvd
Annapolis, MD 21409

aacounty.org/locations/jonas-green-park

Open hours vary with the season; see web site for info

Plenty of free parking on site

Free admission.

Restrooms in the Visitor Center

Handicap accessible

Well-disposed dogs on leashes are welcome; doggie bag dispensers available

Walk 49

Ferry Point Park and Fried Oysters: A Winning Combination

A certain musical pal of mine posted something of interest last Monday. He noted that March 31 was the end of the wild-caught oyster season, so it's time for the Great Chesapeake Bay Oyster Migration, when herds of those tasty bivalves make their way up the C&D Canal to head toward their traditional summering grounds in the cold water off Nova Scotia.

Huh. I thought I knew a lot about oysters, but that was news to me. I wondered why Gerald Winegrad hasn't yet written about it in his excellent column on Chesapeake Bay environmental issues. Still, my friend's mention of oysters made me hanker to slurp some while there still might be a few left, so I headed across the Bay to Kent Narrows, where seafood restaurants line the waterfront like so many cormorants perched on a row of pilings.

Kent Narrows is the strait that separates Kent Island from the mainland of Queen Anne's County and Maryland's Eastern Shore. We visited there on one of those misty days in early April 2024. The "we" of course, refers to me and Millie, the rescue retriever. She needed a walk, so we stopped at a place that we hadn't tried before: Ferry Point Park. I'd driven past the place thousands of times, and I was curious to find out what it was all about.

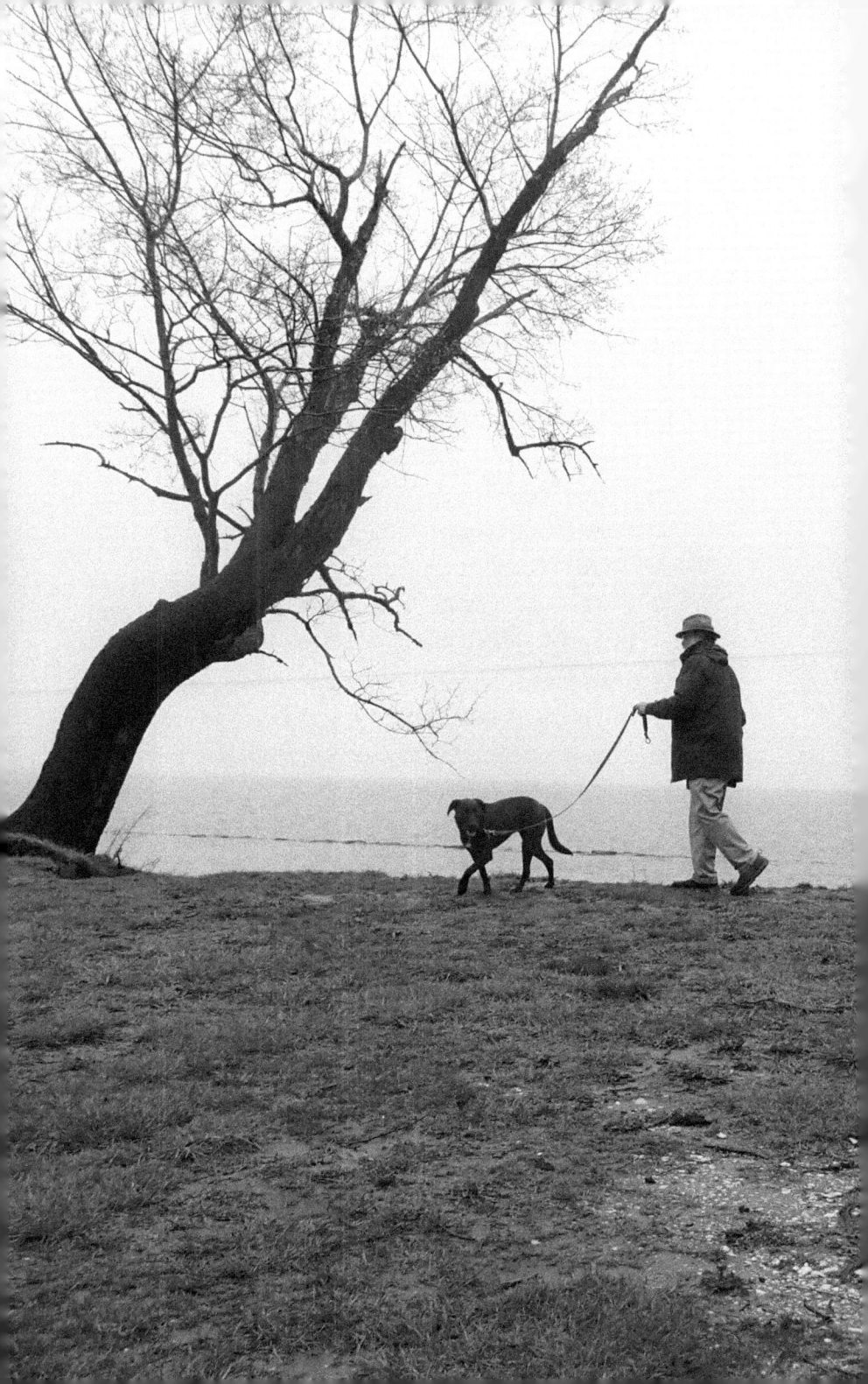

It's only about a half hour drive from our home in Annapolis. Driving across the Bay Bridge, the fog was so thick I couldn't see the tops of the towers, let alone any distance north or south. I knew there were at least six big ships at anchor in the middle of the Bay between the bridge and Thomas Point Shoal Lighthouse, but they were completely invisible.

We parked at the newly renovated Chesapeake Heritage Center, which serves as the Queen Anne County visitor center. Ferry Point Park occupies a 41-acre peninsula of loblolly pine and marsh that extends in a T shape out between Piney Creek and the northern end of the Kent Narrows channel.

In colonial times, the Narrows was so shallow, it was known as the "Wading Place." A ferry launched from this point carried passengers and cargo across the channel to the Eastern Shore. A raised earthen causeway built in 1826 allowed wagons to cross, but it closed the Narrows to all boat traffic. Fifty years later, they dismantled the causeway and dredged the channel. Since then, this stretch of water has been home port for hundreds, if not thousands of working watermen.

Millie led the way along a boardwalk spanning the marsh, then we followed a paved road about a quarter of a mile long that brought us to a lane lined with crushed oyster shell. We followed the lane to the right, which was lined with bristling pines. Red-winged blackbirds flashed their bright shoulder bars through the reeds and filled the air with their warbling trills. An osprey chirruped as it flew overhead and came to rest in its newly formed nest high up in a tree leaning out over the water.

The park has just reopened after being closed for renovation. There are conveniently placed benches along the trail, all of which look new. Fortunately, most of the site has been left in its natural, pristine state. It's not at all difficult to imagine the Monoponson people making a very pleasant living here, fishing and gathering oysters and hunting wild game. That is, until the English showed up.

Curiously, the first settlement in Maryland was not St. Mary's City, but just south of this point on Kent Island, where a Virginian named William Claiborne established a trading post in 1631 to buy beaver furs from the Indians. That was three years before Lord Baltimore's contingent arrived on the *Ark* and the *Dove* to settle Maryland.

It was Claiborne who named the island after his home county back in England. He chafed at Baltimore's claim that the island was in Maryland territory, not Virginia. The two sides even fought over the question in 1635 on the Pocomoke Sound, the first recorded naval battle between Englishmen on the North American continent. Baltimore's forces seized the island in 1638. After losing his claim in court, Claiborne and his family returned to Virginia, and Kent Island became a permanent part of Maryland.

Millie and I met only a couple of other people who braved the weather that day, an older gentleman with a frisky tricolored Australian shepherd pup and a retired couple with a retriever who was nearly identical to Millie, with its short, floppy ears and white blaze on the chest. They were surprised to learn that both Millie and their dog were Labradors mixed with border collies, which explains their high energy and keen intellect.

Millie and I reached the end of the road, which looped around in the woods, then walked back along the beach. It was just past high tide, but there was still a narrow stretch of sand cluttered with intricately sculpted driftwood. One huge log had washed up into the reeds, so smooth and dark it looked from a distance like a beached manatee. Millie enjoyed posing on top of it. A fringe of loblollies decorated the far point, where the crescent-shaped cove came to an end.

I'm sure if it hadn't been drizzling and fog-bound, we'd have had wonderful views across the mouth of the Chester River to Eastern Neck Island on the far side. But the weather only added to the dramatic coastal scenery. We both found it quite enjoyable to walk through it in the light drizzle, but as the rain began to come down harder, we headed back to the car. My curiosity was satisfied, but my appetite for oysters was not.

We stopped at Harris Crab House on the other side of the Narrows. Millie curled up in her bed in the back of the car while I went inside for a plate of fried oysters. They were hot and succulent, encased in a crunchy cornbread crust and dipped in tangy cocktail sauce. It was while I was watching a lone workboat rumbling past in the current and chomping down on the third fried oyster that it hit me: My buddy posted about the Great Chesapeake Bay Oyster Migration on Monday. Monday was April 1. No wonder Gerald Winegrad never wrote about it.

Ferry Point Park
600 Swan Cove Lane
Chester, MD 21619

Open dawn to dusk

Plenty of parking at the Chesapeake Heritage and Visitor Center

Free admission

Restrooms are located inside the Visitor Center

**Compatible dogs on leashes are welcome;
bring your own doggie bags**

Ferry Point Park is a nature park, so the county bans coolers, grills, open fires, shade structures and fishing.

Walk 50

Encountering Genius at Benjamin Banneker Historical Park & Museum

How do you account for genius? Benjamin Banneker had very little formal education, but he became one of early America's most brilliant astronomers. Like George Washington, he was a surveyor, and like Benjamin Franklin, he was an inventor and publisher of almanacs containing no end of useful information. Unlike those other Founding Fathers, Banneker happened to be Black.

To celebrate the great man's 292nd birthday in November 2023, I visited the Benjamin Banneker Historical Park & Museum near Ellicott City with my friend Jon Chapman and my rescue retriever, Millie. This is a Baltimore County Park located on 142 acres in the Patapsco River valley. While we were disappointed that the museum happened to be closed at the time of our visit, we were really there to walk the trails.

If the museum had been open, we would have seen exhibits of Benjamin Banneker's life and legacy. He was born free on November 9, 1731 in a tiny log cabin on this site. His mother was a white indentured servant who attained her freedom and started growing tobacco. She bought an enslaved prince from Senegal named Bannaka, freed him and then married him. After Bannaka died, she married another black man who adopted the Bannaka

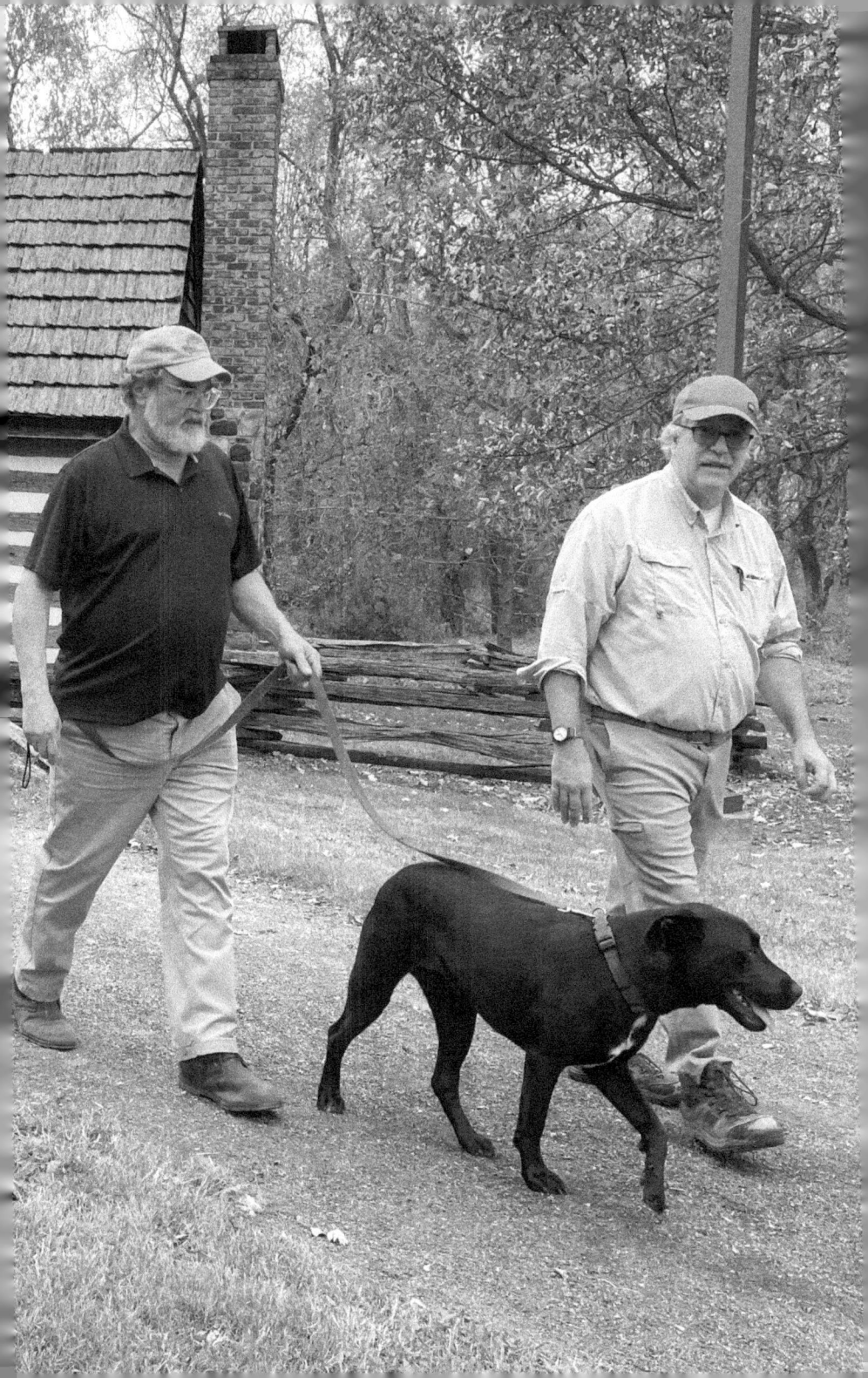

name, and he became Benjamin's father. The name Bannaka eventually morphed into Banneker.

At the age of 21, Banneker disassembled a pocket watch, replicated each part to scale out of carved wood, and constructed a clock that ran until the day he died half a century later. He helped his neighbor Major Andrew Ellicott start the survey of what would become the District of Columbia, using his astronomical skills—and that clock—to position the cornerstone in Alexandria. The stone is still there.

He indulged in such curious pursuits as a study of the 17-year locust. His almanacs contained predictions of sunrises and sunsets, the timing of eclipses, and even the course of tides around the Chesapeake Bay. Banneker also included proverbs, mathematical puzzles, and essays on the evil of slavery. He published six almanacs between 1792 and 1797, by which time they had become bestsellers.

Noted astronomer David Rittenhouse stated that Banneker's work "was a very extraordinary performance, considering the Colour of the Author." To which Banneker replied, "I am annoyed to find that the subject of my race is so much stressed. The work is either correct or it is not. In this case, I believe it to be perfect." That response tells me a lot about the integrity of the man as well as his strength of self-worth and his keen intelligence.

Chapman and I studied the interpretive panels on display outside the museum, then set out on one of several trails. We had found a crude map in a literature dispenser attached to an information kiosk, but it wasn't a lot of help. We strolled around to the back of the museum and found a replica of the log cabin where Banneker lived most of his life, and where he died in 1806 at the age of 74, unmarried and childless.

Unfortunately, the original cabin burned to the ground during his funeral at a nearby church, and most of his journals and other papers were destroyed. We might never know the full depth of that genius.

The day we were there was one of those crazy days this past week when the temperature started out cool and then zoomed way into the 70s. We followed a trail marked with yellow blazes into the woods. We passed what must have been a well or the fountain of a spring. Chapman knows his trees, having recently retired from the Maryland Environmental Trust, where he managed more than 1,300 properties protected with conservation easements statewide.

We were both impressed by the sheer size of the maples in these woods. Two of the biggest have grown together into one massive trunk.

More than once, we became baffled by the few trail signs, none of which seemed to sync with the map. It didn't really matter, since we weren't following any particular agenda, just enjoying being out in the woods on a nice day. Eventually, we found ourselves on the paved Number Nine Trolly Trail that leads down to Ellicott City.

While that town is a perfectly pleasant place to visit, we chose not to go that route, but instead retraced our steps up the hill through the woods and at last found ourselves back at the museum.

Throughout his life, Banneker was a stout abolitionist who abhorred "that State of tyrannical thraldom, and inhuman captivity, to which too many of my brethren are doomed." He wrote a letter to Thomas Jefferson to remind him that there was a time "in which you clearly saw into the injustice of a State of Slavery, and in which you had just apprehensions of the horrors of its condition." Banneker reminded Jefferson of what he had written about "all men are created equal." Did he really mean it?

Banneker sent Jefferson a manuscript copy of his upcoming 1792 almanac. Ironically, Jefferson acknowledged Banneker's plea for universal liberty, though he never acted on it. He did, however, forward the almanac to the Academy of Sciences in Paris, France, where it was well received, much to Banneker's delight.

Throughout the year, the museum celebrates Banneker's legacy with programs and events featuring local historical re-enactors and craftsmen, along with demonstrations of cooking on an open hearth, surveying with 18th-century tools and instruments, gardening, rope-making, and other skills essential to operating a small tobacco farm like the one he inherited.

I'll have to bring Millie back for one of those events, especially the ones featuring the farm animals that would have been raised here. She seemed to have spent our entire afternoon sniffing out their scent from the last time they were there.

Benjamin Banneker Historical Park & Museum
300 Oella Avenue
Catonsville, MD 21228
Museum is open from 10 a.m. to 4 p.m.
Tue.–Sat. The park is open from sunrise to sunset
Plenty of parking on site; free admission to the park
There's a portable toilet in the parking lot
Copacetic dogs on leashes are welcome; bring your own doggie bags

Walk 51

Back Creek by Kayak

Back Creek is an astonishing body of water with a fascinating history. Not really a flowing creek at all but a tidal estuary less than a mile long, Back Creek has more than 1,200 boats of all descriptions filling the slips in a dozen commercial marinas and at scores of private piers. There are more marine-oriented businesses lining its shores than anywhere between Newport, Rhode Island, and Fort Lauderdale, Florida. Where the mouth of the creek opens up onto the Severn River, that's probably the busiest square mile of water anywhere on the East Coast, especially during special events like the annual Blue Angels demonstration.

And yet, there are quiet coves where a paddler can find repose, even with the cacophony of a half-dozen Boeing F/A-18 Super Hornets screaming overhead. I wanted to get out on the water early on the Tuesday in late May 2024, when the jet squadron makes its practice run. If I got out early enough, I could be back home before the practice started. Millie, our wonder retriever, was coming with me as usual, and I didn't want her to get freaked out by the racket. But we got out late and the Angels got out early. Yet to my surprise, Millie wasn't fazed at all when the first jets roared by, seemingly at mast-height. What a good dog. And what a great boat dog.

I had arranged to take out a tandem kayak from Capital SUP's new location at Nautilus Point, the complex in Eastport formerly known as Watergate. Capital SUP's main location is at Quiet Waters Park. They're opening up a third location at the Point Crab House on the Magothy River. When Millie and I arrived at Nautilus Point, the kayak was waiting for us on the bulkhead by Dock C.

I brought the dog mat that Millie uses as a bed from the back of the car and placed it over the bow seat. Millie hopped right on it. The kayak was one of the sit-on-top types, not my favorite, since your butt is bound to get wet, but it's easier to get in and out of than a typical kayak with a cockpit, though there's never any way to do so gracefully, no matter what type of kayak you choose. Millie tested her sea legs as the wake from a passing boat gave us a little rock and roll, but then she settled down on her mat to enjoy the ride.

We paddled across the creek to the wooded bluff with the tall blue water tower poking above the tree line. This is the site of the Ellen O. Moyer Back Creek Nature Park, now under the aegis of the Annapolis Maritime Museum. As the jets rocketed into the stratosphere to spin their looped vapor trails through the sky, several little barn swallows flitted by, and it occurred to me that these birds could achieve much more intricate aerobatic antics than the Blue Angels ever could—tighter turns, more dramatic dives, swifter swoops—and all without the deafening macho mega-decibels.

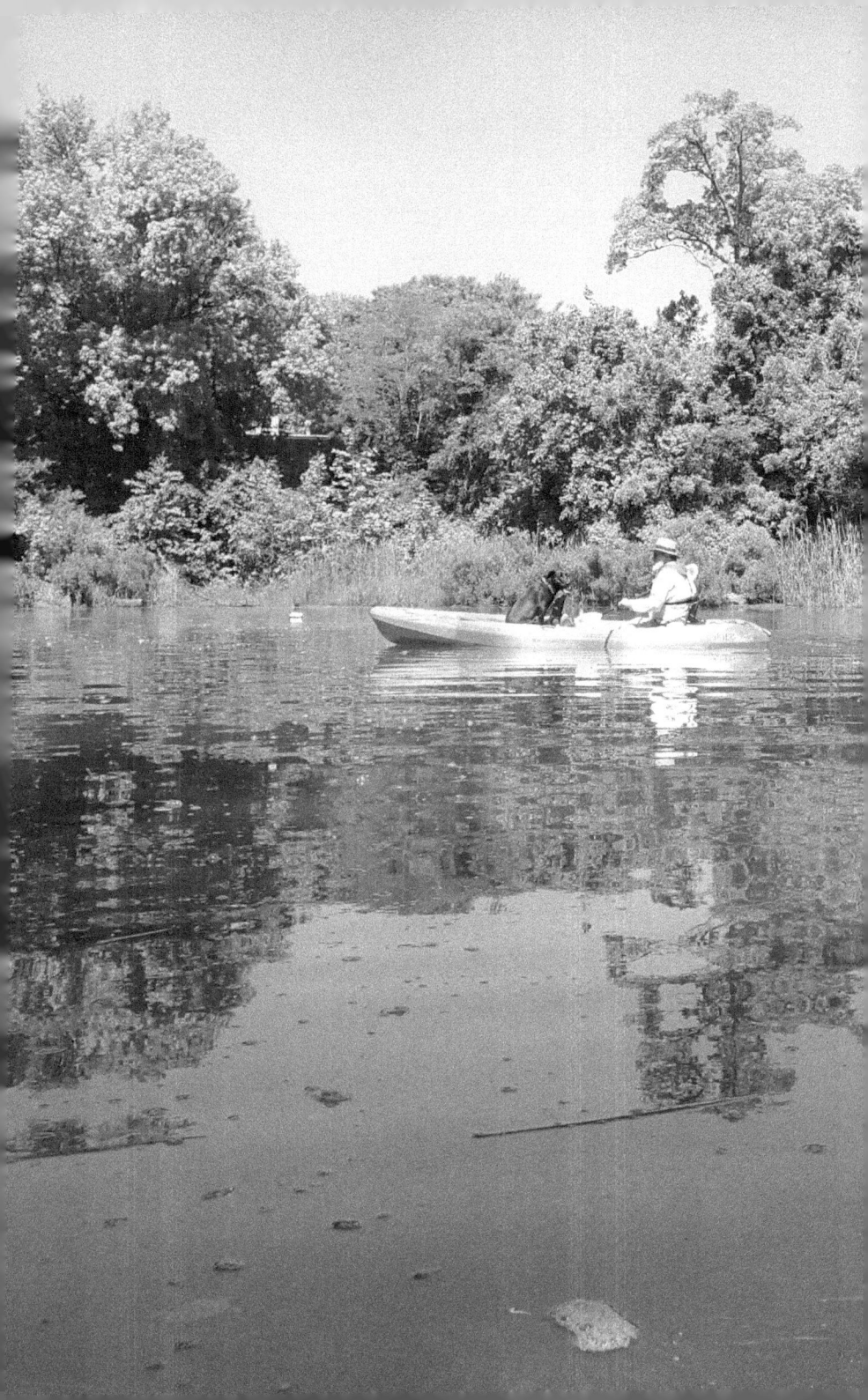

The Angels shared the sky with a number of birds that morning: a laconic great blue heron, a high-flying black vulture, and an osprey or two, none of whom seemed fazed by the air show. A pair of Canada geese paddled by, ushering four newly hatched goslings between them. Apparently, they chose to rear their young here on Back Creek rather than on the icy slopes of western Greenland. Fortunately, Millie opted not to go in swimming with them.

We paddled back across the creek to a secluded unnamed cove tucked in behind Nautilus Point. At the end of this cove is the outfall from the stream restoration project at St. Luke's Church in Eastport. There's a 180-degree viewshed of nothing but trees and marsh back there. It was so serene, you might think you were somewhere on the Eastern Shore.

Back Creek is marked on the oldest maps as Hill's Back Creek. From the mid-1600s to the mid-1700s, the Horn Point peninsula and most of what we now think of as Eastport was owned by the Hill family and used as pastureland for horses and farm stock. In 1761, the land was inherited by Henrietta Margaret Hill. Henrietta, known as Henry, was only 10 years old at the time. In 1774, at the age of 23, she married Benjamin Ogle and would become Maryland's First Lady from 1798 to 1801, when Ogle served as one of the state's early governors.

Ogle died in 1809 in Annapolis, leaving his estate to Henry, who lived until 1815. According to his last wishes,

Benjamin Ogle's body was buried in an unmarked grave. I have no idea where to find Henry's grave, either.

As we passed the street-end park on Sixth Street, I heard someone call out, "Say, is that the famous Millie?" And there, standing on the end of a pier, was my new friend Dan Bornstein, whom I'd met at a recent Maritime Republic of Eastport event. Dan was nice enough to take some photos of Millie and me as we chatted. We made it safely back to the dock as the jets wound up their practice run.

Here are a few tips on paddling around Annapolis city waters:

1

Stay out of the way. Water taxis, tour boats, and gigundo motor yachts are operated by professional captains who just might be able to see you and respond in time if you get in their way, but privately owned boats may not be operated so responsibly—or soberly. Stay out of the channel to be safe. If you do have to cross, watch for traffic and make it quick.

2

Please don't go up Market Slip, known colloquially as Ego Alley. Sure, it's fun to be seen by all the tourists, but the slip can be ridiculously busy with all kinds of boats, all maneuvering in an extraordinarily tight channel. For this reason, I think it's crazy to consider putting a kayak rental operation at City Dock. It's just asking for trouble when you inject inexperienced paddlers into one of the world's busiest harbors.

3

Stay close to shore when you round Horn Point, where it's too shallow for most powerboats to run.

4

Watch the western horizon for storm clouds. Get a weather radar app for your smartphone and keep your phone in a waterproof case or dry bag. I have a dedicated waterproof camera.

5

Always wear a personal floatation device. I prefer the inflatable type. They're so lightweight you hardly notice you're wearing them.

Here are some resources for canoe, kayak, and stand-up paddleboard rentals and guided tours:

Annapolis Canoe & Kayak
annapoliscanoeandkayak.com • 410-263-2303
311 Third Street, (Eastport)
Annapolis, MD 21403

Capital SUP (3 locations:)
Capitalsup.com • 410-919-9402

Quiet Waters Park
600 Quiet Waters Park Rd, Annapolis, MD 21403

Nautilus Point (formerly Watergate)
655 Americana Drive,
Dock C, (Eastport)
Annapolis, MD 21403

Point Crab House
700 Mill Creek Rd.
Arnold, MD 21012

Chesapeake Paddle Sports
chesapeakepaddlesports.com
443-221-9732
629 Deale Rd, Deale, MD 20751

Paddle Annapolis
Paddle-annapolis.com
410-980-3911
326 First Street, (Eastport),
Annapolis, MD 21403

Smithsonian Environmental Research Center
serc.si.edu • 443-482-2200
647 Contees Wharf Rd.
Edgewater, MD 21037

Terrapin Adventures
terrapinadventures.com
301-725-1313
Savage Mill
8600 Foundry Street
Savage, MD 20763

Walk 52

Old Critters Endorse New Living Shoreline at Franklin Point State Park

It was with a little chagrin but no surprise whatsoever that I read recently of the Chesapeake Bay cleanup efforts failing to meet the program's ambitious goals by the 2025 deadline. While this may be true, there are hopeful signs of recovery. For instance, you can now swim in Baltimore Harbor, which just 10 years ago would have been cause for your life insurance company to cancel your double-indemnity policy.

Over the past 30 years, all the environmental groups involved in the Bay's restoration have been applying the method of adaptive management as they evolutionarily discovered which strategies work and which ones don't work so well and how they could be made to work better. This has been a trial-and-error effort out of necessity. Nobody had tried to clean up America's largest estuary before.

During that same period, the population in the Mid-Atlantic region has grown by 15 percent from 37 million to 42 million, meaning there are that many more people living near the Bay, each person flushing toilets six times a day. That's 30 million additional toilet flushes a day. That's a lot of pollution (or: insert your favorite euphemism here) to counteract. And that's just

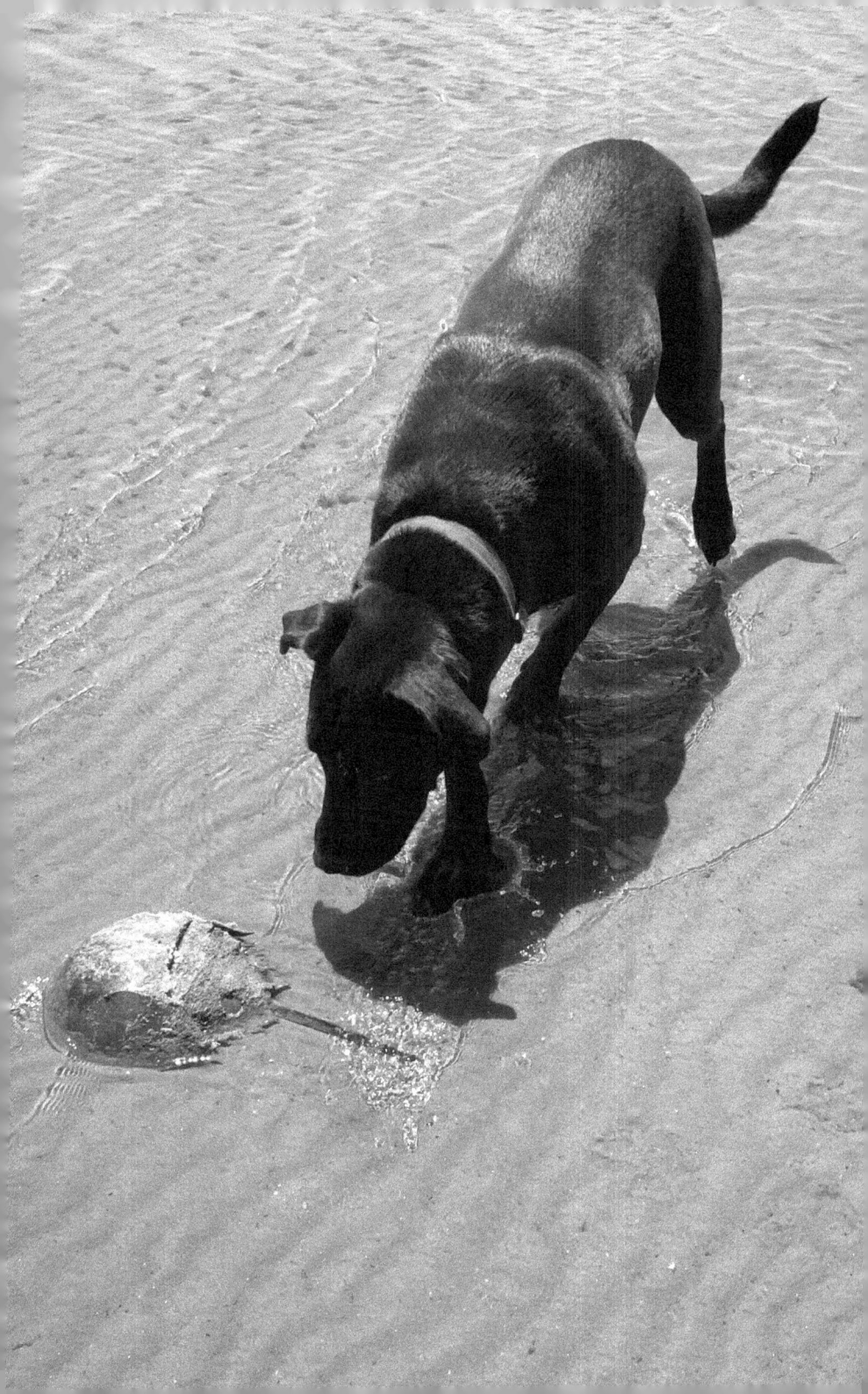

one impact of population growth on the environment. No wonder the program has fallen short of its goals. Still, as I say, there are signs that not all the work has been in vain.

In 2022, I gave a tour of Franklin Point State Park to Maryland State Senator Sarah Elfreth, along with my rescue retriever, Millie. At that time, we walked along the Bayside portion of the park. A true champion of Maryland's environment, the senator was alarmed by the severe erosion there, which had eaten up acres of shoreline and left it in a vast cluster of toppled trees.

This section of the park is on Franklin Point proper, just south of the Columbia Beach neighborhood on the Shady Side Peninsula in southern Anne Arundel County. The severity of the erosion was due to the fact that it faces more or less southeast, and there's nothing but open Bay for 103 miles in that direction. An osprey flying that way that far in a perfectly straight line would wind up on the Virginia bit of the lower Eastern Shore not far from the village of Machipongo.

That means the northwesterly wind and current have 103 miles to build up force. Such lengthy buildup is referred to as "fetch." I told the senator that the Maryland Department of Natural Resources had a project in the works to repair the damage, but it had been dormant nearly a decade. In the ensuing years since that tour, the project suddenly came back to life and a new living shoreline was completed in May 2024.

If you want to see what progress has been made over time in the shoreline protection department, you only need to look at an aerial photograph of this site. Decades ago, the Columbia Beach shoreline was encapsulated in a solid wall of rock. Two saltwater ponds got sealed off from the Bay, causing them to stagnate. This is an early example of how not to do it.

The Franklin Point project connects with the southern tip of the Columbia Beach bulkhead, but instead of a solid wall of rock, there are judiciously placed breakwaters separated by gaps of sandy beach. This living-shoreline strategy allows essential access in and out of the water for terrapins, horseshoe crabs, grandkids, and other wildlife. In this case, the project has created a fairly large crescent-shaped beach, and quite a pleasant one at that.

Millie and I stopped by to inspect the project on one of those cool, breezy days in early July 2024. It was at low tide, and sure enough, Millie discovered with alarm a horseshoe crab up near the damp high tide mark, struggling to inch its way through the sand toward the receding water. Horseshoe crabs, like terrapins, need such a beach to lay their eggs, as they've been doing for the past 445 million years.

When Millie was through with her investigation, I gently picked the critter up by its shell and waded out into the water to let it wiggle away. If you see one stranded up on a beach, don't pick it up by the tail, or "telson." It can snap off easily, and the crab needs it for navigation. The presence of this particular horseshoe crab meant that the new beach has the seal of approval from Maryland's oldest living fossil.

The water in the cove between the stone breakwaters was shallow and still clear. Millie frolicked in the gentle waves. The view from there is impressive. On a clear day like this, you can see the pine tree fringe of Jefferson Island nearly nine miles across the Bay. Just offshore, you can see a line of stakes that comprise a pound net, replete with a regiment of cormorants perched on the tops of the posts, waiting for a free meal at the waterman's expense.

Millie and I had the whole beach to ourselves, outside of the osprey circling overhead. The habitat has quite a coastal feel, with a forest of windblown loblolly pines, hollies and sweet gum trees. Volunteers had planted native grasses that looked green and vibrant even with the drought we'd been experiencing. The planted areas have been roped off until the plants get established. Their roots will help hold the new sand in place, and they'll help absorb excess stormwater runoff before it washes into the Bay.

We walked along the high breakwater and saw where it connects with the original stone bulkhead that runs all the way down to the end of the point, about 300 yards further south. I'd be thrilled if some stellar volunteers were to cut a new trail running through the forest down to the tip of the point, and then create some sort of pedestrian ferry across the back channel to connect with the main section of Franklin Point State Park on the mainland of the Shady Side Peninsula.

I was pleased with the results of the new living shoreline and pleased that the DNR had created a new parking area next to the bus turn-around at the end of Columbia Beach Road. The stroll down a lane lined with pine trees leads a short distance to the beach. Most of all, I was pleased that the horseshoe crabs have a new beach where they can crawl up and lay their eggs in the sand, just as they've done for so many millennia. Build it and they will come. See? There are hopeful signs.

Franklin Point State Park
(Bayside section)
End of Columbia Beach Road
Shady Side, MD 20764

From Edgewater, head east on Central Ave., then turn south onto Muddy Creek Road, which becomes West Shady Side Road. Important: You need to pass by the first entrance to Franklin Point State Park on Dent Road and turn right onto Columbia Beach Road. Follow that to the end and park just past the school bus turn-around.

Open dawn to dusk

Free admission

Limited parking available in the lot at the end of Columbia Beach Road

No toilets

Good-natured dogs on leashes are welcome; bring your own doggie bags

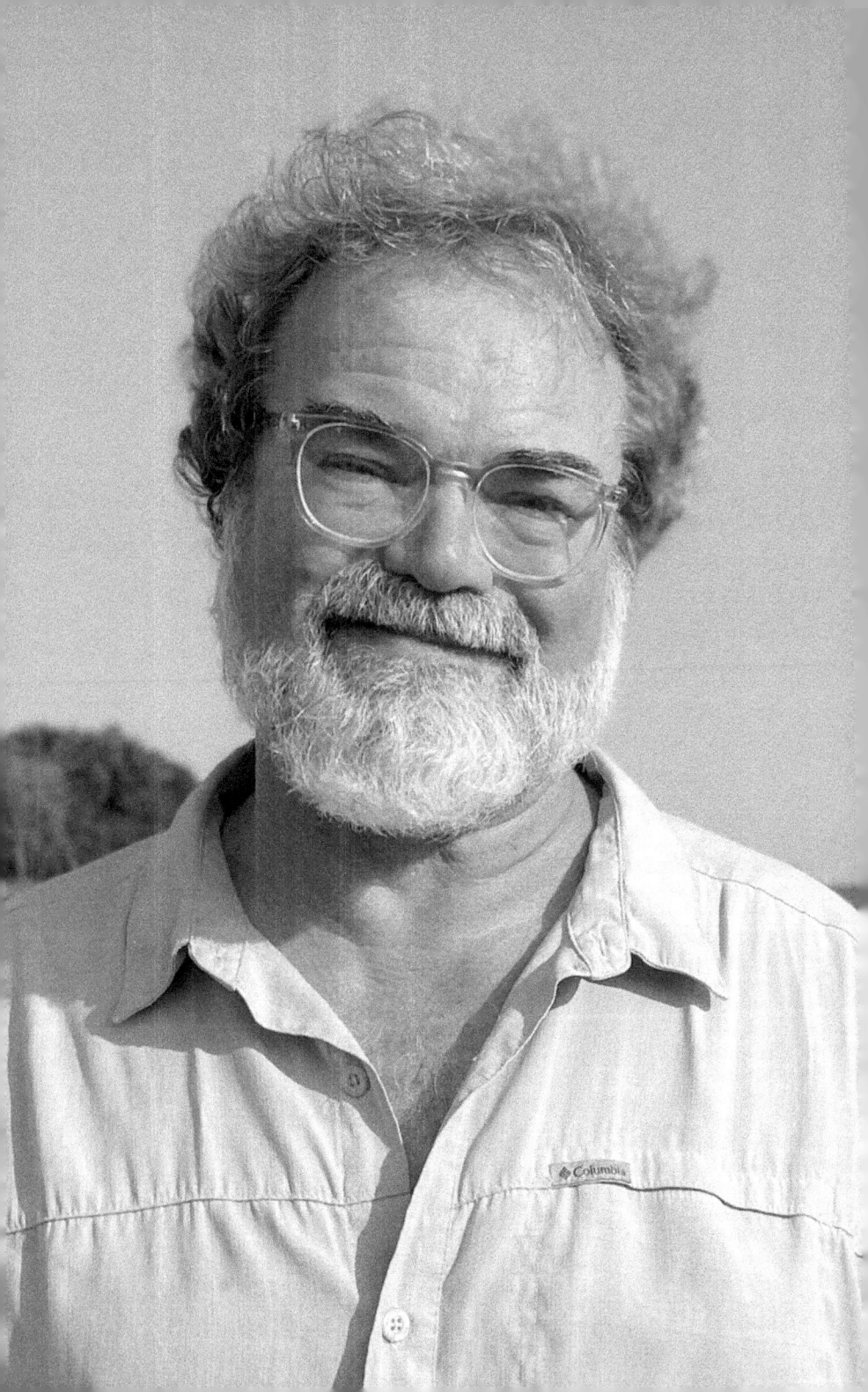

About the Author

A modern-day Chesapeake troubadour, Jefferson Holland is a singer, songwriter, poet, and story-teller, performing all original material inspired by decades of life on the Bay. Jeff has served as the director of the Annapolis Maritime Museum and the Riverkeeper for the West and Rhode Rivers. He co-founded the Chesapeake folk group "Crab Alley" in the 1980s and 90s and founded "Them Eastport Oyster Boys" with partner Kevin Brooks in 1992. Jeff has written dozens of songs and recorded four CDs. In 1994, he was appointed the Poet Laureate of Eastport and published the children's book, *Chessie the Sea Monster that Ate Annapolis*. Currently, in between performances, Jeff writes an outdoor adventure column in the *Annapolis Capital* newspaper. In 2024, he was appointed Poet Laureate of Annapolis by Mayor Gavin Buckley. He lives in Annapolis with his partner, Louise White, and Millie the wonder retriever.

Photo Captions

A note on the photographs in this book:

I took most of these pix myself, using my iPhone mounted on a small tripod. Early on, I relied on the self-timer, but then discovered a Bluetooth remote shutter. Eventually, I bought an Olympus Tough TG-6 point-and-shoot camera. It's compact, waterproof, and has a limited zoom feature. Best of all, it links by GPS with my iPhone, which serves as a remote shutter. I can set up a shot and click the shutter from 120 feet away. Now and then a walking companion or a kind passer-by will snap a pic or two.

Foreword: Jeff and Millie, shortly after Louise and I adopted her. She was about six months old and this was her first long-ish walk with us. *(Photo by Louise White)*

Page 1: Jeff and Bonnie, the beautiful Irish setter. *(Photo by Louise White)*

Page 7: Visitors at Franklin Point State Park admire the view of the channel winding through a salt marsh between Deep Creek and the open Chesapeake Bay.

Page 12: Bonnie leads Dave Isbell on a saunter through the Odenton Natural Area.

Page 18: Fred Shaffer of Crofton uses a spotting scope to spot all the diving ducks bobbing in the Bay at Fort Smallwood Park.

Page 26: Bonnie leads Dave Isbell across the little bridge that spans the headwaters of Broad Creek at Annapolis Waterworks Park.

Page 33: Jeff takes a solitary walk in the rain at Beverly Triton Nature Park.

Page 40: Louise follows Bonnie through a gully on the Forked Creek Trail in Arnold.

Page 47: Visitors walk along the living shoreline at Jack Creek Park. Note the sky in the early stages of the pandemic: curiously clear of any pollution and (somewhat eerily) not a jet contrail to be seen.

Page 55: Three-year-old Greta Marie rides her 'baby elephant' as her mom, Genevieve Mason, and her baby brother look on.

Page 62-63: Fishermen relax in the early spring sunshine on the beach at Sandy Point State Park.

Page 68: Jeff and Bonnie on the banks of Harness Creek at Quiet Waters Park.

Page 75: Jeff casts a fly line into the muddy waters of the Patuxent River at Patuxent Wetlands Park.

Page 80: A young man and his little boy came walking along the lane hand-in-hand, inspiring visions of Sheriff Andy Taylor and Opie on their way to the fishing hole.

Page 87: Environmentalist Tom Guay looks out over the head of the Severn River.

Page 94: Jack Neil and his son Devin on a walk around Spriggs Farm Park. Jack was one of the community leaders who created the foundation to preserve the farm from development and make it accessible to the public.

Page 100: After Bonnie's passing, Jeff got his "doggie fix" by paroling pooches from the SPCA. This is Loki Loc, a Plott hound. Plott hounds originated in North Carolina, where they were bred to hunt bears.

Page 108: Loki Loc searches for bears in the marsh at the headwaters of Spa Creek at Truxtun Park.

Page 115: Louise looks out over the reservoir on a trail at Annapolis Waterworks Park.

Page 122: Jeff and Max explore the trails at Bacon Ridge. Max, another SPCA parolee, is mostly bulldog, a beefy 90-pound bundle of laid-back sweetness.

Page 132: Athena, a German shepherd mix borrowed from the SPCA, leads Jeff along the boardwalk over Galloway Marsh at Jug Bay's Glendenning Nature Preserve. *(Louise White photo)*

Page 136-137: Jeff looks for eagles on the boardwalk across the marsh to Hog Island at the Smithsonian Environmental Research Center. From a distance, the tree line of the island resembles the form of a sleeping hog.

Page 142: Tom Guay and his dog, Mahki, joined Jeff on a chilly mid-winter trek around Greenbury Point. Here, they're spotting diving ducks cavorting in the Severn River.

Page 150: Paul Spadaro, president of the all-volunteer Magothy River Association, led the effort to restore Beachwood Park and make it accessible to the public.

Page 157: Cody Boy, a purebred Alaskan husky borrowed from the SPCA for the afternoon, lets Jeff take a needed break on their winter trek along Morning Choice Trail at the Patapsco Valley State Park.

Page 164-165: Dr. Geoffrey "Jess" Parker, the forest ecologist at the Smithsonian Environmental Research Center, walks alongside a submerged trail at Corcoran Woods, a 215-acre tract of forest next to Sandy Point State Park.

Page 170: Louise and the newly adopted pup, Millie, overlook the Patuxent River at Davidsonville Park.

Page 177: Millie poses at the prow of the deadrise workboat *Miss Lonesome* at the Back Creek Nature Park.

Page 185: Millie leads Jeff on the path by the salt pond at Terrapin Nature Park on Kent Island.

Page 190: Jeff and Millie walk along the edge of a bluff overlooking the Patapsco River at Weinberg Park.

Page 196: Millie tests the waters at Valentine Creek. At this point, she's shown interest in wading, but she still hasn't figured out what the webbing between her toes is for, so she hasn't actually gone swimming yet.

Page 202: Midshipman Eve Warden, class of 2023, who missed her two mutts back home in Phoenix, Arizona, gets her "doggie fix" as Millie wiggles with glee.

Page 209: Millie gets nose-to-nose with a sheep at Kinder Farm Park.

Page 217: Millie and Jeff commune at the amphitheater behind St. Luke's Church in Eastport.

Page 223: Millie and Jeff take a winter walk through the Magothy Greenway Natural Area with environmentalist Tom Guay and his protégé, Jack Beckham.

Page 229: Millie leads Jeff and (then) Maryland State Senator, and now Congresswoman, Sarah Elfreth along a path through the pines at Franklin Point State Park.

Page 238: Yong Kim, who lives nearby and visits the Downs Memorial Park almost every day, said, "My day doesn't start until I take Coco for a ride."

Page 240: Jeff uses a piece of driftwood as an improvised bat to hit a tennis ball for Millie to fetch. This is one of Millie's favorite pastimes.

Pages 248-249: Millie leads Jeff past the Hooper Island draketail workboat on display at the Annapolis Maritime Museum in Eastport. The boat is called *Peg Wallace*, in honor of the woman who founded the museum in the year 2000.

Page 257: Jeff hits a tennis ball for Millie at Quiet Waters Park's doggie beach on the South River. Millie figured out what those webs between her toes were for when she was about a year old, and she's been an enthusiastic swimmer ever since.

Page 263: Millie and Louise walk through the Helen Avalynne Tawes Garden in Annapolis with Ranger Jay Myers and Suzanne Weber, the horticulturist for both the Tawes Garden and Sandy Point State Park.

Pages 270-271: Lois Findlay and her dog, Bella, lead Jeff and Millie across a boardwalk at a stream restoration project recently completed along the Broadneck Trail. Bella and Millie could be twins; both are a mix of Labrador retriever and border collie.

Page 277: Jeff, Louise, and Millie walk past the William Brown House at Historic London Town and Gardens. The large brick Georgian house was built as a tavern around 1760.

Page 283: Jeff contemplates the grave of Annapolis artisan John Shaw, who died in 1793.

Page 290:	Commodore Waddel's monument.
Page 293:	Jeff and Millie gaze out over Annapolis Harbor, a sea of shimmering silver with the morning sun silhouetting the sailboats in the mooring field.
Page 298:	Millie proves she's a great boat dog, providing the perfect ballast for Jeff's canoe as they paddle the Rhode River. Jon Chapman's ahead in the kayak.
Page 305:	Jeff leads his granddaughter, Lyla, along the edge of the Severn River at Elktonia Park.
Page 311:	Millie and Jeff take a snowy walk at Chesapeake Bay Foundation's headquarters at the end of the Annapolis Neck Peninsula.
Page 317:	Jeff and Millie take a stroll at Jonas and Catharine Green Park, with the academic buildings of the U.S. Naval Academy on the horizon across the Severn River.
Page 322:	Millie and Jeff wander along the foggy shore at Ferry Point Park on Kent Narrows.
Page 328:	Jon Chapman, Jeff, and Millie walk past the reconstructed cabin of a genius inventor at Benjamin Banneker Historical Park & Museum.
Page 335:	Jeff and Millie kayak along a secluded cove in the upper reaches of Back Creek.
Page 342:	Millie's intrigued by the horseshoe crab that got stuck in the sand at high tide.

Maps

The following pages contain maps to help you locate the general locations of the parks mentioned in this book. In this day of cellphone navigation, of course, you will probably be relying on your phone to get where you are going. However, for handy book reference, these maps will help you get an idea where the parks are located.

The maps are organized in three sections roughly following the book's table of contents, with the third map a close-up of the Annapolis parks.

Walk 1	Scoping the Scoters at Thomas Point Park	1
Walk 2	Winter Wandering at Franklin Point State Park	6
Walk 3	Sauntering Around the Odenton Natural Area	13
Walk 4	Fort Smallwood Park: An Ageless Attraction	19
Walk 5	Ease Your Anxiety with a Good Walk at Annapolis Waterworks Park	25
Walk 6	Walkin' in the Rain at Beverly Triton Nature Park	32
Walk 7	Discovering a Pocket Wilderness in Arnold	39
Walk 8	You Don't Know Jack Creek	46
Walk 9	Riding Baby Elephants at Patuxent Research Refuge	53
Walk 10	A Solitary Beach Walk at Sandy Point State Park	60
Walk 12	Delving into the Historic Depths at Wooton's Landing Wetlands Park	73
Walk 13	Hooking Sea Monsters at South River Farm Park	81
Walk 14	Discovering Sources at Severn Run Natural Environmental Area	87
Walk 15	Spritely Whimsy of Spriggs Farm Park	93
Walk 16	Keeping Broad Creek Trail Safe from Bears	101
Walk 18	Waterworks Park Redux	115
Walk 41	Tour a Restored Stream at Broadneck Trail	268
Walk 45	Paddling the Rhode River	299

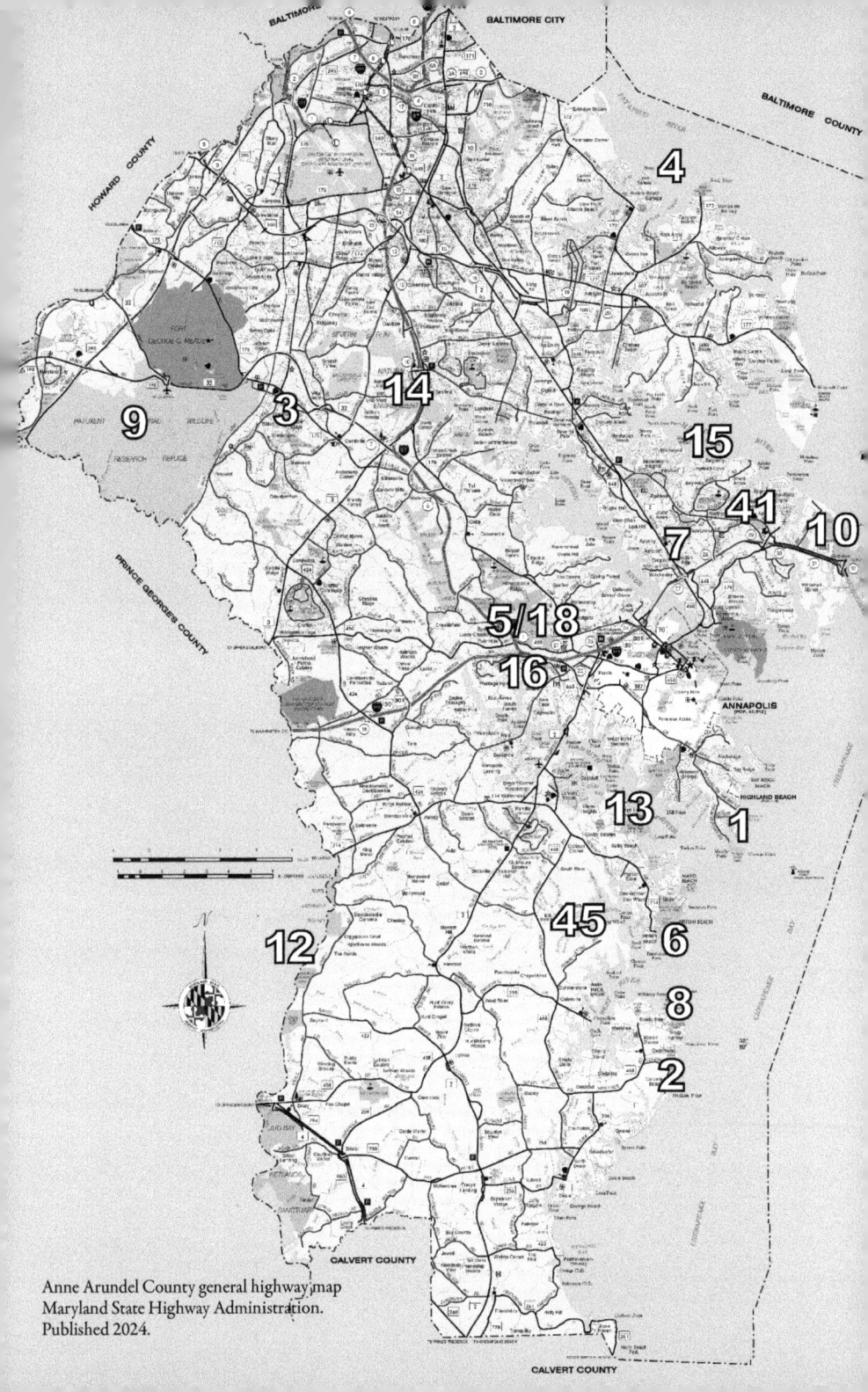

Anne Arundel County general highway map
Maryland State Highway Administration.
Published 2024.

Walk 19	Chillin' Out with Max at Bacon Ridge............................	121
Walk 20	The Goddess of Glendening Nature Preserve at Jug Bay...	129
Walk 21	Dogless on the Hog Island Trail at Smithsonian Environmental Research Center.......	136
Walk 23:	Thank Volunteers for Beachwood Park.......................	149
Walk 24	Mushing on Morning Choice Trail	155
Walk 25	Walking with Giants at Corcoran Woods	162
Walk 26	Meet Millie at Davidsonville Park................................	171
Walk 28	Taking a Turn Around Terrapin Nature Park.............	184
Walk 29	Searching for Palm Trees at Weinberg Park................	191
Walk 30	Nursing a Broken Heart at Valentine Creek Trail......	197
Walk 32	Kinder Farm Park: A Literal Kinder-garten	208
Walk 34	Magothy Greenway Natural Area: a Wonderful Wilderness..	221
Walk 35	Exploring Franklin Point State Park with Senator Sarah	227
Walk 36	What's Up at Downs Memorial Park	234
Walk 37	Millie Runs Happily Amok at Matapeake Dog Park	241
Walk 49	Ferry Point Park and Fried Oysters: A Winning Combination	321
Walk 50	Encountering Genius at Benjamin Banneker Historical Park & Museum	327
Walk 52	Old Critters Endorse New Living Shoreline at Franklin Point State Park	340

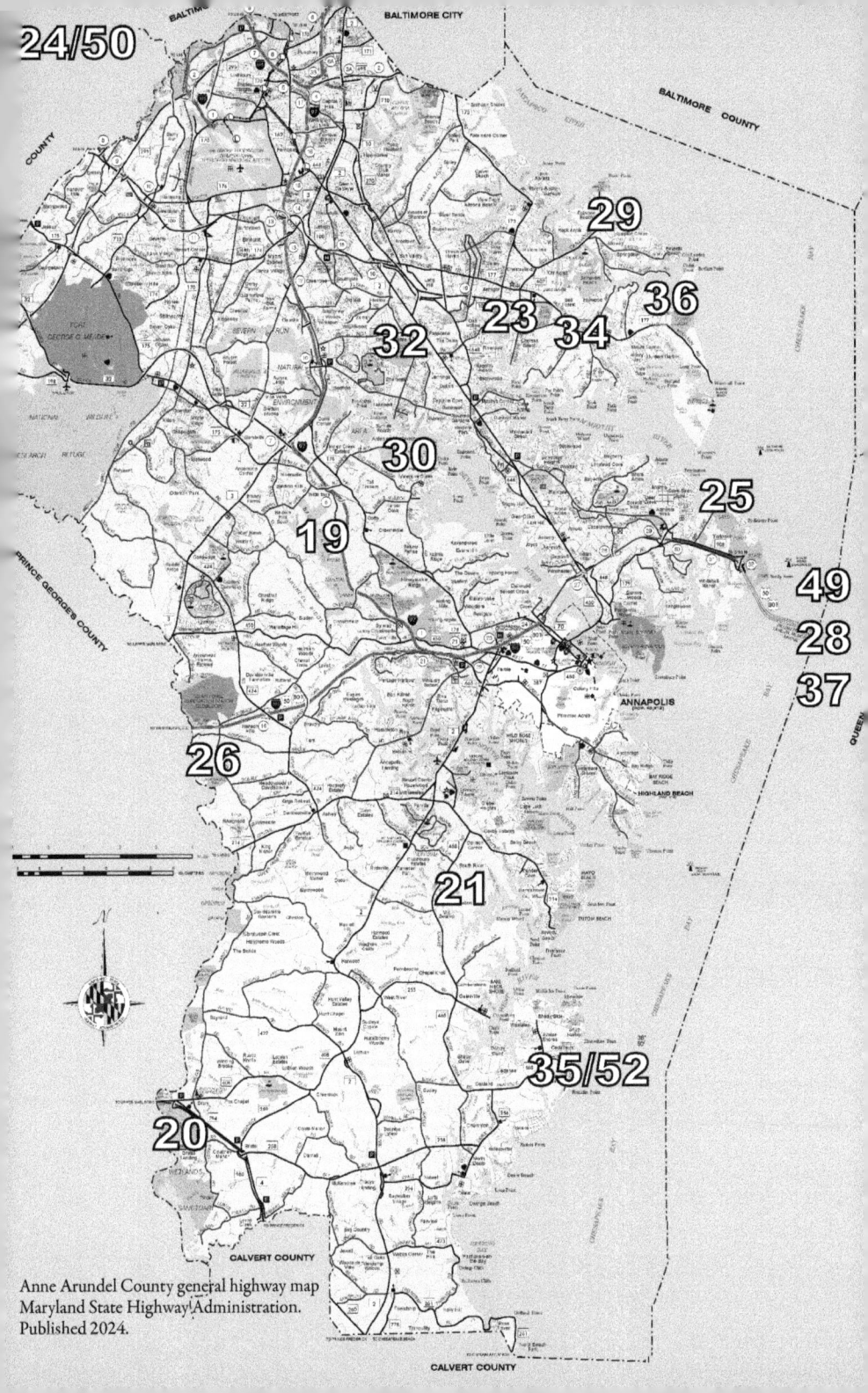

Anne Arundel County general highway map
Maryland State Highway Administration.
Published 2024.

Walk 11	Requiem for a Red Dog at Quiet Waters Park............67
Walk 17	Trekking Through Truxtun Park................................109
Walk 22	What's Towering over Greenbury Point.....................143
Walk 27	Back Creek Nature Park: A Hidden Gem in Annapolis 177
Walk 31	Patrolling the Yard at the United States Naval Academy................................203
Walk 33	St. Luke's Restoration of Nature.................................215
Walk 38:	Stroll Horn Point on the Eastport Walking Tour........24
Walk 39	Doggie Parks for the Dog Days of Summer...............257
Walk 40	Hooray for Butterflies at Tawes Garden 262
Walk 42	Smelling the Begonias at Historic London Town and Gardens......................276
Walk 43	Who's Who at St. Anne's Cemetery.............................282
Walk 44	A Free Morning at Annapolis City Dock...................291
Walk 46	Elktonia Beach: Walking a New Park with a New Walking Buddy 304
Walk 47	Chasing the Chill at Chesapeake Bay Foundation....310
Walk 48	Discovering History at Jonas and Anne Catharine Green Park 315
Walk 51	Back Creek by Kayak 333

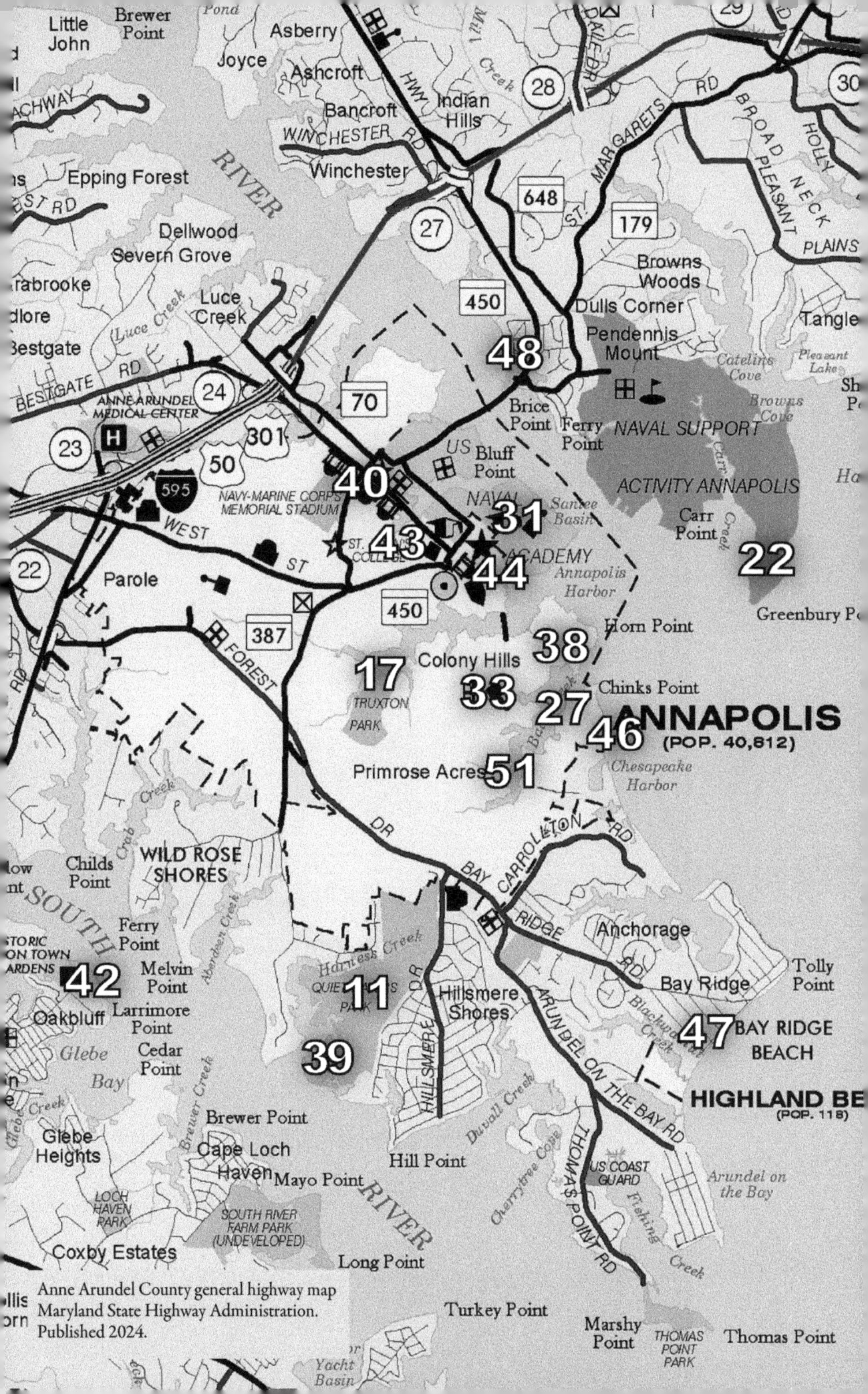

Anne Arundel County general highway map
Maryland State Highway Administration.
Published 2024.

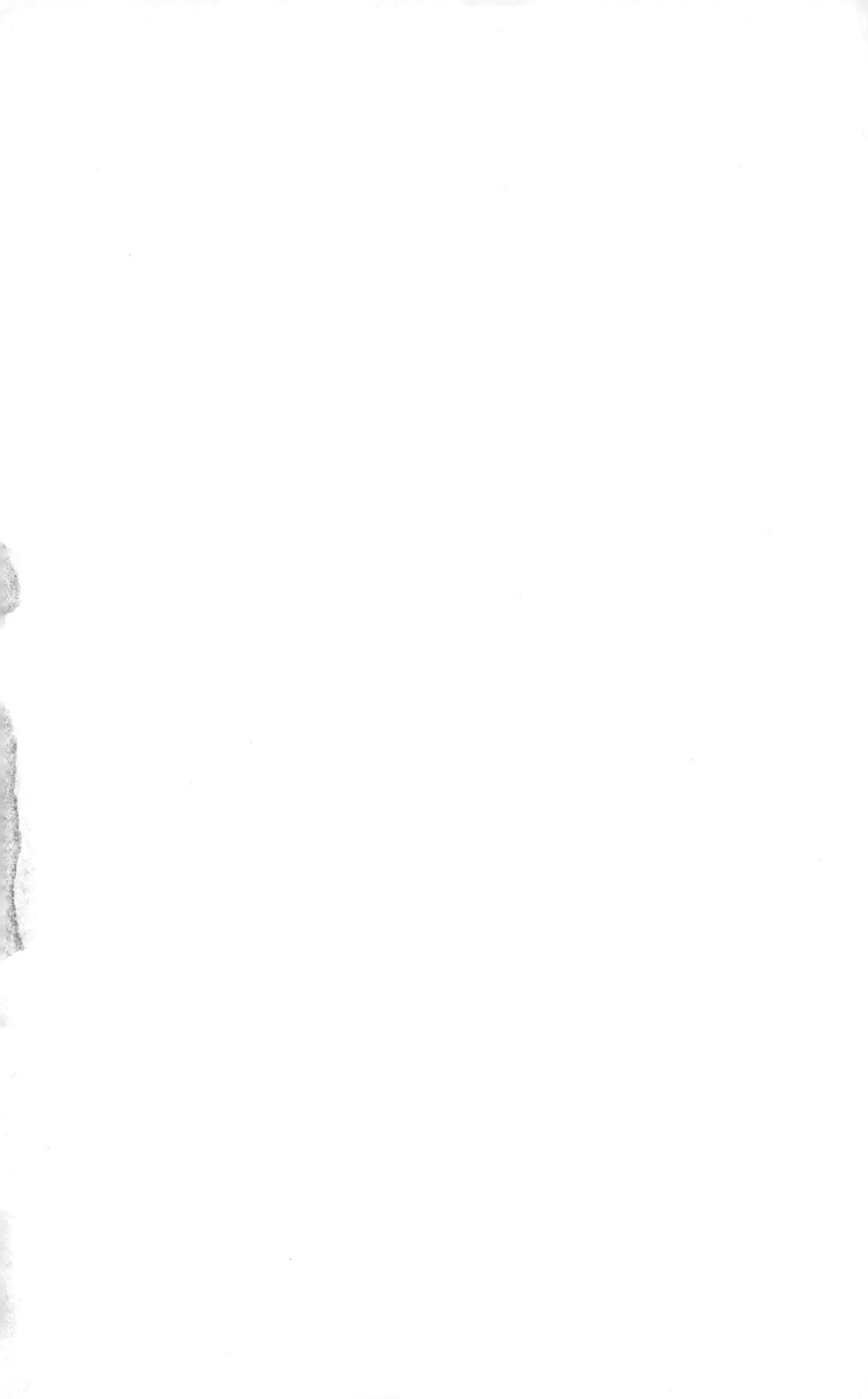

Milton Keynes UK
Ingram Content Group UK Ltd.
UKHW020125021224
451695UK00019B/288

9 798988 299851